# Distribution and Treatment of Infectious Diseases:

## Challenges for Developed and Developing Nations

Hiba Hamdar
*Medical Learning Skills Academy, Lebanon*



IGI Global
Scientific Publishing
Publishing Tomorrow's Research Today

Vice President of Editorial — Melissa Wagner
Director of Acquisitions — Mikaela Felty
Director of Book Development — Jocelynn Hessler
Production Manager — Mike Brehm
Cover Design — Jose Rosado

Published in the United States of America by
IGI Global Scientific Publishing
701 East Chocolate Avenue
Hershey, PA, 17033, USA
Tel: 717-533-8845
Fax: 717-533-7115
Website: https://www.igi-global.com E-mail: cust@igi-global.com



Library of Congress Cataloging-in-Publication Data

Names: Hamdar, Hiba, 1995- editor http://id.loc.gov/rwo/agents/n2025015099
Title: Distribution and treatment of infectious diseases : challenges for developed and developing nations / edited by Hiba Hamdar.
Description: Hershey, PA : IGI Global Scientific Publishing, [2026] | Includes bibliographical references and index. | Summary: "The aim of this book is to examine the diseases and infections in the developed and developing world, prevalence, epidemiology, distribution, pathophysiology, symptoms and signs, risk factors, diagnosis, challenges, lack of knowledge of antibiotic usage, management, and research strategies as a future plan to eliminate the infection or reduce its prevalence"-- Provided by publisher.
Identifiers: LCCN 2024058252 (print) | LCCN 2024058253 (ebook) | ISBN 9798369319901 hardcover | ISBN 9798369366516 paperback | ISBN 9798369319918 ebook
Subjects: LCSH: Communicable diseases--Epidemiology http://id.loc.gov/authorities/subjects/sh2009120850 | Communicable diseases--Treatment
Classification: LCC RA643 .D58 2025 (print) | LCC RA643 (ebook) | DDC 362.1969--dc23/eng/20250403
LC record available at https://lccn.loc.gov/2024058252
LC ebook record available at https://lccn.loc.gov/2024058253

British Cataloguing in Publication Data
A Cataloguing in Publication record for this book is available from the British Library.

# Table of Contents

# Detailed Table of Contents


*Layal Bassam Msheik, Faculty of Medical Sciences, Lebanese University, Beirut, Lebanon*
*Ahmad Saifan, Faculty of Medical Sciences, Lebanese University, Beirut, Lebanon*
*Ahmad Afyouni, Faculty of Medical Sciences, Lebanese University, Beirut, Lebanon*
*Zeinab Kazan, Faculty of Medical Sciences, Lebanese University, Beirut, Lebanon*
*Rim Awada, Faculty of Medical Sciences, Lebanese University, Beirut, Lebanon*
*Mohammad Barakat, Faculty of Medical Sciences, Lebanese University, Beirut, Lebanon*

This chapter explores infections, emphasizing microorganisms, their forms, and environmental impact, especially in low-income countries. It delves into infection transmission, their interplay with the environment, and hygiene/sanitation effects. Prevalence and epidemiology in low-income countries are analyzed, showcasing their impact on public health. Challenges faced by both income groups, like healthcare limitations, socioeconomic factors, and access issues, are examined. Cultural/societal influences, misconceptions, and traditional healing practices are explored. Strategies for low-income countries include affordable healthcare, immunization promotion, antimicrobial resistance combat, and community-based interventions. The chapter stresses empowering local communities, enhancing health education, and fostering awareness. The conclusion advocates for a comprehensive global approach to combat infections, especially in resource-limited settings."

Pathogenic therapy in infectious disease is linked to the treatment of infectious diseases such as diarrhea, cholera, and other diseases that affect the intestines and cause an imbalance in body fluids and important minerals such as sodium, potassium, calcium, chloride and other minerals that play a strong vital role in transmitting signals, Nervousness, muscle contraction, hormone secretion, and other essential functions, the occurrence of any imbalance in their levels leads to disturbances in the electrical balance, such as muscle spasms or breathing and heart rhythm disturbances, which may lead to low or high blood pressure or cardiac arrest. Previous studies have shown that the survival rate for cholera and diarrhea patients has become more than 99% thanks to these treatments and studies. Therefore, rehydration and electrolyte balance are important for normal physiological functions and require appropriate therapy when disrupted by environmental factors or illness. This chapter's knowledge helps us understand the importance of this type of treatment and health guidelines.



One of the most significant developments in medical history was the discovery of antibiotics and their subsequent large-scale manufacture in the early 1900s. In the history of medical pharmacotherapy, antibiotics caused absolute mortality reductions. Since antibiotics were so effective at eliminating harmful germs, many people thought that infectious diseases would eventually disappear from all human societies. The rise and quick spread of infections resistant to antibiotics, particularly those resistant to several drugs, lead to multidrug resistance. In this chapter, we will discuss the importance and classification of antibiotics according to different points of view, their complications, and finally, the problem that faces our world now is antibiotic resistance and how to reduce it.

Influenza, generally known as flu, is a viral respiratory disease. It can cause symptoms like fever, cough, sore throat, body aches, and fatigue. Researching treatments for influenza is important to develop effective antiviral medications and vaccines to prevent its spread and reduce its impact on public health. Influenza is typically a self-limiting illness, and most people recover during a week or two without any complications. It's worth noting that while influenza can cause significant illness and even death, it is distinct from the common cold, which is caused by different viruses and typically produces milder symptoms. This chapter provides Epidemiology, symptoms, prevention, advancements and future directions of Influenza.



Adenoviruses, respiratory syncytial viruses, and parainfluenza viruses are among the major causes of respiratory infections, which are a serious global health concern. This thorough analysis examines the virology, clinical presentation, and epidemiology of these viruses, emphasizing the effects they have on a range of demographics, including young children, the elderly, and people with weakened immune systems. In order to address the changing landscape of respiratory viral infections, emphasis is given on recent developments in diagnostics, antiviral treatments, and vaccine development. Through an understanding of the unique characteristics and shared traits of these viruses, this chapter hopes to support ongoing efforts to reduce the global burden of respiratory disorders.

Measles or rubeola is a highly contagious disease, that is often overlooked, keeps possessing global challenges due to its stability outside the body for long periods of time and complications especially in younger kids. Due to its high transmissibility over 90% of people get infected after being exposed to a potential measles risk. It usually spreads through respiratory droplets, aerosol particles and human contact. The measles virus initiates infection by the attachment to SLAM or CD150 receptors which is a lymphoid surface receptor involved in immune cell activation, then it is transmitted to epithelial cells through the use of CD46. Manifestations of measles are often associated with high fevers, rashes and koplik spots. Currently numerous diagnostic approaches are being employed to detect measles, some of them being serologic techniques that work on detecting IgM or IgG antibodies. Although no cure has been found to treat measles, few strategies have been developed in order to combat symptoms such as the use of vitamin A and vaccinations.



This chapter provides a comprehensive exploration of rubella, encompassing its definition, epidemiology, risk factors, pathogenesis, signs and symptoms, as well as diagnosis and treatment modalities. It delves into the challenges posed by rubella in both developed and developing countries, addressing issues such as misinformation, high birthrates, and healthcare infrastructure constraints. Furthermore, the abstract outlines potential solutions to these challenges, emphasizing the importance of strengthening immunization programs, improving healthcare infrastructure, and implementing targeted educational initiatives. The holistic approach presented here aims to contribute to a deeper understanding of rubella and offers insights into effective strategies for minimizing its impact on global health.


*Rahma Mahmoud Saad, Faculty Of Medicine, Modern University For Technology And Information-MTI, Cairo, Egypt*
*Ahmed Tharwat Al-Namrouti, Faculty of Medicine, Galala University, Suez, Egypt*
*Esraa Y. Salem, Faculty of Medicine, Modern University for Technology and Information (MTI), Cairo, Egypt*
*Karim S. Shata, Faculty of Medicine, Cairo University, Cairo, Egypt*
*Shahd Gamal Abdelsamad, Faculty of Medicine, Ain Shams University, Cairo, Egypt*
*safaa AlMawas, Faculty of Medicine, Mansoura University, Mansoura, Egypt*

Poliomyelitis, also known as polio, is a highly contagious disease that affects children under the age of five, mostly transmitted through the fecal-oral route by contaminated water and food. It is caused by three different types of wild polioviruses (WPV), a non-enveloped, single-stranded RNA virus, and can cause a range of symptoms and signs, from a mild flu-like illness to acute flaccid paralysis in severe cases. People have been plagued by this illness for many generations, which has resulted in global epidemics and high rates of morbidity and mortality. Nonetheless, vaccinations like the live Sabin vaccine and the inactivated Salk vaccine, which were developed in the 20th century, have been crucial in both lowering the disease's occurrence and eliminating it. Numerous challenges have been faced in the fight to eradicate polio, such as outbreaks of vaccine-derived poliovirus (VDPV) and resistance. Despite all these challenges, there is still a worldwide responsibility and constant cooperation to work toward a world free of polio.

*Ala'a Fawaz, Lebanese University, Lebanon*
*Fatima Al Amin, Faculty of Medical Sciences, Lebanese University, Beirut, Lebanon*
*Fatima Ahmad Mroueh, Lebanese University, Beirut, Lebanon*
*Zeinab Karaki, Lebanese University, Beirut, Lebanon*
*Zahraa Awada, Lebanese University, Beirut, Lebanon*
*Jina Hasan, Lebanese University, Beirut, Lebanon*

Rabies is a fatal neurological infection caused by the Rabies Virus (RABV) and transmitted through wild animals and unvaccinated pets via saliva contact, especially through bites. The virus enters the CNS, and after a certain incubation period, it causes encephalitic or paralytic symptoms. Diagnosis relies on clinical evaluation and specialized assays, though no effective treatment exists once symptoms appear. Rabies has a variety of risk factors primarily including lack of post-exposure prophylaxis (PEP) and unvaccinated dogs. Transmission routes vary by virus strain and exposure type, affecting incubation periods. Symptoms of this infection include prodromal signs like pruritus and fever, with furious and paralytic forms defining the disease. Prevention involves vaccination—pre-exposure prophylaxis (PrEP) for high-risk individuals and postexposure prophylaxis (PEP) for suspected exposures. However, no effective treatment exists once symptoms manifest. Recent advancements in diagnostic tools and vaccine development aim to enhance detection and preventive strategies..

This chapter delves into Coxsackie and Echovirus, pervasive enteroviruses causing a range of illnesses from mild to severe. It examines their molecular biology, epidemiology, and impact on global health, particularly in vulnerable populations like neonates. The discussion includes transmission methods, clinical challenges, and the dire need for effective treatments and preventive measures. The absence of vaccines and the difficulties in managing outbreaks, especially in underprivileged areas, are also highlighted.

Plague, a vector-borne illness caused by Yersinia pestis, is a serious threat to the public's health, particularly in light of its previous human outbreaks in Africa, Asia, and South America. Transmission occurs mostly by infected flea bites, causing typical painful, swollen lymph nodes known as buboes, followed by septicemic pathogen propagation. However, droplet inhalation following intimate contact with diseased mammals causes primary pneumonic plague. Clinical manifestations include bubonic and pneumonic forms, septicemia, and in rare cases, pharyngitis and meningitis. Early diagnosis and the immediate initiation of treatment can decrease mortality rate in bubonic plague and septicemic plague to 5-50%; however, a delay in treatment can be life threatening. Majority of cases can be successfully managed with antibiotics. This chapter covers current knowledge of Y. pestis, the most important current technologies and criteria for laboratory diagnosis of plague, main challenges experienced in underdeveloped nations, and the current novel research approaches.

# Preface

## INTRODUCTION

Infectious diseases have long posed a formidable challenge to human health and global development, and this challenge continues today with renewed complexity. As Editor of this volume, *Distribution and Treatment of Infectious Diseases: Challenges for Developed and Developing Nations*, my goal has been to assemble a comprehensive reference that not only details the current state of infectious diseases but also bridges the disparities between the experiences of developed and developing nations. The book is driven by a central aim: to explore the epidemiology, prevalence, symptoms, diagnosis, risk factors, and management of major infections, while also addressing gaps in antibiotic knowledge, challenges in treatment, and opportunities for future research and global cooperation.

This volume recognizes that while the burden of infectious diseases is a universal concern, its impact is not evenly distributed. Developed nations benefit from advanced healthcare systems, sanitation infrastructure, and widespread vaccination programs. Yet even these countries are grappling with new issues, such as rising antimicrobial resistance, vaccine hesitancy, and global disease transmission facilitated by modern travel. On the other hand, developing countries often face more acute challenges—ranging from inadequate healthcare infrastructure and limited vaccine access to poverty and the presence of endemic tropical diseases.

Our intent in curating this book is to offer an inclusive, multidimensional exploration of infectious diseases. We emphasize the importance of localized challenges and solutions, while also promoting shared understanding across borders. Addressing infectious diseases demands nuanced, context-specific strategies. Success will depend on improved disease surveillance, equitable access to medical innovations, targeted public health interventions, and coordinated international efforts.

The contributors to this volume have been carefully and systematically selected for their expertise and the diversity of their perspectives, ensuring a global and interdisciplinary conversation. This book is intended for a broad audience that includes medical students, researchers, physicians, infectious disease specialists, and public health professionals. It may also serve as a valuable resource in academic and medical institutions across disciplines. We hope it will introduce new readers to this vital area of study, broaden engagement with emerging global health issues, and serve as a foundation for meaningful collaboration and innovation in infectious disease research and treatment.

Constructing a reference of this scale and scope has been a challenging yet rewarding endeavor. I am deeply grateful to the contributors whose insights, research, and commitment to public health have shaped this volume. It is my hope that this book will serve as a catalyst for continued dialogue, deeper understanding, and actionable progress in the global effort to combat infectious diseases.

## ORGANIZATION OF THE BOOK

This volume begins by laying a foundational understanding of infectious diseases and their broader social, ecological, and biological contexts. Chapter 1, "Infection, Infectious Process (Definition, Forms) and the Role of Microorganisms, Macro Organisms, and Environment," explores the essential definitions, classifications, and transmission pathways of infections. With particular attention to low-income countries, the chapter discusses how environmental factors, hygiene, sanitation, and socio-cultural norms influence the prevalence and spread of infectious diseases. The authors emphasize the importance of community engagement, education, and context-specific interventions to reduce infection rates, especially in resource-constrained settings. The chapter sets the stage for the book's global perspective on disease distribution.

Chapter 2, "Pathogenetic Therapy in Infectious Diseases: Rehydration and Correction of Electrolytes Disbalance," turns our attention to therapeutic responses, focusing on the physiological disruption caused by infections like cholera and diarrheal diseases. It highlights the critical importance of fluid replacement and electrolyte therapy in preventing life-threatening complications such as cardiac arrest and respiratory failure. This chapter presents both clinical insight and practical guidelines, showcasing how such therapies have achieved remarkable survival rates, particularly in outbreak-prone regions.

Building upon therapeutic considerations, Chapter 3, "Antibacterial Therapy in Infectious Diseases," revisits one of the most transformative discoveries in modern medicine—the development and use of antibiotics. This chapter offers a comprehensive overview of antibiotic classifications, their historic role in reducing mortality, and the mounting global crisis of antibiotic resistance. The authors analyze contemporary challenges in antimicrobial stewardship and emphasize the urgency of global collaboration to reduce misuse and overuse, especially in settings with limited diagnostic resources.

The discussion of specific infectious agents begins in Chapter 4, "Influenza Virus," which presents an in-depth analysis of this globally prevalent respiratory illness. While generally self-limiting, influenza poses serious health risks, especially for vulnerable populations. The chapter outlines current treatments, vaccination strategies, and epidemiological trends, while also addressing distinctions between influenza and common cold viruses. It provides valuable insight into public health approaches and ongoing vaccine research.

Complementing the discussion on influenza, Chapter 5, "Parainfluenza, Adenoviruses, and RS-Viruses," broadens the focus to other prominent viral causes of respiratory illness. These infections are particularly severe in pediatric and immunocompromised populations. The chapter examines virology, clinical outcomes, and progress in diagnostics and vaccine development, offering a panoramic view of the viral respiratory disease landscape and the evolving response from the medical and research communities.

Chapter 6, "Measles," examines one of the most contagious diseases in human history. This chapter delves into the pathophysiology of measles, its complications, and the global challenges surrounding its control despite the availability of vaccines. It discusses diagnostic methods such as serologic testing and the role of vitamin A supplementation in treatment. By highlighting the persistent gaps in vaccine coverage and public health education, the chapter reinforces the need for comprehensive immunization strategies.

In Chapter 7, "Rubella," the authors provide a detailed account of rubella's clinical and epidemiological profile, with special emphasis on its risks during pregnancy and its broader social implications. The chapter discusses disparities in healthcare access, cultural attitudes toward vaccination, and infrastructure deficiencies in both developed and developing contexts. A call is made to strengthen routine immunizations and deploy educational campaigns that confront misinformation and cultural barriers.

Continuing with vaccine-preventable illnesses, Chapter 8, "Poliomyelitis: A Global Perspective on the Challenges and Progress in Developing and Developed Countries," offers a historical and contemporary overview of the global fight against polio. The authors discuss the biology of polioviruses, the global success of vaccination campaigns, and the setbacks posed by vaccine-derived strains and public resistance. This chapter underscores the importance of sustained international cooperation and vigilant public health efforts in the near-eradication of a once-devastating disease.

Chapter 9, "Rabies," provides a sobering look at one of the deadliest known viral infections—an illness that remains universally fatal once clinical symptoms appear. This chapter outlines the transmission of Rabies Virus (RABV), most commonly via the saliva of infected animals through bites, and its insidious progression from incubation to severe neurological symptoms. While post-exposure prophylaxis (PEP) can be highly effective if administered promptly, rabies continues to exact a heavy toll in regions with insufficient healthcare infrastructure. The chapter also reviews recent developments in diagnostic tools and vaccine technology, offering hope for better surveillance and prevention in high-risk areas.

Chapter 10, "Unraveling Coxsackie and Echovirus," explores the wide-reaching implications of these enteroviruses, which range from benign febrile illnesses to severe complications, particularly in neonates and immunocompromised individuals. The authors present a layered understanding of their molecular biology and transmission, while confronting the global public health challenges posed by the absence of vaccines and limited treatment options. The chapter is especially attentive to the impact on vulnerable populations and the need for innovative solutions in under-resourced settings.

With Chapter 11, "Unveiling the Plague," we revisit one of history's most feared pandemics, now understood through the lens of modern microbiology and global health research. Caused by *Yersinia pestis* and transmitted primarily through fleas and infected animals, plague persists as a zoonotic threat. This chapter examines the pathology of bubonic, septicemic, and pneumonic forms of the disease, emphasizing early diagnosis and antibiotic intervention. It also highlights new diagnostic methods, current treatment guidelines, and the unique challenges in managing outbreaks in rural or poorly equipped healthcare environments.

Chapter 12, "Decoding Cholera," focuses on *Vibrio cholerae*, a pathogen that remains a critical concern in the developing world due to its rapid dehydration effect and potential for widespread outbreaks. The chapter explains the bacterium's mechanism of action, diagnostic techniques, and clinical management, underscoring the life-saving importance of immediate rehydration therapy. It also reviews the role of oral cholera vaccines and advances in outbreak response, demonstrating how a combination of public health infrastructure and biomedical innovation can mitigate cholera's impact.

Chapter 13, "M. Lyme," centers on Lyme disease, a complex tick-borne illness caused by *Borrelia burgdorferi*. The chapter contextualizes its emergence in the U.S. and the global diversity in its clinical presentation due to varying spirochete strains. With special attention to diagnostic ambiguities, the authors discuss the chronic effects of untreated Lyme disease, emphasizing the need for more reliable testing, public awareness, and support for research. The disease's persistence despite advances in science makes it a formidable public health challenge even in developed nations.

In Chapter 14, “Lassa Fever,” the discussion turns to a highly lethal viral hemorrhagic fever endemic to parts of West Africa. The chapter presents a detailed overview of Lassa virus transmission, often from rodents to humans, and its severe impact on populations with limited access to healthcare. With no approved vaccines or definitive treatments, the chapter underscores the urgency of investment in research and global preparedness. Importantly, it also warns of the disease's potential for international spread, reinforcing the need for coordinated surveillance and containment strategies.

Chapter 15, “Dengue and Dengue Hemorrhagic Fever,” shifts the lens toward vector-borne illness in tropical and subtropical regions. The authors examine the epidemiology and socioeconomic disparities that influence Dengue's spread and severity. The chapter details prevention efforts, diagnosis, and treatment options while highlighting the limitations of current healthcare systems in endemic regions. Through a global perspective, the authors advocate for future research, cross-border cooperation, and integrative strategies to combat the ongoing burden of Dengue fever and its severe forms.

Finally, Chapter 16, “Hepatic Encephalopathy,” introduces a neuropsychiatric disorder not primarily infectious, but deeply entwined with infectious risk through hepatic dysfunction. The chapter dissects the intricate pathophysiology of hepatic encephalopathy, often triggered by cirrhosis, infections, or metabolic stress. With emphasis on prevention, early detection, and therapeutic interventions—from diet to liver transplantation—the chapter provides a multidisciplinary view on managing this debilitating condition. It serves as a poignant reminder of the interconnectedness of chronic disease and infection in shaping global health outcomes.

## CONCLUSION

As this volume draws to a close, it becomes evident that the fight against infectious diseases remains one of the most pressing global health imperatives of our time. From ancient scourges like plague and rabies to persistent modern threats such as dengue, cholera, and Lyme disease, each chapter of this book has offered critical insights into the biology, transmission, diagnosis, treatment, and prevention of these conditions. More importantly, it has underscored the vast inequalities that exist between developed and developing nations in terms of healthcare access, infrastructure, public health literacy, and disease response capacity.

The diversity of pathogens presented here—viral, bacterial, and vector-borne—demonstrates not only the complexity of infectious disease management but also the interconnectedness of environmental, socioeconomic, and cultural factors. While medical science continues to advance in diagnostics, therapeutics, and vaccination strategies, the practical implementation of these breakthroughs remains uneven across the globe.

A central theme that emerges is the urgent need for collaborative, interdisciplinary, and cross-sectoral approaches. Whether combating antimicrobial resistance, addressing vaccine hesitancy, or managing outbreaks in under-resourced settings, a coordinated effort involving governments, health institutions, researchers, and communities is essential. Furthermore, the importance of health education, timely intervention, and equitable healthcare delivery cannot be overstated.

We hope that this reference book serves not only as an academic resource but also as a catalyst for continued inquiry, policy innovation, and global cooperation. By bridging knowledge gaps and highlighting both challenges and triumphs, we aim to inspire collective action toward a healthier, more resilient world—one where the burden of infectious diseases is no longer defined by geography or income, but met with unity, science, and compassion.

# Chapter 1
# Infection, Infectious Process (Definition, Forms) and the Role of Microorganisms, Macro Organisms, and Environment

**Layal Bassam Msheik**
*Faculty of Medical Sciences, Lebanese University, Beirut, Lebanon*

**Ahmad Saifan**
*Faculty of Medical Sciences, Lebanese University, Beirut, Lebanon*

**Ahmad Afyouni**
*Faculty of Medical Sciences, Lebanese University, Beirut, Lebanon*

**Zeinab Kazan**
https://orcid.org/0009-0002-9138-1154
*Faculty of Medical Sciences, Lebanese University, Beirut, Lebanon*

**Rim Awada**
*Faculty of Medical Sciences, Lebanese University, Beirut, Lebanon*

**Mohammad Barakat**
https://orcid.org/0000-0001-7254-083X
*Faculty of Medical Sciences, Lebanese University, Beirut, Lebanon*

## ABSTRACT

*This chapter explores infections, emphasizing microorganisms, their forms, and environmental impact, especially in low-income countries. It delves into infection transmission, their interplay with the environment, and hygiene/sanitation effects. Prevalence and epidemiology in low-income countries are analyzed, showcasing their impact on public health. Challenges faced by both income groups, like health-*

DOI: 10.4018/979-8-3693-1990-1.ch001

*care limitations, socioeconomic factors, and access issues, are examined. Cultural/ societal influences, misconceptions, and traditional healing practices are explored. Strategies for low-income countries include affordable healthcare, immunization promotion, antimicrobial resistance combat, and community-based interventions. The chapter stresses empowering local communities, enhancing health education, and fostering awareness. The conclusion advocates for a comprehensive global approach to combat infections, especially in resource-limited settings."*

## INTRODUCTION

When infectious agents enter the body, they induce infection (Barreto, Teixeira, & Carmo, 2006). Infections have significant rates of death and morbidity (Straif-Bourgeois, Ratard, & Kretzschmar, 2014). Agents can be spread by an animal host, an infected human, a vector, or an inanimate environment (Barreto et al., 2006). Microbes are found in all environments, including human bodies. These microorganisms are useful; for example, in the gastrointestinal system, they inhibit pathogen colonization. Most bacteria are beneficial to us, but some can cause illness. This infection will cause sickness if it destroys any of the body's structures or alters the individual's normal biological function (Drexler & Institute of, 2010). The infectious process begins with a pathogen entering a host and then attaching and invading host tissues, where it multiplies. The infection is dealt with by the host's immune system, and the outcome might range from asymptomatic to severe illness. Pathogens are often transferred to new hosts, and while successful resolution results in immunity, some infections may become chronic or return over time. Understanding this pathway is critical for infectious disease management and prevention (Zachary, 2017). The pathogen, host, and environment are the three components of infection. Environmental variables impact vulnerability and susceptibility to infection. This can occur as a result of causing physiologic changes in individuals, such as malnutrition-induced immunosuppression (van Seventer & Hochberg, 2017). For a variety of causes, developing nations face a double burden of communicable and noncommunicable illnesses, with a worrying trend (Boutayeb, 2010). Because infectious illness death rates are greater in less developed nations (Straif-Bourgeois et al., 2014). Poverty, conflicts, and natural disasters are the causes of such increased vulnerability and rates. The inability of individuals to access and get appropriate health care as a result of either poor economic performance or inadequate public health infrastructure is a major concern in such nations (Macfarlane, Racelis, & Muli-Musiime, 2000). This chapter aims to investigate the crucial role of microorganisms in infectious illnesses in developing nations, as well as to emphasize the particular environmental issues they confront. We will review the considerable health costs faced by these illnesses, examine the underlying environmental variables that contribute to their spread, and provide viable solutions and interventions to reduce the effects of infectious diseases in these susceptible areas.

## DISCUSSION

### Microorganisms: The Key Players in Infection

#### What are Microbes?

Microbes, found in water, soil, and air, are essential for human health and can cause illness. Common types include bacteria, viruses, fungi, and protozoa (Sharma & Gilbert, 2018). Viruses, nonliving and lacking organelles, have a nucleic acid core enclosed in a protein shell, with some having an additional lipid envelope, requiring infiltrating a host for replication (Taylor, 2021). Bacteria, single-celled prokaryotes, differ in existence, survival, and metabolism, with many naturally occurring in our normal flora, and only 1% being harmful (Sharma & Gilbert, 2018). Protozoa, eukaryotes with a complex interior structure, are one-cell eukaryotes with sophisticated metabolic functions (Yaeger, 1996). Fungi and microorganisms are eukaryotes, primarily aerobic, heterotrophic with chitinous cell walls, ergosterol-containing plasma membranes, 80S rRNA, and tubulin-based microtubules (McGinnis & Tyring, 1996).

#### Microbial Pathogenesis

For infection to occur a pathogen must cross a barrier to colonize the host (Chaffey, 2003). Microbes enter the body through the alimentary, respiratory, urogenital, and integumentary systems, as well as the ear and eye (Zachary, 2017). Portals in the body, including the small intestine, use various mechanisms to prevent pathogen entry, including mucus layers and cilia for respiratory cells (Chaffey, 2003; Zachary, 2017). Microbes have target cells to infect (Zachary, 2017). Many infections, such as Vibrio cholerae and Bordetella pertussis, infect their hosts without penetrating host cells, whereas others are intracellular (Chaffey, 2003). Target cells of intracellular pathogens have certain receptors that can bind to ligands expressed on microbes (Zachary, 2017). Following this contact, the pathogen enters by phagocytosis (large bacteria) or endocytosis (viruses). The primary goal of this entrance for viruses is to regulate the metabolism of these cells and utilize them to multiply and disseminate to other tissues (Chaffey, 2003). Others function without penetrating cells, mainly by producing toxins in bacteria that can produce several toxins (Forbes,

2020). Toxins range in size from tiny molecules to big proteins and interfere with the regular functioning of the host's metabolism (Marshall, Warrington, Watson, & Kim, 2018). Pathogens spread after colonization and proliferation, using cellular invasion or enzyme production to break down host tissues and overcome barriers (Zachary, 2017).

## Host-Microbe Interaction

An interaction happens when a pathogen comes into touch with the host. As previously stated, this interaction begins with colonization, invasion, replication, toxin generation, and host defense (Sen, Nayak, & De, 2016). Innate immunity comprises physical barriers such as skin, chemical barriers such as temperature, and immune cell recruitment (Marshall et al., 2018). Epithelial cells in entrance portals serve as the primary defense against pathogen penetration due to their presence of occluding junctions and anchoring connections to the basement membrane and ECM (Zachary, 2017). Pathogens enter the body after bleaching these barriers to be in touch with innate immunity, attracting neutrophils for phagocytosis and inflammation. They are recognized by pattern recognition receptors (PRRs) binding to pathogen-associated molecular patterns (Marshall et al., 2018). The complement system is an important component in this step by acting as opsonin, cytokines, or killing pathogens directly (Turvey & Broide, 2010). After a few hours, macrophages are recruited and persist for a longer time (Chaplin, 2010). Macrophages release cytokines for cell recruitment, inflammation, and anti-inflammatory effects, such as tumor necrosis factor (TNF), interleukin 1 (IL-1), and interleukin 6 (IL-6) during bacterial infection, enhancing cell recruitment and inflammation (Marshall et al., 2018). Several opsonins aid in macrophage phagocytosis including antibodies receptors, C3b, PRRs that bind to antibodies-antigen complex, C3b and PAMPs respectively (Zachary, 2017) (Figure 1). Dendritic cells are the primary antigen-presenting cells (APCs) that activate adaptive immunity. T cells that express the T Cell Receptor (TCR) are the major components of adaptive immunity. These cells require the signal from APCs to be activated. T cells are classified into two types: T helper or T4 cells and cytotoxic T cells (T8). T 4 will either differentiate into T helper 1 (Th1) or T helper 2 (Th2). T8 and macrophage are activated by Th1 cells to fight intracellular infections. Th2 is activated, however, against extracellular pathogens such as bacteria and parasites. They primarily stimulate B cells, which develop into plasma cells and release antibodies (Bonilla & Oettgen, 2010). Antigenic variation via mutation, phagocytosis resistance, immunological suppression like human immunodeficiency virus (HIV), and antibiotic resistance are among strategies by which microbes might evade immunity (Scully, Georgakopoulou, & Hassona, 2017).

*Figure 1. Phagocytosis and opsonins*

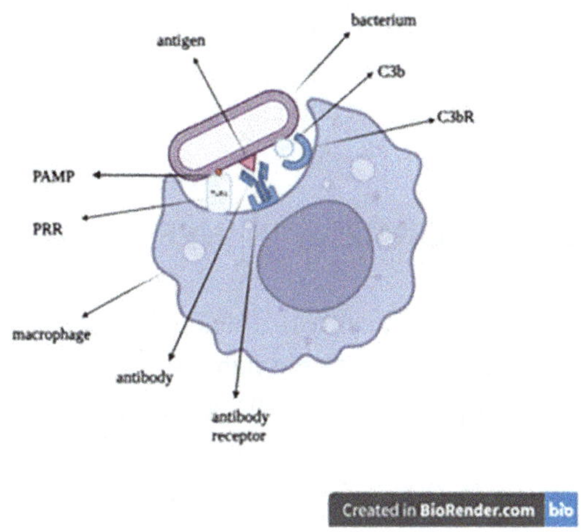


## FORMS OF INFECTION

Acute inflammation is the tissue's local reaction to infection; its principal clinical signs are induced by changes in the diameter and flow of blood vessels, an increase in vascular permeability, and the recruitment of leukocytes (Kushner, 1982). There is a rise in particular types of proteins that indicate inflammation; these proteins include erythrocyte sedimentation rate (ESR), CRP, procalcitonin (PCT), serum amyloid A (SAA) protein, fibrinogen, ferritin, and alpha-1 antitrypsin. Cytokines are secreted by macrophages and monocytes (Macfarlane et al., 2000) . An acute infection that the host and therapeutic interventions are unable to treat sets in motion a series of events that eventually lead to chronic illness. The inflammatory nidus is confined by host responses. Friable granulations deteriorated into necrotic debris, and exposed tissues dried up. Microorganisms attach and easily adhere to nonviable tissue and prosthetic surfaces. The host's weakened immune system, antimicrobial resistance, poor wound healing, and pathogen attachment to themselves and wound surfaces via a strong, tenacious biofilm are all variables that contribute to this outcome (Cierny & DiPasquale, 2006). The incubation time for latent infections may be greatly extended due to the host's resistance to the infection or the presence of environmental variables that are unfavorable to the pathogen, such as cold climate. As the environment changes, illnesses appear. A change in the pathogenicity of the pathogen while remaining in healthy tissues may also cause a previously latent disease to exhibit sickness symptoms. Latent infection may imply low pathogen levels (Steiner & Kennedy, 1995). Nosocomial infections, on the other hand, are acquired when a patient is hospitalized. They are an issue because they typically afflict the sick or handicapped, and the organisms that cause them are frequently resistant to commonly used treatments. A nosocomial infection can occur anywhere on the body, causing organ failure, sepsis, and even death (Johnson, 2002).

## ROLE OF THE ENVIRONMENT IN INFECTION

Environmental factors significantly influence the transmission of infectious diseases. Studies have shown that climatic elements such as temperature, humidity, wind speed, and rainfall play a pivotal role in disease transmission, with some research establishing their connection with the spread of infections (Mwiinde, Siankwilimba, Sakala, Banda, & Michelo, 2022). These climate-related variables can impact the viability and persistence of pathogens in the environment. For instance, temperature and humidity can affect the survival of specific infectious agents like COVID-19 (Buckee, Noor, & Sattenspiel, 2021).

Additionally, the transmission of vector-borne diseases like malaria is closely tied to specific geographic regions, influencing the distribution of disease vectors (van Seventer & Hochberg, 2017). The social environment also plays a role in shaping disease transmission dynamics (Buckee et al., 2021). High population density has been identified as a risk factor for disease transmission, as it increases the potential for close contact and facilitates rapid infection spread (Ganasegeran, Jamil, Ch'ng, Looi, & Peariasamy, 2021). Moreover, international travel, in particular, has been linked to the global dissemination of diseases, highlighting its role in infectious disease transmission (Buckee et al., 2021).

Furthermore, the built environment, including healthcare settings, is critical for infection control. Proper sanitation, ventilation, and hygiene within healthcare facilities are essential to prevent healthcare-associated infections and reduce the risk of disease transmission (Collins, 2008).

Zoonotic diseases are infections transmitted from animals to humans. Those diseases may be caused by various agents, with viruses being particularly prominent in their emergence. Nowadays, a concerning surge in viral zoonotic diseases had emerged, including Ebola virus, SARS-CoV-2, and polioviruses (Marie & Gordon, 2023). The factors contributing to zoonotic transmission are multifaceted. In fact, global changes like climate change, deforestation, habitat destruction, intensified agriculture, and increased travel and trade have been shown to disrupt the delicate equilibrium between humans, animals, and the environment, making the risk of zoonotic infections more than ever (Elsohaby & Villa, 2023).

Importantly, environmental reservoirs play a pivotal role in the long-term presence and spread of disease-causing agents. Soil, water, and air act as reservoirs for diverse pathogens, creating a substantial threat to human well-being. These settings can host disease-causing agents, encompassing bacteria, viruses, and fungi, thereby establishing them as potential origins of infections. To illustrate, consider tetanus and botulism, caused by environmental pathogens like Clostridium tetani and C. botulinum, which persist in the soil. Similarly, Legionella pneumophila serves as another instance, inhabiting freshwater rivers as an environmental pathogen (van Seventer & Hochberg, 2017).

It is worth mentioning that a substantial health burden is linked to inadequate hygiene, sanitation, and water access, but it can be significantly reduced through well-established, cost-effective measures. These interventions offer benefits that extend beyond health, surpassing the initial costs. While hygiene, sanitation, and water supply are critical components of development, global policies concerning drinking water and sanitation often fall short of the needed ambition. Even in developed nations, hygiene, sanitation, and water supply remain important factors in public health. To make significant strides in health improvement, the active participation of healthcare professionals in promoting and advancing hygiene, sanitation, and water supply is indispensable (Bartram & Cairncross, 2010).

## PREVALENCE OF INFECTION

In low-income countries, the prevalence and epidemiology of infectious diseases paint a challenging landscape. These nations often bear a higher burden of infectious diseases compared to their high-income counterparts. The overview of disease prevalence reveals a stark reality, with conditions such as malaria, tuberculosis, and diarrheal diseases affecting a significant portion of the population. The impact on public health is substantial, leading to increased mortality, morbidity, and reduced overall life expectancy. The burden of infectious diseases in these countries places immense strain on healthcare systems and contributes to a cycle of poverty and ill health (Shears, 2007).

### Challenges

Controlling infectious diseases is a complex problem that presents a wide range of challenges for both industrialized and developing countries, necessitating the development of comprehensive policies that take into account a variety of sociological, medical, and economic considerations.

## Challenges in Developing Countries

During epidemics or pandemics, low- and middle-income countries (LMICs) face challenges in healthcare facilities due to inadequate infrastructure, lack of healthcare professionals, and the absence of essential resources like personal protective equipment (PPE). Hand hygiene programs also face difficulties due to a lack of basic infrastructure, insufficient supply of soaps and alcohol-based hand rubs, and low awareness and compliance (Angrup, Kanaujia, Ray, & Biswal, 2020).

Antimicrobial resistance is a growing problem in infection control, worsened in LMICs by factors such as rising antibiotic use, lax control over-the-counter sales, high hospital infection rates, limited infection control strategies, insufficient surveillance programs, and lack of microbiology labs. Additionally, there is a lack of stewardship programs, medical personnel with the necessary training, and inadequate availability and support for bioinformatics. National surveillance systems are often lacking in LMICs due to inaccurate information and a lack of established reporting standards. External variables like political and economic interests also affect surveillance operations, making transparent data not only modified but also not readily available (Vilar-Compte, Camacho-Ortiz, & Ponce-de-León, 2017). Moreover, drug shortages pose a serious threat to patient safety, leading to under- or non-treatment and errors when using alternative drugs. This is a result of the minimal manufacturing capacities of LICs and the persistent pharmaceutical trade deficits (Sabogal De La Pava & Tucker, 2022). Vaccination in LMICs is challenging due to vaccine shortages, uneven access and distribution, poor vaccination knowledge, and lack of cold chain infrastructure and technologies. There are significant disparities in vaccination rates between high- and low-income nations, making global infection management more challenging (Moyazzem Hossain, Abdulla, & Rahman, 2022).

## Challenges in Developed Countries

Globalization's rapid evolution and complexity pose significant challenges to our understanding of the world. One example is the spread of infectious diseases, which often result in medication resistance and resurgence of previously under-controlled infections. The increasing number of infected contacts due to commerce and travel has made traditional quarantine methods outdated and surveillance more difficult. It should also be noted that migrants to high-income countries have higher rates of illness and mortality from infectious diseases, making them one of the most vulnerable populations (Frenk, Gómez-Dantés, & Knaul, 2011). Antimicrobial resistance (AMR) threatens global public health systems, resulting in severe infections, extended hospital stays, higher medical expenses, and treatment failures. Travelers often return home colonized and infected, facilitating the spread of AMR through modern travel routes (Dadgostar, 2019) . Vaccination reluctance is a major concern, as lower vaccination rates could lead to more hospital admissions and deaths in both vaccinated and unvaccinated populations (Olivera Mesa et al., 2022). In high-income nations, aging is a significant challenge in infection control, as it alters innate and adaptive immunity, making older people more susceptible to infections. Additionally, diminished renal function with age may make antibiotic therapy less effective, leading to more expensive acute bacterial infections in the elderly (Kline & Bowdish, 2016). Social factors, such as work-related restrictions on quarantine, difficulty finding private childcare, and discrimination, also increase the susceptibility of racial and ethnic minorities to infections. Low-income groups in high-income nations also experience higher levels of psychological stress, which compromises their immunity and increases their susceptibility to illness (Quinn & Kumar, 2014).

## Treatment and Prevention

The main focus concerning prevention of infectious diseases lies in Low-income countries where access to medical care is not always accessible, acceptable, or affordable (Ozawa, Shankar, Leopold, & Orubu, 2019). Some challenges affect the decision to seek care in these settings (gender, marital status, health status, education, employment) (Srivastava & McGuire, 2015).

A systematic review by Bright et al. identified strategies to enhance healthcare access, targeting both supply and demand aspects. Supply-side approaches include bringing healthcare services closer to communities and implementing school programs, while demand-side strategies involve health promotion and education to improve accessibility and acceptability. Notably, text messages and proximity to services consistently prove effective in improving healthcare utilization (Bright, Felix, Kuper, & Polack, 2017).

Vaccination represents a significant breakthrough in the prevention of infectious illnesses: it decreases the likelihood of complications and death when a person is later exposed to the infectious agent (Canouï & Launay, 2019). Findings suggest that it provide equity and sustainability, and increases productivity gains in the long term by increasing cognitive outcomes in later childhood. Moreover, vaccination can provide "herd protection" by preventing infection transmission from vaccinated to unvaccinated individuals hence reducing disease incidence in unvaccinated individuals (Deogaonkar, Hutubessy, van der Putten, Evers, & Jit, 2012).

Additionally, many strategies and initiatives must be undertaken to increase vaccination rates. To enhance HPV vaccination rates in low-income countries, leveraging school-based delivery methods by effectively coordinating between the health and education sectors should be a central strategy. Simultaneously, addressing concerns about the associated costs, and ensuring sustainability and rumors and misinformation proactively must be integrated into the vaccination campaign (Tsu, LaMontagne, Atuhebwe, Bloem, & Ndiaye, 2021).

The WHO has deployed many plans to combat AMR. The Global Action Plan for Antimicrobial Resistance (GAP-AMR) is designed to safeguard the effectiveness of antimicrobial treatments and the prevention of infectious diseases. It emphasizes responsible antimicrobial use with appropriate accessibility and quality controls. Among its five primary objectives, one focuses on improving the effectiveness of antimicrobial drug utilization in both human and animal health, necessitating the establishment of robust regulatory systems to achieve this goal (Khouja, Mitsantisuk, Tadrous, & Suda, 2022).

Many community-based interventions have shown an important impact in confronting infections spread within any population. For instance, nutrition projects that emphasize household food production and nutrition education lead to a significant reduction in the incidence of respiratory infections and diarrheal infections, as well as pneumonia and severe pneumonia (English et al., 1997). In addition, in a study by Meyers et al. surveillance systems relying upon community-based or crowd-sourced have shown a correlation with hospital data in the same community. These systems can complement traditional facilities-based data sources to keep public health responses in the loop of any spread of an infection, especially in resource-limited settings (Meyers et al., 2016). Moreover, in the context of health, educational programs play a pivotal role in uplifting low-income communities by fostering knowledge and raising awareness about the transmission and prevention of diseases, equipping people with the tools they need to protect themselves and their communities, thus creating a foundation for healthier populations (Beks et al., 2022). Additionally, access to clean water ensures that people can maintain proper personal hygiene, such as handwashing, which is one of the most effective ways to prevent the transmission of diseases. New approaches relying on household treatment devices that are lower in cost in comparation to traditional approaches show a decrease in the concentrations of chemical and microbial contaminants (Mwabi et al., 2011).

Moreover, Beks, H et.al examined the use of information and communications technology (ICT) in delivering health programs in high-income countries during the COVID-19 pandemic. It found 83 diverse ICT-based programs across 19 countries, demonstrating that nurse and allied health ICT programs were effective, sometimes even more so than in-person programs. The study encourages healthcare professionals to build on this knowledge, collaborate with consumers, and develop innovative ICT-based programs in community health settings (Beks et al., 2022).

A project evaluation of Drinking Water Supply, Sanitation, and Hygiene (WASH) Promotion Interventions in Two Slum Communities in Central Uganda has demonstrated substantial enhancements in the WASH conditions of the slums, marked by a significant rise in piped water usage, a noteworthy reduction in the reliance on unsafe water sources, and a substantial decrease in haphazard solid waste disposal (Musoke et al., 2018).

These WASH interventions can substantially decrease the risk of infections spreading within a community. The presence of beneficial household WASH practices was linked to a substantial decrease in the long-term likelihood of severe cholera in an urban slum in Dhaka. Specifically, individuals residing in households with superior WASH practices, comprising roughly one-third of the population, experienced a noteworthy 47% reduction in the risk of severe cholera (Kang et al., 2022).

On another note, education plans can have a noteworthy effect on having better health outcomes. In an Randomized Controlled Trial conducted in China, the groups of children having more frequent health education sessions showed a significant decrease in hospitalization compared to other groups with less frequent sessions (Liping, 2015).

## CONCLUSION

In conclusion, understanding infections requires a holistic approach that integrates knowledge of microorganisms, their varied forms, and the dynamic interplay with the environment. Particularly, in low-income countries, where challenges in healthcare infrastructure, socioeconomics, and cultural factors persist, a comprehensive strategy involving accessible healthcare, robust vaccination initiatives, and community empowerment is imperative. By addressing these complexities collaboratively on a global scale, we can navigate the intricate landscape of infections and work towards a healthier, more resilient world.

## REFERENCES


Angrup, A., Kanaujia, R., Ray, P., & Biswal, M. (2020). Healthcare facilities in low- and middle-income countries affected by COVID-19: Time to upgrade basic infection control and prevention practices. *Indian Journal of Medical Microbiology*, *38*(2), 139–143. DOI: 10.4103/ijmm.IJMM_20_125 PMID: 32883925

Barreto, M. L., Teixeira, M. G., & Carmo, E. H. (2006). Infectious diseases epidemiology. *Journal of Epidemiology and Community Health*, *60*(3), 192–195. DOI: 10.1136/jech.2003.011593 PMID: 16476746

Bartram, J., & Cairncross, S. (2010). Hygiene, sanitation, and water: Forgotten foundations of health. *PLoS Medicine*, *7*(11), e1000367. DOI: 10.1371/journal.pmed.1000367 PMID: 21085694

Beks, H., King, O., Clapham, R., Alston, L., Glenister, K., McKinstry, C., Quilliam, C., Wellwood, I., Williams, C., & Wong Shee, A. (2022). Community Health Programs Delivered Through Information and Communications Technology in High-Income Countries: Scoping Review. *Journal of Medical Internet Research*, *24*(3), e26515. DOI: 10.2196/26515 PMID: 35262498

Bonilla, F. A., & Oettgen, H. C. (2010). Adaptive immunity. *The Journal of Allergy and Clinical Immunology*, *125*(2, Suppl 2), S33–S40. DOI: 10.1016/j.jaci.2009.09.017 PMID: 20061006

Boutayeb, A. (2010). The Burden of Communicable and Non-Communicable Diseases in Developing Countries. In Preedy, V. R., & Watson, R. R. (Eds.), *Handbook of Disease Burdens and Quality of Life Measures* (pp. 531–546). Springer New York. DOI: 10.1007/978-0-387-78665-0_32

Bright, T., Felix, L., Kuper, H., & Polack, S. (2017). A systematic review of strategies to increase access to health services among children in low and middle income countries. *BMC Health Services Research*, *17*(1), 252. DOI: 10.1186/s12913-017-2180-9 PMID: 28381276

Buckee, C., Noor, A., & Sattenspiel, L. (2021). Thinking clearly about social aspects of infectious disease transmission. *Nature*, *595*(7866), 205–213. DOI: 10.1038/s41586-021-03694-x PMID: 34194045

Canouï, E., & Launay, O. (2019). Histoire et principes de la vaccination. *Revue des Maladies Respiratoires*, *36*(1), 74–81. DOI: 10.1016/j.rmr.2018.02.015 PMID: 30579659

Chaffey, N. (2003). Alberts, B., Johnson, A., Lewis, J., Raff, M., Roberts, K. and Walter, P. Molecular biology of the cell. 4th edn.

Chaplin, D. D. (2010). Overview of the immune response. *The Journal of Allergy and Clinical Immunology, 125*(2, Suppl 2), S3–S23. DOI: 10.1016/j.jaci.2009.12.980 PMID: 20176265

Cierny, G., 3rd, & DiPasquale, D. (2006). Treatment of chronic infection. *J Am Acad Orthop Surg, 14*(10 Spec No.), S105-110. DOI: 10.5435/00124635-200600001-00025

Collins, A. S. (2008). Advances in Patient Safety Preventing Health Care–Associated Infections. In Hughes, R. G. (Ed.), *Patient Safety and Quality: An Evidence-Based Handbook for Nurses*. Agency for Healthcare Research and Quality (US).

Dadgostar, P. (2019). Antimicrobial Resistance: Implications and Costs. *Infection and Drug Resistance, 12*, 3903–3910. DOI: 10.2147/IDR.S234610 PMID: 31908502

Deogaonkar, R., Hutubessy, R., van der Putten, I., Evers, S., & Jit, M. (2012). Systematic review of studies evaluating the broader economic impact of vaccination in low and middle income countries. *BMC Public Health, 12*(1), 878. DOI: 10.1186/1471-2458-12-878 PMID: 23072714

Drexler, M., & Institute of, M. (2010) *What You Need to Know About Infectious Disease*. Washington (DC): National Academies Press (US) Copyright © National Academy of Sciences.

Elsohaby, I., & Villa, L. (2023). Zoonotic diseases: Understanding the risks and mitigating the threats. *BMC Veterinary Research, 19*(1), 186. DOI: 10.1186/s12917-023-03736-8 PMID: 37789313

English, R. M., Badcock, J. C., Giay, T., Ngu, T., Waters, A. M., & Bennett, S. A. (1997). Effect of nutrition improvement project on morbidity from infectious diseases in preschool children in Vietnam: Comparison with control commune. *BMJ (Clinical Research Ed.), 315*(7116), 1122–1125. DOI: 10.1136/bmj.315.7116.1122 PMID: 9374884

Forbes, J. D. (2020). Clinically Important Toxins in Bacterial Infection: Utility of Laboratory Detection. *Clinical Microbiology Newsletter, 42*(20), 163–170. DOI: 10.1016/j.clinmicnews.2020.09.003 PMID: 33046946

Frenk, J., Gómez-Dantés, O., & Knaul, F. M. (2011). Globalization and infectious diseases. *Infect Dis Clin North Am, 25*(3), 593-599, viii. DOI: 10.1016/j.idc.2011.05.003

Ganasegeran, K., Jamil, M. F. A., Ch'ng, A. S. H., Looi, I., & Peariasamy, K. M. (2021). Influence of Population Density for COVID-19 Spread in Malaysia: An Ecological Study. *International Journal of Environmental Research and Public Health, 18*(18), 9866. Advance online publication. DOI: 10.3390/ijerph18189866 PMID: 34574790

Johnson, J. A. (2002). Nosocomial infections. *The Veterinary Clinics of North America. Small Animal Practice, 32*(5), 1101–1126. DOI: 10.1016/S0195-5616(02)00038-4 PMID: 12380168

Kang, S., Chowdhury, F., Park, J., Ahmed, T., Tadesse, B. T., Islam, M. T., Kim, D. R., Im, J., Aziz, A. B., Hoque, M., Pak, G., Khanam, F., Ahmmed, F., Liu, X., Zaman, K., Khan, A. I., Kim, J. H., Marks, F., Qadri, F., & Clemens, J. D. (2022). Are better existing WASH practices in urban slums associated with a lower long-term risk of severe cholera? A prospective cohort study with 4 years of follow-up in Mirpur, Bangladesh. *BMJ Open, 12*(9), e060858. DOI: 10.1136/bmjopen-2022-060858 PMID: 36130764

Khouja, T., Mitsantisuk, K., Tadrous, M., & Suda, K. J. (2022). Global consumption of antimicrobials: Impact of the WHO Global Action Plan on Antimicrobial Resistance and 2019 coronavirus pandemic (COVID-19). *The Journal of Antimicrobial Chemotherapy, 77*(5), 1491–1499. DOI: 10.1093/jac/dkac028 PMID: 35178565

Kline, K. A., & Bowdish, D. M. E. (2016). Infection in an aging population. *Current Opinion in Microbiology, 29*, 63–67. DOI: 10.1016/j.mib.2015.11.003 PMID: 26673958

Kushner, I. (1982). The phenomenon of the acute phase response. *Annals of the New York Academy of Sciences, 389*(1), 39–48. DOI: 10.1111/j.1749-6632.1982.tb22124.x PMID: 7046585

Liping, Z. (2015). Relationship between health education plan and hospitalization frequency in the children with respiratory tract infection. *Pakistan Journal of Pharmaceutical Sciences, 28*(1, Suppl), 393–395. PMID: 25631503

Macfarlane, S., Racelis, M., & Muli-Musiime, F. (2000). Public health in developing countries. *Lancet, 356*(9232), 841–846. DOI: 10.1016/S0140-6736(00)02664-7 PMID: 11022943

Marie, V., & Gordon, M. L. (2023). The (Re-)Emergence and Spread of Viral Zoonotic Disease: A Perfect Storm of Human Ingenuity and Stupidity. *Viruses, 15*(8), 1638. Advance online publication. DOI: 10.3390/v15081638 PMID: 37631981

Marshall, J. S., Warrington, R., Watson, W., & Kim, H. L. (2018). An introduction to immunology and immunopathology. *Allergy, Asthma, and Clinical Immunology : Official Journal of the Canadian Society of Allergy and Clinical Immunology, 14*(2), 49. DOI: 10.1186/s13223-018-0278-1 PMID: 30263032

McGinnis, M. R., & Tyring, S. K. (1996). Introduction to Mycology. In S. Baron (Ed.), *Medical Microbiology*. Galveston (TX): University of Texas Medical Branch at Galveston Copyright © 1996, The University of Texas Medical Branch at Galveston.

Meyers, D. J., Ozonoff, A., Baruwal, A., Pande, S., Harsha, A., Sharma, R., Schwarz, D., Schwarz, R. K., Bista, D., Halliday, S., & Maru, D. S. (2016). Combining Healthcare-Based and Participatory Approaches to Surveillance: Trends in Diarrheal and Respiratory Conditions Collected by a Mobile Phone System by Community Health Workers in Rural Nepal. *PLoS One, 11*(4), e0152738. DOI: 10.1371/journal.pone.0152738 PMID: 27111734

Moyazzem Hossain, M., Abdulla, F., & Rahman, A. (2022). Challenges and difficulties faced in low- and middle-income countries during COVID-19. *Health Policy OPEN, 3*, 100082. DOI: 10.1016/j.hpopen.2022.100082 PMID: 36405972

Musoke, D., Ndejjo, R., Halage, A. A., Kasasa, S., Ssempebwa, J. C., & Carpenter, D. O. (2018). Drinking Water Supply, Sanitation, and Hygiene Promotion Interventions in Two Slum Communities in Central Uganda. *Journal of Environmental and Public Health, 3710120*, 1–9. Advance online publication. DOI: 10.1155/2018/3710120 PMID: 29623096

Mwabi, J. K., Adeyemo, F. E., Mahlangu, T. O., Mamba, B. B., Brouckaert, B. M., Swartz, C. D., Offringa, G., Mpenyana-Monyatsi, L., & Momba, M. N. B. (2011). Household water treatment systems: A solution to the production of safe drinking water by the low-income communities of Southern Africa. *Physics and Chemistry of the Earth Parts A/B/C, 36*(14), 1120–1128. DOI: 10.1016/j.pce.2011.07.078

Mwiinde, A. M., Siankwilimba, E., Sakala, M., Banda, F., & Michelo, C. (2022). Climatic and Environmental Factors Influencing COVID-19 Transmission-An African Perspective. *Tropical Medicine and Infectious Disease, 7*(12), 433. Advance online publication. DOI: 10.3390/tropicalmed7120433 PMID: 36548688

Olivera Mesa, D., Hogan, A. B., Watson, O. J., Charles, G. D., Hauck, K., Ghani, A. C., & Winskill, P. (2022). Modelling the impact of vaccine hesitancy in prolonging the need for Non-Pharmaceutical Interventions to control the COVID-19 pandemic. *Communications Medicine, 2*(1), 14. DOI: 10.1038/s43856-022-00075-x PMID: 35603311

Ozawa, S., Shankar, R., Leopold, C., & Orubu, S. (2019). Access to medicines through health systems in low- and middle-income countries. *Health Policy and Planning*, *34*(Supplement_3), iii1–iii3. DOI: 10.1093/heapol/czz119 PMID: 31816069

Quinn, S. C., & Kumar, S. (2014). Health inequalities and infectious disease epidemics: A challenge for global health security. *Biosecurity and Bioterrorism*, *12*(5), 263–273. DOI: 10.1089/bsp.2014.0032 PMID: 25254915

Sabogal De La Pava, M. L., & Tucker, E. L. (2022). Drug shortages in low- and middle-income countries: Colombia as a case study. *Journal of Pharmaceutical Policy and Practice*, *15*(1), 42. DOI: 10.1186/s40545-022-00439-7 PMID: 35698240

Scully, C., Georgakopoulou, E. A., & Hassona, Y. (2017). The Immune System: Basis of so much Health and Disease: 3. Adaptive Immunity. *Dental Update*, *44*(4), 322–324, 327. DOI: 10.12968/denu.2017.44.4.322 PMID: 29172358

Sen, R., Nayak, L., & De, R. K. (2016). A review on host-pathogen interactions: Classification and prediction. *European Journal of Clinical Microbiology & Infectious Diseases*, *35*(10), 1581–1599. DOI: 10.1007/s10096-016-2716-7 PMID: 27470504

Sharma, A., & Gilbert, J. A. (2018). Microbial exposure and human health. *Current Opinion in Microbiology*, *44*, 79–87. DOI: 10.1016/j.mib.2018.08.003 PMID: 30195150

Shears, P. (2007). Poverty and infection in the developing world: Healthcare-related infections and infection control in the tropics. *The Journal of Hospital Infection*, *67*(3), 217–224. DOI: 10.1016/j.jhin.2007.08.016 PMID: 17945396

Srivastava, D., & McGuire, A. (2015). Patient access to health care and medicines across low-income countries. *Social Science & Medicine*, *133*, 21–27. DOI: 10.1016/j.socscimed.2015.03.021 PMID: 25829195

Steiner, I., & Kennedy, P. G. (1995). Herpes simplex virus latent infection in the nervous system. *Journal of Neurovirology*, *1*(1), 19–29. DOI: 10.3109/13550289509111007 PMID: 9222339

Straif-Bourgeois, S., Ratard, R., & Kretzschmar, M. (2014). Infectious Disease Epidemiology. In Ahrens, W., & Pigeot, I. (Eds.), *Handbook of Epidemiology* (pp. 2041–2119). Springer New York. DOI: 10.1007/978-0-387-09834-0_34

Taylor, M. W. (2021). National implementation of HPV vaccination programs in low-resource countries: Lessons, challenges, and future prospects. *Preventive Medicine*, *144*, 106335. DOI: 10.1016/j.ypmed.2020.106335 PMID: 33678232

Turvey, S. E., & Broide, D. H. (2010). Innate immunity. *The Journal of Allergy and Clinical Immunology*, *125*(2, Suppl 2), S24–S32. DOI: 10.1016/j.jaci.2009.07.016 PMID: 19932920

van Seventer, J. M., & Hochberg, N. S. (2017). Principles of Infectious Diseases: Transmission, Diagnosis, Prevention, and Control. In Quah, S. R. (Ed.), *International Encyclopedia of Public Health* (2nd ed., pp. 22–39). Academic Press. DOI: 10.1016/B978-0-12-803678-5.00516-6

Vilar-Compte, D., Camacho-Ortiz, A., & Ponce-de-León, S. (2017). Infection Control in Limited Resources Countries: Challenges and Priorities. *Current Infectious Disease Reports*, *19*(5), 20. DOI: 10.1007/s11908-017-0572-y PMID: 28401447

Yaeger, R. G. (1996). Protozoa: Structure, Classification, Growth, and Development. In S. Baron (Ed.), *Medical Microbiology*. Galveston (TX): University of Texas Medical Branch at Galveston Copyright © 1996, The University of Texas Medical Branch at Galveston.

Zachary, J. F. (2017). Mechanisms of Microbial Infections1. *Pathologic Basis of Veterinary Disease*, 132 - 241.e131.

# Chapter 2
# Pathogenetic Therapy in Infectious Diseases:
## Rehydration and Correction of Electrolytes Disbalance

**Fatima M. Abbas**
*Cairo Univercity, Egypt*

**Shahd M. Mosa**
*Cairo Univercity, Egypt*

**M. Atef El-Badawy**
*Cairo University, Egypt*

**Habiba Y. Essa**
*Cairo Univercity, Egypt*

**Aya Sanad Abousaad**
*Cairo Univercity, Egypt*

## ABSTRACT

*Pathogenic therapy in infectious disease is linked to the treatment of infectious diseases such as diarrhea, cholera, and other diseases that affect the intestines and cause an imbalance in body fluids and important minerals such as sodium, potassium, calcium, chloride and other minerals that play a strong vital role in transmitting signals, Nervousness, muscle contraction, hormone secretion, and other essential functions, the occurrence of any imbalance in their levels leads to disturbances in the electrical balance, such as muscle spasms or breathing and heart rhythm disturbances, which may lead to low or high blood pressure or cardiac arrest. Previous studies have*

DOI: 10.4018/979-8-3693-1990-1.ch002

*shown that the survival rate for cholera and diarrhea patients has become more than 99% thanks to these treatments and studies. Therefore, rehydration and electrolyte balance are important for normal physiological functions and require appropriate therapy when disrupted by environmental factors or illness. This chapter's knowledge helps us understand the importance of this type of treatment and health guidelines.*

## INTRODUCTION

An infectious disease is one that develops when pathogenic agents or germs (such as viruses, bacteria, protozoans, or fungus) enter the body and begin to grow and reproduce there, (Wayne & Bolker, 2023). Which can cause a lot of symptoms like vomiting, fever, diarrhea, or sweating, (World Health Organization, 2020) (Morgenstern & Thoma, 2018). These symptoms can affect the balance of the body even after the treatment of the infection. So pathogenetic therapy is very important for the patient, (Gusev, Sarapultsev, & Chereshnev, 2021).

## PATHOGENETIC THERAPY IN INFECTIOUS DISEASES

Pathogenetic therapy in infectious diseases involves measures to help the body overcome the disease by eliminating or moderating its effects, supporting the healing process, or preventing complications. This can include drug treatments that target specific bacteria, increase effective drug concentration, and reduce the dosage of antibiotics, thus improving antibacterial efficacy and slowing down the development of drug resistance. Recent advances in immunotherapies have also shown promise in disease management by targeting and manipulating components of the immune system to eliminate pathogens, (Gusev, Sarapultsev, & Chereshnev, 2021) (Shang *et al.,* 2020).

In the context of the 2019 novel coronavirus disease, the optimal therapy is being explored based on the understanding of the disease's pathogenesis, (Cloeckaert & Kuchler, 2020).

Implementing pathogenetic therapy in infectious diseases faces several challenges.

## Challenges Pathogenetic Therapy in Infectious Diseases

### Lack of Funding

There is a dramatic lack of public, private, and corporate funding in many areas of infectious diseases research, which can hinder the development and implementation of new treatments, (Gusev, Sarapultsev, & Chereshnev, 2021).

### Complexity of Host-Pathogen Interactions

The genetic complexity of the individual host, the adaptive potential of pathogens, and spatiotemporal disease dynamics make it difficult to develop efficient therapies, (Gusev, Sarapultsev, & Chereshnev, 2021).

### Polymicrobial Infections

These infections challenge the host's immune defense capacity at all stages by activating pathogen-specific immune responses, making it difficult to develop effective therapies, (Shang *et al.,* 2020).

### Antimicrobial Resistance

The development of antimicrobial resistance (AMR) poses a serious threat to global public health, as conventional antibiotics are increasingly less effective against drug-resistant bacteria, (Cloeckaert & Kuchler, 2020).

### Limited Pipeline of New Antibiotics

The development and deployment of novel antimicrobial drugs are slow, as few new antibiotics are being developed over time, and even fewer of them can reach the market, (Cloeckaert & Kuchler, 2020).

To overcome these challenges, researchers are exploring alternative therapeutic strategies, such as pathogen-oriented therapy (POT), which aims to target specific bacteria, increase effective drug concentration, and reduce the dosage of antibiotics, thus improving antibacterial efficacy and reducing the development of drug resistance, (Cloeckaert & Kuchler, 2020). However, more research funding, collaboration, and innovative approaches are needed to address these challenges and implement effective pathogenetic therapies in infectious diseases.

# DEHYDRATION AND REHYDRATION IN INFECTIOUS DISEASES

## Dehydration in Infectious Diseases

Dehydration often happens when you have an Infection in your digestive system, such as cholera, typhoid, dysentery, or rotavirus. These infections can make you have a lot of:

- Diarrhea, vomiting. These can make you lose a lot of water and electrolytes very quickly, (World Health Organization, 2020) (Morgenstern & Thoma, 2018).
- Fever, when you have a high fever, you may become more dehydrated. This can get worse if you also have diarrhea and vomiting, (World Health Organization, 2020) (Morgenstern & Thoma, 2018).
- Sweating. You sweat out water, especially when it is hot or when you work out hard, (Centers for Disease Control and Prevention, 2020) (Weisz, 2020).
- Urination. You pee out water, especially if you have a condition that makes you pee more, such as diabetes or kidney disease, (Centers for Disease Control and Prevention, 2020) (Weisz, 2020).
- Medications. Some medicines can make you lose water, such as diuretics, antihistamines, or blood pressure medications, (Centers for Disease Control and Prevention, 2020) (Weisz, 2020).
- Not drinking enough water. You may not drink enough water because you are ill, busy, or do not have access to clean drinking water, (Centers for Disease Control and Prevention, 2020) (Weisz, 2020).

Dehydration can affect how your body works and make you have symptoms like thirst, dry mouth, tiredness, dizziness, headache, confusion, and more. If you don't get treatment for dehydration, it can cause very serious problems, such as kidney failure, seizures, shock, and death, (Centers for Disease Control and Prevention, 2020) (Weisz, 2020). That's why it's very Important to prevent and treat dehydration by drinking enough fluids, preferably water or oral rehydration solution (ORS). ORS Is a mix of clean water, sugar, and salt that can help you replace the fluids and electrolytes you lost, (World Health Organization, 2020). If you are very dehydrated, you may need to get fluids through a vein, (Weisz, 2020).

## Rehydration in Infectious Diseases

So, Rehydration is an essential treatment for infectious diseases that cause fluid and electrolyte loss due to diarrhea, vomiting, or fever, such as cholera, which can result in severe dehydration and death. Rehydration replenishes the body's water and salt balance and reduces symptoms such as weak pulse, low blood pressure, unconsciousness, breathing problems, sunken eyes, and kidney failure. The way to rehydrate a person varies depending on how dehydrated they are, what caused their illness, and what resources are at hand. For mild to moderate dehydration, oral rehydration therapy (ORT) is advised, which means drinking ORS that have glucose and electrolytes like sodium, potassium, chloride, and bicarbonate. ORS can be made by mixing oral rehydration salts (a packet of glucose and electrolytes) with 1 liter of clean water. A simple way to estimate how much ORS drink for older children and adults is 100 ml every 5 minutes, until they feel better, (Guerrant *et al.,* 2001).

For babies and young children, ORS can be given by spoon, cup, or syringe, and the amount should be based on how thirsty and how much urine they have. If ORS is not available, water, fruits, and vegetables with high water content can be consumed, but tea, coffee, and sugary drinks should be avoided, (ETHealthWorld, 2021).

For severe dehydration or shock, intravenous fluid therapy (IVT) is needed, which means giving fluids through a vein, usually in a hospital. The kind and amount of fluid depends on how the person is doing and why they are dehydrated. For example, for cholera, the World Health Organization (WHO) suggests giving Ringer's lactate solution or normal saline solution as the first fluid. The speed of fluid delivery should be adjusted by the person's vital signs, urine amount, and mental state, (Guerrant *et al.,* 2001) (Longo, 2020).

## ELECTROLYTE IMBALANCES

Electrolytes are ionized salts that are found in blood and body fluids and play a necessary role in maintaining physiological balance of the body, (Spence, 1999) (Asima *et al.,* 2015). The occurrence of any disorder in them leads to many risks, and one of the most important factors that lead to electrolyte disorders is infection with infectious diseases (Asima *et al.,* 2015), and Electrolyte imbalances can be caused by various factors, including fluid loss due to vomiting, diarrhea, or sweating, certain medications, and underlying medical conditions such as kidney disease and heart problems too, (Song *et al.,* 2023). Additionally, research has shown that infectious diseases can impact the body's electrolyte balance, leading to disturbances in water and electrolyte levels, (Gonzalez, Finberg, & Bluestein, 1964). The symptoms of electrolyte imbalances can range from muscle aches and weakness to more severe complications such as seizures and coma, (Song *et al.,* 2023). The most important electrolytes that are severely affected in the event of an infection and causes the symptoms mentioned are: Sodium $Na^+$ is the most important cation in the body. It is responsible for the distribution of body fluids, blood pressure, and the body electrical activity, (Fox, 2013). When an imbalance in its concentration occurs, it leads to an imbalance in the entire body. For example, but not limited to, when its concentration decreases, you suffer from hyponatremia, one of its most important symptoms like headache, confusion, nausea, vomiting, etc., (Sahay & Sahay, 2014) (Królicka *et al.,* 2020). Magnesium is the fourth most important ion in the human body. It is involved in the composition of more than 300 enzyme systems that regulate various chemical reactions and helps balance blood pressure, (Asima *et al.,* 2015) (Rude, 2010) (Rude, 2012). It also plays a role in the functioning of muscles and nerves, and an imbalance in its concentration, such as a decrease, for example, leads to: vomiting, fatigue, weakness, muscle contraction and spasm, (Rude, 2012), Calcium(Ca), which is one of the most abundant ions in the body, is stored in the bones and is responsible for the strength of the bones, teeth, and other parts of the body. An imbalance in its concentration causes many changes, such as muscle spasm, osteoporosis, etc., (Asima *et al.,* 2015) and Potassium (K), which is known as the heart mineral, has a direct effect on its cells. It also has an important role in regulating the activity of heart muscle and nervous system signals, and any imbalance in its concentration leads to increased heart rate, feebleness, and tiredness, (Asima *et al.*, 2015). A study conducted at King Abdulaziz Hospital in Jeddah found that the prevalence of electrolyte imbalance in hospitalized patients with infectious diseases was high, especially at admission and during the hospital stay, (Albeladi *et al.,* 2022). Another study focused on patients with severe COVID-19 and highlighted the occurrence of electrolyte imbalances in this specific patient population, (Lippi, South, & Henry, 2020).

Electrolyte imbalances are frequently observed in infectious disease patients and can have significant implications for their prognosis and treatment.

## CORRECTION OF ELECTROLYTES DISBALANCE

It's important to note that the specific approach to correcting electrolyte imbalances may vary based on the type and severity of the imbalance, as well as the patient's overall health status. Therefore, healthcare professionals should carefully assess each patient's condition and tailor the correction of electrolyte imbalance to their individual needs, (Hoque, 2023). Medical treatments for electrolyte imbalances depend on the type and severity of the imbalance. In minor cases, dietary changes may be sufficient to correct the imbalance. However, in more severe cases, medical interventions may be necessary. Some medical treatments for electrolyte imbalances include:

## Electrolyte Replacement Therapy

This involves giving the patient more of the deficient electrolyte, which can be administered orally, intravenously, or through supplements, (Healthline, n.d.).

## IV Fluids

Intravenous fluids can help rehydrate the body and restore electrolyte balance, typically through sodium chloride, (Healthline, n.d.).

## Medications

Certain medications can help restore electrolyte balance quickly, such as calcium gluconate, magnesium sulfate, and potassium chloride, (Healthline, n.d.).

## Supplements

Supplements can help replace depleted electrolytes on a short- or long-term basis, depending on the underlying cause of the imbalance. Examples include calcium, magnesium, potassium, and phosphate binders, (Healthline, n.d.).

## Dialysis

In severe cases, dialysis may be necessary to filter out the electrolyte, (Healthline, n.d.).

## Dietary Changes

Can play a crucial role in correcting electrolyte imbalances. Here are some foods rich in specific electrolytes that can help address imbalances, (Hoque, 2023):

### Common Sources of Electrolytes in our Diet

- Bananas that Rich in potassium, which is essential for maintaining electrolyte balance, (Weaver, 2013).
- Coconut water: Contains potassium, sodium, and magnesium, making it a natural source of electrolytes, (Hoque, 2023).

- Leafy green vegetables: Good sources of calcium and magnesium, important electrolytes for muscle function and hydration, (Hoque, 2023).
- Yogurt: Contains calcium and potassium, which are important electrolytes for muscle and nerve function, (Weaver, 2013).
- Nuts and seeds: Provide magnesium, a key electrolyte involved in hydration and muscle function, (Akram *et al.,* 2020).

## CONCLUSION

Pathogenetic therapy, focusing on rehydration and electrolyte balance, has revolutionized the treatment of infectious diseases like diarrhea and cholera. Its success, with survival rates exceeding 99%, underscores the critical role of proper fluid and electrolyte levels in maintaining vital bodily functions.

Understanding the profound impact of proper hydration and electrolyte balance underscores the importance of both preventive measures and effective rehydration therapy during illness. These insights guide healthcare professionals in formulating appropriate treatment plans and individuals in adopting health guidelines to maintain optimal electrolyte levels.

In conclusion, pathogenetic therapy is not just a treatment for infectious diseases; it's a cornerstone of maintaining overall health and well-being. Recognizing the delicate balance of fluids and electrolytes empowers us to prioritize hydration and responsible electrolyte intake, thereby safeguarding against a multitude of potential health complications.

## REFERENCES


Akram, M., Munir, N., Daniyal, M., Egbuna, C., Găman, M. A., Onyekere, P. F., & Olatunde, A. (2020). Vitamins and Minerals: Types, sources and their functions. Functional Foods and Nutraceuticals: Bioactive Components, Formulations and Innovations, 149-172.

Albeladi, F. I., Salem, I. M. W., Albandar, A. A., Almusaylim, H. A., & Albandar, A. S. (2022). Electrolyte imbalance in infectious disease patients at King Abdulaziz Hospital, Jeddah. *Journal of Taibah University Medical Sciences*, *17*(2), 256–263. DOI: 10.1016/j.jtumed.2021.09.010 PMID: 35592808

Asima, R. A. N. I., Akhtar, S., Nawaz, S. K., Irfan, S., Sadia, A. Z. A. M., & Arshad, M. (2015). Electrolyte disturbance and the type of malarial infection. *Iranian Journal of Public Health*, *44*(11), 1492. PMID: 26744706

. Centers for Disease Control and Prevention. (2020, December 4). Global WASH (water, sanitation & hygiene).

Cloeckaert, A., & Kuchler, K. (2020). Grand Challenges in Infectious Diseases: Are We Prepared for Worst-Case Scenarios? *Frontiers in Microbiology*, *11*, 613383. DOI: 10.3389/fmicb.2020.613383 PMID: 33329504

. ETHealthWorld. (2021, March 26). Hydration: An important step to recovery from illness. ET HealthWorld.

Fox, M. (2013). Importance of Sodium. *Living Strong Foundation*. Available from: https://www.livestrong.com/article/499403-importance-of-sodium/

Gonzalez, C. F., Finberg, L., & Bluestein, D. D. (1964). Electrolyte concentration during acute infections: Observations in infants and children. *American Journal of Diseases of Children*, *107*(5), 476–482.

Guerrant, R. L., Van Gilder, T., Steiner, T. S., Thielman, N. M., Slutsker, L., Tauxe, R. V., Hennessy, T., Griffin, P. M., DuPont, H., Bradley Sack, R., Tarr, P., Neill, M., Nachamkin, I., Reller, L. B., Osterholm, M. T., Bennish, M. L., & Pickering, L. K. (2001). Practice guidelines for the management of infectious diarrhea. *Clinical Infectious Diseases*, *32*(3), 331–351. DOI: 10.1086/318514 PMID: 11170940

Gusev, E., Sarapultsev, A., Hu, D., & Chereshnev, V. (2021). Problems of pathogenesis and pathogenetic therapy of COVID-19 from the perspective of the general theory of pathological systems (general pathological processes). *International Journal of Molecular Sciences*, *22*(14), 7582. DOI: 10.3390/ijms22147582 PMID: 34299201

· Healthline. (n.d.). *Electrolyte Imbalance: Types, Symptoms, Causes, and More.*

Hoque, M. (2023). A Review on Different Dietary Sources of Important Vitamins and Electrolytes. *International Journal of Research Publication and Reviews*, *4*(8), 731–736. DOI: 10.55248/gengpi.4.823.50408

Królicka, A. L., Kruczkowska, A., Krajewska, M., & Kusztal, M. A. (2020). Hyponatremia in infectious diseases—A literature review. *International Journal of Environmental Research and Public Health*, *17*(15), 5320. DOI: 10.3390/ijerph17155320 PMID: 32718076

Lippi, G., South, A. M., & Henry, B. M. (2020). Electrolyte imbalances in patients with severe coronavirus disease 2019 (COVID-19). *Annals of Clinical Biochemistry*, *57*(3), 262–265. DOI: 10.1177/0004563220922255 PMID: 32266828

. Longo, D. L. (2020, October 29). How Cholera Is Treated. Verywell Health.

Morgenstern, J., & Thoma, B. (2018). Infectious diarrheal disease and dehydration. In Tintinalli, J. E., Ma, O. J., Yealy, D. M., Meckler, G. D., Stapczynski, J., Cline, M., & Thomas, S. (Eds.), *Tintinalli's emergency medicine: A comprehensive study guide* (9th ed.). McGraw-Hill Education.

Rude, R. K. (2010). Magnesium. In: *Encyclopedia of Dietary Supplements*. Eds, Coates PM, Betz JM, Blackman MR, Cragg GM, Levine M, Moss J, White JD. 2nd ed, NY: Informa Healthcare; New York, pp. 527– 37. [Google Scholar]

Rude, R. K. (2012). Magnesium. In Ross, A. C., Caballero, B., Cousins, R. J., Tusker, K. L., & Ziegler, T. R. (Eds.), *Modern nutrition in health and disease* (11th ed., pp. 159–175). Lippincott Williams & Wilkins. [Google Scholar]

Sahay, M., & Sahay, R. (2014). Hyponatremia: A practical approach. *Indian Journal of Endocrinology and Metabolism*, *18*(6), 760. DOI: 10.4103/2230-8210.141320 PMID: 25364669

Shang, Z., Chan, S. Y., Song, Q., Li, P., & Huang, W. (2020). *The strategies of pathogen-oriented therapy on circumventing antimicrobial resistance*. Research. DOI: 10.34133/2020/2016201

Song, H. J. J. M. D., Chia, A. Z. Q., Tan, B. K. J., Teo, C. B., Lim, V., Chua, H. R., Samuel, M., & Kee, A. (2023). Electrolyte imbalances as poor prognostic markers in COVID-19: A systemic review and meta-analysis. *Journal of Endocrinological Investigation*, *46*(2), 235–259. DOI: 10.1007/s40618-022-01877-5 PMID: 36070177

Spence, T. H. (1999). The Truth about Salt. Available from: http://www.pensgard.com/nutrition/13_Salt_Good.htm

Wayne, M., & Bolker, B. (2023). *Infectious disease: a very short introduction*. Oxford University Press.

Weaver, C. M. (2013). Potassium and health. *Advances in Nutrition*, *4*(3), 368S–377S. DOI: 10.3945/an.112.003533 PMID: 23674806

. Weisz, A. (2020, July 14). Dehydration and infections. Weisz Concierge Medical

. World Health Organization. (2020, December 2). Diarrhoeal disease.

# Chapter 3
# Antibacterial Therapy in Infectious Diseases

**Hla I. Dewidar**
*Cairo Univercity, Egypt*

**Mariam Gomaa**
*Ain Shams University, Egypt*

**Yara Ashraf Abouzeid**
*Ain Shams University, Egypt*

**Yasmine Ashraf**
*Cairo Univercity, Egypt*

**Gana Mohamed Morsy Emam**
*Cairo Univercity, Egypt*

## ABSTRACT

*One of the most significant developments in medical history was the discovery of antibiotics and their subsequent large-scale manufacture in the early 1900s. In the history of medical pharmacotherapy, antibiotics caused absolute mortality reductions. Since antibiotics were so effective at eliminating harmful germs, many people thought that infectious diseases would eventually disappear from all human societies. The rise and quick spread of infections resistant to antibiotics, particularly those resistant to several drugs, lead to multidrug resistance. In this chapter, we will discuss the importance and classification of antibiotics according to different points of view, their complications, and finally, the problem that faces our world now is antibiotic resistance and how to reduce it.*

DOI: 10.4018/979-8-3693-1990-1.ch003

# INTRODUCTION

## An Overview of the Development of Antibiotics

The use of antibacterial combinations for the treatment of infections originated more than 2,000 years ago. A number of ancient cultures, including the Greeks and Egyptians, mostly used plant and mold extracts and materials (Adeyemi, Akinyamoju, & Kolude, 2018) (Aminov, 2010), the discovery of antibiotics inspired hope that infections could be managed and avoided. Accordingly, with the observation of the antimicrobial potential of penicillin, clinical trials on humans using penicillin started in 1940. Antibiotics were once thought to be organic substances produced by one type of bacterium that is poisonous to other bacteria, (Schlegel & Zabrosch, 1993) (Denyer, Hodges, & Gorman, 2004). Besides, they are substances produced by different microorganisms (fungi, bacteria), which hinder the development of other microorganisms and ultimately cause them to dissipate from the system. The discovery of antibiotics inspired hope that infections could be managed and avoided. Nevertheless, in developing nations with limited resources, infections persist to be the leading cause of death. Antimicrobial therapy can be categorized as either killing microorganisms or inhibiting their development; thus, in the medical treatment of microbial diseases, antibiotics, which are chemotherapeutic drugs, have been proven to be a highly effective tool, (Sengupta, Chattopadhyay, & Grossart, 2013).

# CLASSIFICATION OF ANTIBIOTICS

*Figure 1. Antibiotics classification*

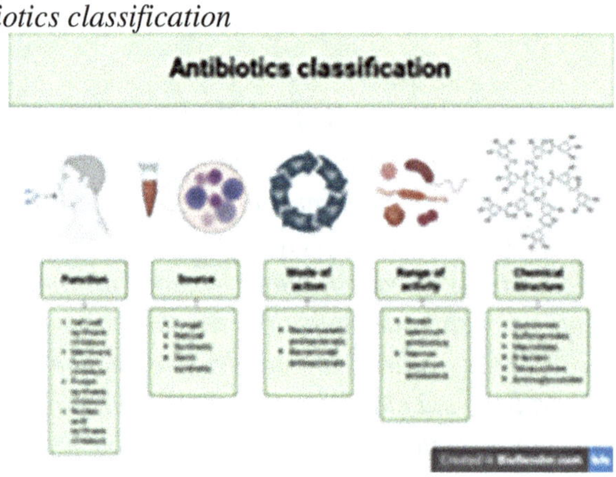

The subclass of antibiotics known as antibacterial has been categorized in several ways in the past. Based on the kind of action, source, range of activity, chemical structure, and function, antibacterial agents are categorized into five groups, as indicated in Figure (1), to make it easier to understand, (Adzitey, 2015).

## Classification Based on Type of Action

The majority of antibiotic classes possess antibacterial characteristics that specifically target bacterial structure or metabolic processes. The processes by which antibiotics function are as follows:

i. suppression of the formation of cell walls
ii. Deterioration of cell membrane function or structure
iii. Preventing the structure and function of nucleic acids
iv. Preventing the production of proteins
v. Obstructing important metabolic processes

## Grouping Based on the Nature of the Source of Antibacterial Agents

Three groups of antibiotics can be identified according to the source that they derive from: (i) natural substances originating from microorganisms; (ii) semisynthetic materials, which are structurally altered natural products; and (iii) synthetic products. Compared to natural antibiotics (benzylpenicillin, cephalosporins, and gentamicin), which have an extreme drawback of high toxicity, semisynthetic (ampicillin and amikacin) and synthetic (moxifloxacin and norfloxacin) have a more significant therapeutic impact and less toxicity, (Oloke, 2000) (Pancu *et al.*, 2021).

## Grouping According to Chemical Structure

Given the antimicrobial family includes a wide range of members with unique chemical structures and therapeutic activities associated with those structures, the chemical structure has been regarded as a trustworthy criterion for differentiating antibiotics. Considering that, the antibiotic classes sulfonamides, quinolones, aminoglycosides, macrolides, tetracyclines, and B-lactam have been introduced.

## Grouping With Respect to the Range of Activity

Antibiotics fall into two categories: broad- or narrow-spectrum, depending on the range of activity they exhibit. While narrow-spectrum antibiotics are restricted to treating a single type of pathogenic bacteria (Gram-positive or Gram-negative bacteria), broad-spectrum medical medicines are effective against a wide range of pathogenic bacteria (both Gram-positive and -negative). Due to their specificity and less bacterial resistance development, narrow-spectrum antibiotics are favored over broad-spectrum ones as the most effective antibacterial agents, according to the available experimental evidence, (Acar, 1997).

## Classification According to the Pharmacological Function

Definitions of antibiotics are based on their pharmacological activities, which can be either bacteriostatic or bactericidal. Antibacterial agents that inhibit or restrict bacterial growth are known as bacteriostatics; on the other hand, compounds known as bactericidal agents kill bacteria by stopping them from developing cell walls, membranes, or proteins. This group includes lipopeptides, macrolides, ansamycins, quinolones, streptogramins, B-lactams, and aminoglycosides. Conversely, the inhibitory phenomena of the bacteriostatic drug include the inhibition of bacterial metabolic pathways or protein production. Differentiating between bacteriostatic and bactericidal medications might be difficult because the former simply inhibit the growth of harmful germs. This is particularly relevant because some bacteriostatic therapies have the potential to function as bactericidal agents when used in high dosages, (Aminov, 2010). Bacteriostatic antibacterials include sulfonamides, which act to reduce folate production in its early stages, and macrolides, such as azithromycin which prevent the bacterial cells from synthesizing proteins. Similarly, minocycline, tetracycline, and doxycycline are all members of the tetracycline drug class.

# MODE OF ACTIONS

## Antibacterial Agents That Attack Cell Wall

Bacterial cell walls include peptidoglycan, which are long sugar polymers cross-linked by trans glycosidases to form glycan strands. Peptide chains form the bonds between individual peptides by growing from the sugars in the polymers. When penicillin-binding proteins (PBPs) are present, glycine monomer cross-links the peptide chain's D-alanyl-alanine region. This crosslinking reinforces the cell wall. In another word, the crosslink that binds polypeptides to each polysaccharide strand's

N-acetyl muramic acid (NAM) is what links the glycan polysaccharide strands, following the transfer of N-acetylglucosamine UDP-NAG and uridine diphosphate UDP-NAM-pentapeptide from the cytoplasm to the external side of the cell membrane by the membrane-bound acceptor bactoprenol, PBPs attached to the cell membrane as DD-peptidases catalyzed trans glycosylation and transpeptidation processes to accumulate peptidoglycan, (Garde, Chodisetti, & Reddy, 2021).

Glycopeptides and β-lactams prevent the formation of cell walls. They perform this by attaching PBPs as a substrate and directly or indirectly limiting the polymerization of peptidoglycan, which has a high affinity for β-lactams. These drugs function as structural analogs of acyl-D-alanyl-D-alanine, which attach to PBP's active site and acts as a substrate within the transpeptidation process. These antibiotics prevent transpeptidation by deactivating PBPs' transpeptidase domain, (Marschall, Cryle, & Tailhades, 2019).

β-lactams operate by covalently and irreversibly attaching to penicillin-binding proteins (PBPs). In order to prevent peptidoglycan production, D, D-transpeptidases and D, D-carboxypeptidases coordinate to establish links with nearby peptidoglycan peptide chains, which is demonstrated by the PBP. Different chemical structures of distinct β-lactam molecules affect how much of an affinity they have for specific PBPs, which leads to variations in their overall antibacterial activity. β-lactam antibiotics selectively acylate a necessary serine monomer with a β-lactam core, so targeting PBP at the molecular level. After the acylation phase, the amide linkage breaks, and the β-lactam ring opens, causing a stable acyl–enzyme complex (AEC), (Baran, Kwiatkowska, & Potocki, 2023).

The glycopeptide antibiotics are another significant class of antibacterial agents with medical significance that have activities result in the inhibition of cell wall production. Nevertheless, by focusing on lipid II, glycopeptide antibioticsunlike β-lactams, limit the synthesis of peptidoglycans by Gram-positive bacteria. Vancomycin's mechanism of action, for instance, is dependent on attatch to the D-Ala-D-Ala terminus of the peptidoglycan (PG) cell wall precursor Lipid II (undecaprenyl-diphospho-N-acetylmuramoyl-[N-acetylglucosamine]) -l-alanyl-γ-d-glutamyl-l-lysyl-d-alanyl-d-alanine). The binding pocket in the vancomycin molecular structure, which takes on a structure equivalent to the spatial organization of D-Ala-D-Ala, acts as what leads to their high-affinity binding. The newly created complex is stabilized by the ability of each antibiotic molecule to make five hydrogen bonds with related groups in the single carboxyl, single amino, and three amide groups of the D-Ala-D-Ala dipeptide. By inhibiting PBP activity and preventing Lipid II from crosslinking into mature peptidoglycan, this link delays the maturation of the peptidoglycan layer. In the end, this leads to bacterial cell death by osmotic shock, (Wang *et al.,* 2018).

## Antibacterial Agents That Inhibit the Protein's Synthesis

The information contained in bacterial DNA is first used in a process called transcription to produce messenger RNA (mRNA), which is subsequently translated by a different process called translation. The macromolecule that makes the proteins found in m-RNA is called a ribosome. Cytoplasmic elements and ribosomes facilitate the synthesis of proteins. The 30S and 50S ribonucleoprotein subunits of the bacterium produce the two halves of the 70S ribosome. Antibacterial agents act on 30S or 50S subunit of the bacterium's ribosome, that stops the cell from producing proteins, (Kapoor, Saigal, & Elongavan, 2017).

## Antibacterial Agents That Inhibit the Nucleic Acids' Synthesis

### Inhibition DNA Synthesis or Replication

The bacteria's DNA gyrase enzyme, which nicks double-stranded DNA, adds negative supercoils followed by reconnecting the nicked ends, which is suppressed by the fluoroquinolones (FQ). This is needed to stop the strands from excessively optimistic supercoiling when they divided apart for transcription or Replication to occur. Two A subunits and two B subunits in DNA gyrase, DNA is nicked by subunit A, negative supercoils are added by subunit B, and the strands are resealed by subunit A. The FQs bind to the A subunit very strongly, meddling with its strand function of cutting and resealing. Topoisomerase IV, which nicks and splits the daughter DNA strand after DNA replication, is the primary effector in Gram-positive bacteria. Greater efficacy against Gram-positive bacteria might be attributed to an increased affinity for this enzyme. Topoisomerase II is present in animal cells rather than DNA gyrase or topoisomerase IV. Because of its extremely low affinity for FQ, this enzyme poses little threat to cells, (Brar *et al.,* 2020).

### Inhibition the Synthesis of Bacterial RNA

The most significant class of antibacterial compounds in this group are the rifamycins, which are members of the naturally occurring ansamycin antibiotic family and its semisynthetic variations rifampicin, rifabutin, rifapentin, and rifaximin are among those whose precursor is rifamycin SV.

The bactericidal activities of rifamycins are attributed to the occurrence of a macrocyclic ring that particularly targets the β-subunit of bacterial DNA-dependent RNA polymerase (RNAP) at its catalytic core. Such attachment prevents the newly produced RNA from expanding by inhibiting RNAP's transcriptional activity at the transcriptional initiation step. The bacteria are killed by this sudden decrease in protein synthesis, (Adams *et al.*, 2021).

## Antibacterial Agents That Disrupt the Integrity of the Cell Membrane

Cyclic lipopeptides are one class of antibacterial drugs that disrupt cell membrane of bacteria. In terms of cyclic lipopeptide antibiotics, daptomycin is the most well-known example. It was initially extracted from the "fermentation medium" of the soil bacteria Streptomyces roseosporus. A 13-amino-acid peptide attached to a decanoyl side chain makes up the daptomycin molecule. This relationship requires the presence of calcium ions because they mask the anionic nature of daptomycin and change its physicochemical features. Particles that breach the inner membrane, attach to the negatively charged phosphatidylglycerol groups, and neutralize them are created when Ca2+ and diphosmycin combine. After being introduced into the membrane, the Ca2+–daptomycin complex goes through phosphatidylglycerol-dependent oligomerization. When these elements combine, membrane channels are produced. This leads to ions—mainly potassium and sodium—leaking out and a drop in the transmembrane potential in addition to endangering the membrane's integrity. This causes the disruption of membrane-associated processes, ultimately culminating in the disintegration of bacterial cells, (Huang, 2020).

In general, the Paenibacillus polymyxa subspecies produces polymyxins, which are cationic peptide antibiotics that cause chemical imbalances in Gram-negative bacteria's outer cell membrane. Because of their amphipathic nature, these chemicals have surface-activating properties. The polymyxin molecule's core is created from joining a cyclic heptapeptide with a linear tripeptide side chain. The latter is connected to a branching fatty acid chain made up of seven to nine carbon atoms by means of an α-amide. Divalent magnesium and calcium ions are competitively shifted as a result of this interaction, stabilizing the structural configuration of monolayer LPS molecules. As a result, outer membrane becomes more permeable, making it easier for succeeding antibiotic molecules to enter. Polymyxins can also be damaging to the inner membrane, causing it to lose its structural integrity, allowing internal components to leak out and ultimately leading to the death of bacterial cells.

Furthermore, polymyxins have been shown to promote the integration of the membrane's inner and outer leaflets, which in turn promotes the passage of phospholipids between the two membranes. Such changes in the lipid makeup the both membranes lead to an osmotic imbalance and cell lysis, (Yin *et al.*, 2020).

Collistin, a cationic peptide, binds to lipid A in lipopolysaccharide and permeabilizes the outer membrane, which results in the death of cells, (Andrade *et al.*, 2020). ipopeptides, such as daptomycin, insert into the cell membrane and produce depolarization, which lowers ATP synthesis and ultimately results in cell death.

## Antibacterial Agents That Interfere With Metabolic Pathways

Antibiotics can also function as antimicrobial agents by interfering with vital metabolic processes. One of the most prevalent instances is the inhibition of folic acid production by the cell of bacteria, which is mostly brought about by sulfonamides either by itself or with trimethoprim because of their synergistic impact.

The structural analogs of para-aminobenzoic acid (PABA), which is imposrtant to bacteria to produce folate, are found in sulfonamides. They are a part of the class of broad-spectrum bacteriostatic antibiotics. Sulfonamides exert their antimetabolite effects by competing with PABA for the dihydropteroate synthase (DHPS) active site. The latter is catalyst that, through condensation with 7,8-dihydro-6-hydroxymethylpterine pyrophosphate (DHPPP), transforms PABA into dihydropteric acid, the precursor of dihydrofolic acid. The amount of metabolically active tetrahydrofolic acid is decreased by sulfonamide-dependent suppression of dihydrofolic acid production. Bacterial growth is inhibited when folate stocks are low because the manufacture of purines, pyrimidines, and certain amino acids reqired for the synthesis of DNA and proteins is impeded. Pyrimidines (trimethoprim) inhibit dihydrofolate reductase later on, which lowers dihydrofolic acid to tetrahydrofolic acid using NADPH as an electron donor that can then be transformed to the various forms of tetrahydrofolate cofactors and sulfonamides compete with dihydropteroate synthase, (Nunes *et al.*, 2020).

*Table 1.*

| **β-Lactams (penicillins, cephalosporins, cephamycins,carbapenems, monobactams)** | **Target peptidoglycan crosslinking by preventing penicillin-binding proteins from crosslinking the cell wall's peptide chain, which causes the cell to lyse.** |
|---|---|
| Glycopeptides (vancomycin, teicoplanin, oritavancin, and telavancin) | Suppress the synthesis of peptidoglycan by attaching to D-alanyl-D-alanine in the peptide chain to prevent cross-linking. |
| Aminoglycosides (Gentamicin, streptomycin, kanamycin) | interact with the 16S rRNA's 30S ribosomal subunit, resulting in misreading, shortened proteins, and cellular death; positively charged, attach to the outer membrane, increasing accumulation through pores, (Baquero & Levin, 2021). |

continued on following page

*Table 1. Continued*

| | |
|---|---|
| Macrolides (azithromycin, erythromycin) and Lincosamides (clindamycin) | Target the 50S ribosomal subunit's 23S rRNA to stop protein translation, which shortens peptide chains, (Jednačak, Mikulandra, & Novak, 2020). |
| Oxazolidinones (linezolid) and streptogramins (dalfopristin) | Restrict translation by attaching to the 50S subunit's 23S rRNA and blocking the synthesis of a functional 70S subunit, (Foti *et al.*, 2021). |
| Phenols (chloramphenicol) | Bind to the A site of the 50S ribosomal subunit to block translation and prevent new proteins' synthesis, (Schwarz *et al.*, 2016). |
| Tetracyclines (Tigecycline, tetracycline) | bind to the 30S ribosomal subunit's 16S rRNA to inhibit translation by preventing tRNA from attaching to 30S at the A site, (Markley & Wencewicz, 2018). |
| Quinolones and fluoroquinolones (ciprofloxacin) | Stop DNA gyrase and topoisomerase IV from replicating DNA, as they are responsible for strand cutting, ligation, and DNA supercoiling. |
| Rifamycin (rifampicin) | Inhibit transcription through binding to RNA polymerase, thereby blocking DNA-dependent RNA synthesis. |

## PNEUMONIA

Acute respiratory disease that affects the lower respiratory tract is called pneumonia. Worldwide, infections of the lower respiratory tract are responsible for a disproportionate number of deaths. According to Hirschtick *et al.* (1995) and the World Health Organisation (2008), pneumonia is a frequent lung disease that greatly increases rates of death and morbidity. It is more common in extremely stressful environments. They pose a serious threat to public health as well. There are three different types of pneumonia that might happen: ventilator-associated pneumonia (VAP), hospital-acquired pneumonia (HAP), and community-acquired pneumonia (CAP), (Maruyama *et al.,* 2019). Pneumonia tends to be more severe in children under five, adults over 65, those with certain diseases like heart failure, diabetes, or COPD, or those whose immune systems have been compromised by HIV/AIDS, chemotherapy (a cancer treatment), organ or bone marrow stem cell transplant procedures, (Zanfardino *et al.,* 2019). According to Biscevic-Tokic *et al.* (2013), common signs of pneumonia include fever, chills, a cough that produces phlegm, chest pain, and shortness of breath. Predisposing variables include malnutrition, overcrowding, and the undeveloped immune systems of children. According to Reynolds *et al.* (2010), smoking is the single biggest preventable risk factor for adults. The primary causes of HAP and VAP are gram-negative bacteria, including *Pseudomonas aeruginosa, Enterobacterales*, and *Acinetobacter,* (Koulenti *et al.,* 2009) (Lanks, Musani, & Hsia, 2019). Conversely, the primary cause of community-acquired pneumonia (CAP) is *Streptococcus pneumoniae,* (Bassetti *et al.,* 2022). The most common cause of bacterial pneumonia is *streptococcus pneumoniae*, an extracellular pathogen identified by a thick polysaccharide capsule, (Tuomanen, Austrian, & Masure, 1995). The diagnosis is supported by radiographic evidence of recent consolidation, (Pates, Periselneris, & Brown, 2023). India, Nigeria, Indonesia, Pakistan, and China accounted for almost 54% of the world's cases of severe pneumonia and clinical pneumonia in 2015. India accounted for 32 percent of all clinical pneumonia episodes in developing countries between 2000 and 2015; nevertheless, throughout that same period, the incidence of pneumonia decreased by just 3 percent, (McAllister *et al.,* 2019).

## Treatment of Pneumonia

Function of Toll-like receptor 4 (TLR4) in pneumonia caused by Gram-negative bacteria (GNB)

Leucine-rich repeats (LRRs) are found in the extracellular domain of TLR4, a transmembrane protein that is linked to MD2 molecules. Approximately two to six hours following intracerebral hemorrhage, there is a considerable rise in TLR4 expression at both mRNA and protein levels. After an hour of exposure to LPS, autologous human alveolar macrophages and monocytes showed increased TLR4 RNA expression.

By attaching to GNB's lipopolysaccharide (LPS), LR4 is able to recognize foreign pathogens. Induce nonspecific immunological response by stimulating the generation of antimicrobial peptides, which activates the nuclear factor-KB (NF-KB) pathway in macrophages. Interactions between LPS and (LBP, MD2, CD14, TLR4) are moderate. By identifying LPS, TLR4, MD2, and CD14 combine to form trimeric receptor complexes. In the outer membrane of GNB, LPS activates TLR4, and complex LPS/MD2/TLR4 activation starts intracellular signalling pathways.

## Antagonists

Oxymatrine: Reducing the expression of TLR4,
Function: Reactions that reduce inflammation
Ginkgolide B: Diminishing apoptosis in neural cells
Function: Blocking the TLR4 signalling cascade
Celastrol and wogonoside: Preventing the Activation of MAPKs
Function: Angiogenesis mediated by TLR4
Lipid A that has been monophosphorylated: Restore antigen display
Function: dampening inflammatory lung lesions
Curcumin: Inhibits TLR4 homodimerization

Function: Blocks TLR4 signalling pathway
Shogaol: Preventing homodimerization of TLR4
Function: TLR4 signalling pathway blockade
Isoliquiritigenin: Preventing homodimerization of TLR4
Function: TLR4 signalling pathway blockade
TLR4 antibody: Preventing microglial activation brought on by hemin
Function: Blocking the TLR4 signalling pathway, (Ding & Liu, 2019).

## ADVERSE EFFECTS AND COMPLICATIONS OF ANTIBIOTIC USAGE

Along with contributing to their therapeutic function, side effects of antibiotics might cause reactions in the patients. Antibiotics have extremely few adverse effects and are generally safe when taken as prescribed. These harmful effects, however, can differ substantially across antibiotics and patients and can range from moderate responses to allergens to serious adverse consequences, (Thong, 2010). Furthermore, a patient's capacity to endure and finish the course may be hampered by a variety of antibiotics. Few people who have experienced an allergic reaction to any antibiotic in the past are not advised to have the same treatment. A skin rash and an allergic reaction known as anaphylaxis, that might give rise to issues with breathing and enlargement of the lips, tongue, and face, are examples of Indications that can accompany allergic reactions. Major antibiotics, including Penicillin, Cephalosporin, Aminoglycosides, Erythromycin, Tetracycline, Quinolones, Ciprofloxacin, and others, can induce several adverse consequences, including nausea, vomiting, gastrointestinal discomfort, anorexia, reactions to hypersensitivity, and more, (Mittal *et al.,* 2020). In addition to these side effects, there are other detrimental effects of antibiotics in individuals with varying conditions.

### Effects of Antibiotics on the Composition of Gut Microbiota

In addition to eliminating the pathogen of interest, broad-spectrum antimicrobial agents also decrease the variety of the gut microbiota. This has adverse effects on the host and will be discussed in more detail in the sections that follow, (Patangia *et al.,* 2022).

## How Antibiotics Affect Pregnancy and Breastfeeding

Using antibiotics during pregnancy or after giving birth can change the bacteria that live in the gut and the baby's resistome, (Wong *et al.,* 2020). Researchers looked at the temporal effects of cefoperazone when given throughout the peripartum phase in an interleukin 10 (IL-10)-deficient murine version of colitis on the microbiota of the mother and the offspring to better understand the possible effects of antibiotic administration on offspring during pregnancy. Children born to dams exposed to cefoperazone had changed their intestinal microbiota throughout adulthood and were more vulnerable to both chemically and dynamically caused colitis, (Miyoshi *et al.,* 2017). A further investigation showed that taking antibiotics while pregnant can change the types of microbes that live in the vaginal area before birth, (Stokholm *et al.*, 2014). The microbiota in milk is influenced by the use of antibiotics by mothers during breastfeeding, and this can have an impact on the makeup of microorganisms in the infant's gut, (Hermansson *et al.,* 2019).

## The Effect of Antibiotics Given to Newborns Directly on Their Gut Microbiome

Due to their medical circumstances, premature newborns are frequently treated with antibiotics, and in the NICU, antibiotics are one of the most routinely administered medications, (Gasparrini *et al.*, 2019). Since many of the antibiotics used for prevention are broad-spectrum, they impact a large percentage of the intestinal bacterium community, changing the early development sequence in numerous ways. A decrease in bacterial diversity and abundance of species, as well as an increase in antibiotic resistance genes, were found in the guts of extremely premature newborns who were given antibiotics for an extended period, according to reports, (Zwittink *et al.,* 2018). The gut flora of premature babies can change after either a short or long period of antibiotic treatment. As a result of these shifts, the relative abundance of *Enterococcus* has increased while that of *bifidobacteria* and *Bacteroidetes* has decreased, (Zwittink *et al.,* 2018) (Del Fiol *et al.,* 2018).

## UTILIZATION OF ANTIBIOTICS HAS ADDITIONAL SIDE EFFECTS IN SEVERAL CASES

### Antibiotics and Microbial Balance

Research has shown that an elevated risk of obesity has been linked to antibiotic use, (Kasai *et al.*, 2015). Although findings are contradictory, some research has linked obesity to a higher ratio of Firmicutes to Bacteroidetes rather than specific quantities, (Schwiertz *et al.*, 2010) (Candon *et al.*, 2015). Research in male rodents found a connection between variations in microbial colonization caused by antibiotics and type 1 diabetes. Experimental type 1 diabetes in neonatal nonobese mice was induced by the administration of either vancomycin alone or a combination of broad-spectrum antibiotics, (McDonald, 2017). The author's investigations have shown that clindamycin, an antibiotic, might modify the microbial population, which can enhance the colonization of dangerous pathogens like C. difficile, which can cause diarrhea and colitis. This alteration, in turn, increases the risk of antibiotic-associated diarrhea (AAD), (Zhu, Huang, & Yang, 2022).

## ANTIBIOTIC RESISTANCE

Antibiotic resistance is a developing global issue in which medicines are no longer functional in treating the transmissible illnesses for which they were developed. After the World Health Organization (WHO) issued a warning that we are "Accelerating depletion of available antibiotics," concerns about the global dissemination of antibiotic-resistant microorganisms skyrocketed. Nosocomial infections have been on the rise as a result of the growth of drug-resistant bacteria, which has presented a significant challenge to the treatment of clinical infectious disorders, (Murray *et al.*, 2022).

After cardiovascular illnesses and cancer, infections resistant to antibiotics are the third most significant cause of death worldwide, (Founou, Founou, & Essack, 2017). There is the potential for antibiotic resistance to have both therapeutic and preventive effects on human health. Failure of treatment and the occurrence of complications are two clear indicators of therapeutic implication, (Choi & Lee, 2019).

## Antibiotic Resistance Mechanisms

In order to withstand the effects of antibiotic compounds, bacteria can evolve resistance. lessening the absorption of drugs, modifying a medication's target, promoting the ineffectiveness of a drug, and enhancing active drug efflux are four primary pathways for antimicrobial resistance.

### Reducing Drug Absorption

As the main component of the outer membrane of gram-negative bacteria, the greatly modified glycolipid lipopolysaccharide acts as an obstacle to the penetration of many substances, even antibiotics. Because of their inherent resilience, gram-negative bacteria are less susceptible to certain antibiotics. Moreover, alterations in the permeability of outer-membrane proteins, specifically porin proteins, might lead to the emergence of medication resistance. Porins play a crucial role in facilitating the entry of hydrophilic antibiotics, including β-lactams, fluoroquinolones, tetracyclines, and chloramphenicol, into the cell. Antibiotics penetrate bacterial cells and the resulting sensitivity of bacteria to these antibiotics are influenced by the amount and kind of porin proteins, (Ghai & Ghai, 2018). Porin mutations that decrease expression or function can also cause acquired antibiotic resistance. Combining porin mutations with efflux pumps or enzymatic breakdown of drugs increases resistance, (Dutt, D'Souza, & Garg, 2022). Some bacteria, such as Pseudomonas aeruginosa, Staphylococcus aureus, Staphylococcus epidermidis, Streptococcus viridans, Escherichia coli, Klebsiella pneumoniae, Proteus mirabilis, and Enterococcus faecalis, have also demonstrated the ability to resist antibiotics by forming biofilms, (Ashley *et al.*, 2017).

### Modifying a Medication's Target

Bacteria have the ability to modify the targets that are essential for medication engagement such that the drug either fails to attach to the changed target or attaches poorly. This alteration arises from unintentional changes in the gene or genes expressing the medication target protein. For example, Mutations in the quinolone-resistance-determining region (QRDR) of the DNA gyrase (topoisomerase II and topoisomerase IV) can cause gram-positive and gram-negative bacteria to become resistant to fluoroquinolones, (Saha & Sarkar, 2021). Methylation is another target alteration technique that is highly effective in creating resistance. erm, methylases against streptogramin B antibiotics, lincosamides, and macrolides are examples of methylation in both gram-positive and gram-negative bacteria. In a similar vein, resistance in several bacteria, such as Proteus vulgaris, Staphylococcus species, Enterococcus species, Bacillus species, and E. coli, has been connected to methylation of the cfr gene, (Afei & Schito, 2022).

## Medication Inactivation

One of two occurrences can happen when a bacterial species inactivates an antibiotic: It is either the antibiotic is hydrolyzed, or it is modified with a chemical group. This can lead to drug resistance. β-lactamases, which are hydrolyzing enzymes generated by enterobacterales family members, are especially good at turning β-lactam antibiotics inactive. The β-lactamases, which were previously called penicillinases and cephalosporinases, disrupt the binding of penicillin-binding proteins by opening a specific region in the β-lactam ring framework, (Reygaert, 2018). Acetyl, phosphoryl, and adenyl groups are traded most often for medication inactivation. Against aminoglycosides, chloramphenicol, streptogramins, and fluoroquinolones, acetylation is the most common technique, but phosphorylation and adenylation are utilized more against aminoglycosides, (Nikaido & Pagès, 2012).

## Drug Efflux

Cytoplasm membranes include energy-dependent pumping systems that bacteria use to manage antibiotic buildup. Bacteria use efflux pumps to remove metabolites, antibiotics, and quorum-sensing signal molecules to regulate their interior setting. The first plasmid-encoded outflow system for tetracycline removal was discovered in Escherichia coli by researchers. Various gram-positive and gram-negative bacteria with resistant strains and different efflux mechanisms have been discovered since then. Interestingly, numerous efflux systems use chromosomal multidrug efflux mechanisms to guarantee bacterial resistance to drugs, (Blair, Richmond, & Piddock, 2014). In terms of structure and energy source, there are six drug discharge pumps: the ATP-binding cassette (ABC) superfamily, the major facilitator superfamily (MFS), the multidrug and toxic compound extrusion (MATE) family, the small multidrug resistance (SMR) family, the resistance--nodulation-division (RND) superfamily, and the drug metabolite transporter (DMT) superfamily. Most efflux pumps seen in gram-positive bacteria belong to the ABC and MFS families and are encoded by chromosomal genes or carried on plasmids. Members of the RND superfamily, which is made up of a cytoplasmic membrane pump, an outer-membrane protein channel, and periplasmic protein, are the primary clinically relevant efflux systems of gram-negative bacteria, (Brives & Pourraz, 2020).

## REMEDIES FOR ANTIBIOTICS

Researchers are diligently endeavoring to identify viable substitutes for antibiotics, resulting in the identification of the primary alternatives to traditional antibiotic usage.

### Phage Treatment

Viruses known as "bacteria eaters," or bacteriophages as they are sometimes called, are able to infect bacteria. Bacteriophages have certain advantages over antibiotics, including their ease of availability, diversity, auto-dosing, low intrinsic toxic effects, particular host range, absence of antibiotic cross-resistance, and minimal adverse ecological effects. When phages are thought of as antibiotic substitutes, these qualities are highly alluring. However, before phage treatment is used clinically, a number of issues need to be resolved. These issues comprise appropriate phage choice, a restricted host spectrum, an efficient manufacturing process, a likely immunological response, and clinician knowledge. Phage therapy has been successfully used as an alternate therapy for transdermal conditions in situations where antibiotics have been demonstrated to be inefficient, even though it is unlikely to replace antibiotics completely, (Murugaiyan *et al.,* 2022).

### Antiviral Medications

As an alternative to growth inhibition or bacterial death in antibiotic therapy, antivirulence medications target the destructive components of bacteria. Antivirulence medications can inhibit specific bacterial proteins that bacteria employ to attach to host cells and start an infection. Antivirulence medications, thus, neutralize the bacteria and stop the spread of infection. Because they work through another mechanism, it is unlikely that antibiotic resistance would arise against antivirulence medications. In further research, findings have shown that antivirulence medicines minimal disturb the normal microbiome and do not encourage the evolution of drug-resistant bacterial strains over vulnerable ones, unlike standard antibiotics. Antivirulence drugs, however, would work best as adjuvant or combination therapy with antibiotics due to difficulties in development and practical application, (Ghai & Ghai, 2018).

### Lantibiotics and Bacteriocins

The expression "lantibiotic" is used to describe peptides that are encoded by genes and contain specific amino acids, like thioether amino acids lanthionine (Lan) and methyllanthionine (MeLan). These amino acids are made by a process called post-translational modification, which adds the intramolecular cyclic patterns to the peptides that are required for specific exporters and post-translational modification. These chemicals are only made by Gram-positive bacteria and work mostly to stop this type of bacteria from growing. It is also noteworthy that most lantibiotics have some antimicrobial effect. There are two main categories of lantibiotic peptides: type-A and type-B. Nisin, subtilin, and epidermin are examples of type-A lantibiotics; they are elongated, cationic peptides that mainly work by compromising the membrane integrity of the organisms they target. Globular Type-B peptides exert their effects via disrupting enzyme function, such as inhibiting the creation of the cell wall. Mersacidin and actagardine, two duramycins produced by Streptomyces species, are examples of type-B peptides. Nevertheless, other lantibiotics cannot be categorized into either group, indicating that the classification of lantibiotics will inevitably get more intricate with the discovery of further compounds, (Simons, Alhanout, & Duval, 2020).

Bacteriocins are proteinaceous or peptidic toxins generated by bacteria, specifically belonging to the type-A lantibiotic category. These compounds possess the capability to eliminate or hinder closely related bacterial strains or unrelated germs without inflicting damage to the original bacteria due to the presence of unique immune proteins. Significantly, bacteriocins have a wide range of structural and functional variations and are particularly resistant to high temperatures, (Mathur *et al.,* 2018). Bacteriocins have garnered considerable attention for their broad-spectrum antibacterial effects, targeting a range of organisms, including bacteria, parasites, viruses, and even complex systems like biofilms of bacteria, (Sheard *et al.,* 2019). The diverse array of bacteriocins produced by bacteria results in a broad spectrum of biological activity exhibited by these toxins. There is yet hope for the discovery of a great many more bacteriotoxins, in addition to the many different bacteriocins that have already been identified. Bacteriocins are also effective against bacteria that become resistant to other poisons, (Mathur *et al.,* 2018).

## Antimicrobial Peptides (AMPs)

AMPs, which include combinations of AMPs and antibiotics: Naturally occurring antimicrobial peptides (AMPs) typically consist of 10 to 50 amino acids. They have a positive charge overall and exhibit amphipathic properties. AMPs demonstrate antibacterial activity that is comparable to or even superior to that of conventional antibiotics, (Rima *et al.,* 2021). AMPs can selectively attack a diverse array of bacteria, including both Gram-positive and Gram-negative types, using the same processes as standard antibiotics. After entering bacteria's cell wall, AMPs perform enhanced antibacterial activities by specifically attacking the manufacturing of DNA and proteins and/or disrupting the development of the cell wall and barrier, (Li *et al.,*

2018). By combining AMPs with traditional antibiotics, encouraging findings are being achieved through the complementary impact of the two substances, paving the way for the targeted eradication of various bacteria that have developed resistance to antibiotics, (Herman & Herman, 2014).

## Strategies Based on Nanoparticles

NPs are currently being utilized as bacterial proliferation blockers in fields such as coverings for implanted devices/medical products and antibiotic administration. They can also be employed as antibacterial agents directly. The precise mechanism by which NPs exhibit their antibacterial activity is not yet comprehensively known, although three concurrent mechanisms have been postulated. Metal ion release, non-oxidative mechanisms, and oxidative stress are all implicated. These reactions result in (1) the degradation of The bacteria's exterior layer and/or infliction of injury to the entire cell wall, (2) the interaction between components inside and outside the cell and ions from the nanoparticles, (3) the generation of reactive oxygen species through photocatalysis, which harm bacterial building components, (4) the prevention of DNA manufacturing, (5) the suppression of the function of enzymes, and (6) the disruption of energy transduction, (Iwu & Patrick, 2021).

In addition to the alternatives mentioned earlier, in response to the growing problem of antibiotic resistance, the World Health Assembly has put into motion five crucial tactical action plans. Firstly, it is essential to enhance public awareness and comprehension of this problem. Secondly, it is crucial to bolster our knowledge base by conducting surveillance and research activities aimed at combating infections and controlling their spread. This will enable us to develop effective control measures and interventions. Thirdly, the implementation of robust sanitation, personal hygiene, and infection prevention measures is essential. Fourthly, it is imperative to optimize the utilization of antimicrobial agents in both human and animal health. Lastly, sustainable expenditure in the development of new pharmaceuticals, diagnostic tools, and vaccines is crucial.

# CONCLUSION

In conclusion, whenever it comes to treating a wide variety of contagious infections, antibiotics are typically the most effective solution. It is essential to recognize that inappropriately using them has the potential to lead to the development of more severe conditions. The overuse and indiscriminate application of antibiotics without initial consultation with a qualified medical professional is one of the key factors contributing to Antibiotic resistance. Because of this, we must exercise caution and get a comprehensive understanding of this essential drug in order to make maximal use of the advantages it offers while reducing its possible adverse effects.

## REFERENCES


Acar, J. (1997). Broad- and narrow-spectrum antibiotics: An unhelpful categorization. *Clinical Microbiology and Infection*, *3*(4), 395–396. DOI: 10.1111/j.1469-0691.1997.tb00274.x PMID: 11864148

Adams, R. A., Leon, G., Miller, N. M., Reyes, S. P., Thanawastien, A., & Kasting, B. J. (2021). Rifamycin antibiotics and the mechanisms of their failure. *The Journal of Antibiotics*, *74*(11), 11. Advance online publication. DOI: 10.1038/s41429-021-00462-x PMID: 34400805

Adeyemi, B. F., Akinyamoju, A. O., & Kolude, B. (2018). Association of squamous cell carcinoma of the tongue with cigarette and alcohol exposure: A retrospective clinicopathological study. *West African Journal of Medicine*, *35*(2), 117–122. PMID: 30027997

Adzitey, F. (2015). Antibiotic classes and antibiotic susceptibility of bacterial isolates from selected poultry: A mini review. *UDS Space*. http://udsspace.uds.edu.gh/handle/123456789/647

Aminov, R. (2010). A brief history of the antibiotic era: Lessons learned and challenges for the future. *Frontiers in Microbiology*, *1*, 134. Advance online publication. DOI: 10.3389/fmicb.2010.00134 PMID: 21687759

Andrade, F. F., Silva, D., Rodrigues, A., & Pina-Vaz, C. (2020). Colistin update on its mechanism of action and resistance, present and future challenges. *Microorganisms*, *8*(11), 1716. Advance online publication. DOI: 10.3390/microorganisms8111716 PMID: 33147701

Ashley, R. E., Dittmore, A., McPherson, S. A., Turnbough, C. L.Jr, Neuman, K. C., & Osheroff, N. (2017). Activities of gyrase and topoisomerase IV on positively supercoiled DNA. *Nucleic Acids Research*, *45*(16), 9611–9624. DOI: 10.1093/nar/gkx649 PMID: 28934496

Baquero, F., & Levin, B. R. (2021). Proximate and ultimate causes of the bactericidal action of antibiotics. *Nature Reviews. Microbiology*, *19*(2), 2. Advance online publication. DOI: 10.1038/s41579-020-00443-1 PMID: 33024310

Baran, A., Kwiatkowska, A., & Potocki, L. (2023). Antibiotics and bacterial resistance—A short story of an endless arms race. *International Journal of Molecular Sciences*, *24*(6), 5777. Advance online publication. DOI: 10.3390/ijms24065777 PMID: 36982857

Bassetti, M., Magnè, F., Giacobbe, D. R., Bini, L., & Vena, A. (2022). New antibiotics for Gram-negative pneumonia. *European Respiratory Review : an Official Journal of the European Respiratory Society*, *31*(166), 220119. Advance online publication. DOI: 10.1183/16000617.0119-2022 PMID: 36543346

Blair, J. M. A., Richmond, G. E., & Piddock, L. J. V. (2014). Multidrug efflux pumps in Gram-negative bacteria and their role in antibiotic resistance. *Future Microbiology*, *9*(10), 1165–1177. DOI: 10.2217/fmb.14.66 PMID: 25405886

Brar, R. K., Jyoti, U., Patil, R. K., & Patil, H. C. (2020). Fluoroquinolone antibiotics: An overview. *Adesh University Journal of Medical Sciences & Research*, *2*(1), 26–30. DOI: 10.25259/AUJMSR_12_2020

Brives, C., & Pourraz, J. (2020). Phage therapy as a potential solution in the fight against AMR: Obstacles and possible futures. *Palgrave Communications*, *6*(1), 1. Advance online publication. DOI: 10.1057/s41599-020-0478-4

Candon, S., Perez-Arroyo, A., Marquet, C., Valette, F., Foray, A.-P., Pelletier, B., Milani, C., Ventura, M., Bach, J.-F., Chatenoud, L., & Lemoine, R. (2015). Antibiotics in early life alter the gut microbiome and increase disease incidence in a spontaneous mouse model of autoimmune insulin-dependent diabetes. *PLoS One*, *10*(5), e0125448. Advance online publication. DOI: 10.1371/journal.pone.0125448 PMID: 25970503

Choi, U., & Lee, C.-R. (2019). Distinct roles of outer membrane porins in antibiotic resistance and membrane integrity in *Escherichia coli*. *Frontiers in Microbiology*, *10*, 953. Advance online publication. DOI: 10.3389/fmicb.2019.00953 PMID: 31114568

Del Fiol, F. S., Balcão, V. M., Barberato-Filho, S., Lopes, L. C., & Bergamaschi, C. C. (2018). Obesity: A new adverse effect of antibiotics? *Frontiers in Pharmacology*, *9*, 1408. Advance online publication. DOI: 10.3389/fphar.2018.01408 PMID: 30559670

Denyer, S. P., Hodges, N. A., & Gorman, S. P. (Eds.). (2004). *Hugo and Russell's pharmaceutical microbiology* (7th ed.). Blackwell Science., DOI: 10.1002/9780470988329

Ding, J., & Liu, Q. (2019). Toll-like receptor 4: A promising therapeutic target for pneumonia caused by Gram-negative bacteria. *Journal of Cellular and Molecular Medicine*, *23*(9), 5868–5875. DOI: 10.1111/jcmm.14529 PMID: 31350813

Dutt, Y., D'Souza, R., & Garg, M. (2022). The association between biofilm formation and antimicrobial resistance with possible ingenious bio-remedial approaches. *Antibiotics (Basel, Switzerland)*, *11*(7), 930. Advance online publication. DOI: 10.3390/antibiotics11070930 PMID: 35884186

Foti, C., Piperno, A., Scala, A., & Giuffrè, O. (2021). Oxazolidinone antibiotics: Chemical, biological and analytical aspects. *Molecules (Basel, Switzerland)*, *26*(14), 4280. Advance online publication. DOI: 10.3390/molecules26144280 PMID: 34299555

Founou, R. C., Founou, L. L., & Essack, S. Y. (2017). Clinical and economic impact of antibiotic resistance in developing countries: A systematic review and meta-analysis. *PLoS One*, *12*(12), e0189621. Advance online publication. DOI: 10.1371/journal.pone.0189621 PMID: 29267306

Garde, S., Chodisetti, P. K., & Reddy, M. (2021). Peptidoglycan: Structure, synthesis, and regulation. *EcoSal Plus*, *9*(2), ecosalplus.ESP-0010-2020. Advance online publication. DOI: 10.1128/ecosalplus.ESP-0010-2020 PMID: 33470191

Gasparrini, A. J., Wang, B., Sun, X., Kennedy, E. A., Hernandez-Leyva, A., Ndao, I. M., Tarr, P. I., Warner, B. B., & Dantas, G. (2019). Persistent metagenomic signatures of early-life hospitalization and antibiotic treatment in the infant gut microbiota and resistome. *Nature Microbiology*, *4*(12), 12. Advance online publication. DOI: 10.1038/s41564-019-0550-2 PMID: 31501537

Ghai, I., & Ghai, S. (2018). Understanding antibiotic resistance via outer membrane permeability. *Infection and Drug Resistance*, *11*, 523–530. DOI: 10.2147/IDR.S156995 PMID: 29695921

Herman, A., & Herman, A. P. (2014). Nanoparticles as antimicrobial agents: Their toxicity and mechanisms of action. *Journal of Nanoscience and Nanotechnology*, *14*(1), 946–957. DOI: 10.1166/jnn.2014.9054 PMID: 24730311

Hermansson, H., Kumar, H., Collado, M. C., Salminen, S., Isolauri, E., & Rautava, S. (2019). Breast milk microbiota is shaped by mode of delivery and intrapartum antibiotic exposure. *Frontiers in Nutrition*, *6*, 4. Advance online publication. DOI: 10.3389/fnut.2019.00004 PMID: 30778389

Huang, H. W. (2020). DAPTOMYCIN, its membrane-active mechanism vs. that of other antimicrobial peptides. *Biochimica et Biophysica Acta (BBA) -. Biomembranes*, *1862*(10), 183395. Advance online publication. DOI: 10.1016/j.bbamem.2020.183395 PMID: 32526177

Iwu, C. D., & Patrick, S. M. (2021). An insight into the implementation of the global action plan on antimicrobial resistance in the WHO African region: A roadmap for action. *International Journal of Antimicrobial Agents*, *58*(4), 106411. Advance online publication. DOI: 10.1016/j.ijantimicag.2021.106411 PMID: 34371112

Jednačak, T., Mikulandra, I., & Novak, P. (2020). Advanced methods for studying structure and interactions of macrolide antibiotics. *International Journal of Molecular Sciences*, *21*(20), 7799. Advance online publication. DOI: 10.3390/ijms21207799 PMID: 33096889

Kapoor, G., Saigal, S., & Elongavan, A. (2017). Action and resistance mechanisms of antibiotics: A guide for clinicians. *Journal of Anaesthesiology, Clinical Pharmacology*, *33*(3), 300–305. DOI: 10.4103/joacp.JOACP_349_15 PMID: 29109626

Kasai, C., Sugimoto, K., Moritani, I., Tanaka, J., Oya, Y., Inoue, H., Tsumura, M., Takemura, M., Yamauchi, S., Kaneko, M., Kawakami, M., & Yamada, T. (2015). Comparison of the gut microbiota composition between obese and non-obese individuals in a Japanese population, as analyzed by terminal restriction fragment length polymorphism and next-generation sequencing. *BMC Gastroenterology*, *15*(1), 100. Advance online publication. DOI: 10.1186/s12876-015-0330-2 PMID: 26261039

Koulenti, D., Lisboa, T., Brun-Buisson, C., Krueger, W., Macor, A., Sole-Violan, J., Diaz, E., Topeli, A., & Rello, J. (2009). Spectrum of practice in the diagnosis of nosocomial pneumonia in patients requiring mechanical ventilation in European intensive care units. *Critical Care Medicine*, *37*(8), 2360–2368. DOI: 10.1097/CCM.0b013e3181a037ac PMID: 19531951

Lanks, C. W., Musani, A. I., & Hsia, D. W. (2019). Community-acquired pneumonia and hospital-acquired pneumonia. *The Medical Clinics of North America*, *103*(3), 487–501. DOI: 10.1016/j.mcna.2018.12.008 PMID: 30955516

Li, W., Separovic, F., O'Brien-Simpson, N. M., & Wade, J. D. (2018). Covalent conjugation of cationic antimicrobial peptides with a β-lactam antibiotic core. *Peptide Science (Hoboken, N.J.)*, *110*(3), e24059. Advance online publication. DOI: 10.1002/pep2.24059

Markley, J. L., & Wencewicz, T. A. (2018). Tetracycline-inactivating enzymes. *Frontiers in Microbiology*, *9*, 1058. Advance online publication. DOI: 10.3389/fmicb.2018.01058 PMID: 29899733

Marschall, E., Cryle, M. J., & Tailhades, J. (2019). Biological, chemical, and biochemical strategies for modifying glycopeptide antibiotics. *The Journal of Biological Chemistry*, *294*(49), 18769–18783. DOI: 10.1074/jbc.REV119.006349 PMID: 31672921

Maruyama, T., Saida, J., Uchida, T., Imamura, H., Sasaki, T., Toyoda, M., Imoto, N., Sunayama, T., & Minami, S. (2019). A therapeutic strategy for all pneumonia patients: A 3-year prospective multicenter cohort study using risk factors for multidrug-resistant pathogens to select initial empiric therapy. *Clinical Infectious Diseases*, *68*(7), 1080–1088. DOI: 10.1093/cid/ciy631 PMID: 30084884

Mathur, H., Field, D., Rea, M. C., Cotter, P. D., Hill, C., & Ross, R. P. (2018). Fighting biofilms with lantibiotics and other groups of bacteriocins. *NPJ Biofilms and Microbiomes*, *4*(1), 1. Advance online publication. DOI: 10.1038/s41522-018-0053-6 PMID: 29707229

McAllister, D. A., Liu, L., Shi, T., Chu, Y., Reed, C., Burrows, J., Adeloye, D., Rudan, I., Black, R. E., Campbell, H., & Nair, H. (2019). Global, regional, and national estimates of pneumonia morbidity and mortality in children younger than 5 years between 2000 and 2015: A systematic analysis. *The Lancet. Global Health*, *7*(1), e47–e57. DOI: 10.1016/S2214-109X(18)30408-X PMID: 30497986

McDonald, L. C. (2017). Effects of short- and long-course antibiotics on the lower intestinal microbiome as they relate to traveller's diarrhea. *Journal of Travel Medicine*, *24*(Suppl. 1), S35–S38. DOI: 10.1093/jtm/taw084 PMID: 28520993

Mittal, A. K., Bhardwaj, R., Mishra, P., & Rajput, S. K. (2020). Antimicrobials misuse/overuse: Adverse effect, mechanism, challenges and strategies to combat resistance. *The Open Biotechnology Journal*, *14*(1), 107–112. DOI: 10.2174/1874070702014010107

Miyoshi, J., Bobe, A. M., Miyoshi, S., Huang, Y., Hubert, N., Delmont, T. O., Eren, A. M., Leone, V., & Chang, E. B. (2017). Peripartum antibiotics promote gut dysbiosis, loss of immune tolerance, and inflammatory bowel disease in genetically prone offspring. *Cell Reports*, *20*(2), 491–504. DOI: 10.1016/j.celrep.2017.06.060 PMID: 28700948

Murray, C. J. L., Ikuta, K. S., Sharara, F., Swetschinski, L., Aguilar, G. R., Gray, A., Han, C., Bisignano, C., Rao, P., Wool, E., & Naghavi, M. (2022). Global burden of bacterial antimicrobial resistance in 2019: A systematic analysis. *Lancet*, *399*(10325), 629–655. DOI: 10.1016/S0140-6736(21)02724-0 PMID: 35065702

Murugaiyan, J., Kumar, P. A., Rao, G. S., Iskandar, K., Hawser, S., Hays, J. P., Mohsen, Y., Adukkadukkam, S., Abiola, A. W., & Essack, S. Y. (2022). Progress in alternative strategies to combat antimicrobial resistance: Focus on antibiotics. *Antibiotics (Basel, Switzerland)*, *11*(2), 200. Advance online publication. DOI: 10.3390/antibiotics11020200 PMID: 35203804

Nikaido, H., & Pagès, J.-M. (2012). Broad-specificity efflux pumps and their role in multidrug resistance of Gram-negative bacteria. *FEMS Microbiology Reviews*, *36*(2), 340–363. DOI: 10.1111/j.1574-6976.2011.00290.x PMID: 21707670

Nunes, O. C., Manaia, C. M., Kolvenbach, B. A., & Corvini, P. F.-X. (2020). Living with sulfonamides: A diverse range of mechanisms observed in bacteria. *Applied Microbiology and Biotechnology*, *104*(24), 10389–10408. DOI: 10.1007/s00253-020-10982-5 PMID: 33175245

Oloke, J. K. (2000). Activity pattern of natural and synthetic antibacterial agents among hospital isolates. *Microbios*, *102*(403), 175–181. PMID: 10955832

Pancu, D. F., Scurtu, A., Macasoi, I. G., Marti, D., Buzatu, R., Dinu, S., Socoliuc, V., & Dehelean, C. A. (2021). Antibiotics: Conventional therapy and natural compounds with antibacterial activity—A pharmaco-toxicological screening. *Antibiotics (Basel, Switzerland)*, *10*(4), 401. Advance online publication. DOI: 10.3390/antibiotics10040401 PMID: 33917092

Patangia, D. V., Ryan, C. A., Dempsey, E., Ross, R. P., & Stanton, C. (2022). Impact of antibiotics on the human microbiome and consequences for host health. *MicrobiologyOpen*, *11*(1), e1260. Advance online publication. DOI: 10.1002/mbo3.1260 PMID: 35212478

Pates, K. M., Periselneris, J. N., & Brown, J. S. (2023). Pneumonia. *Medicine*, *51*(11), 763–767. DOI: 10.1016/j.mpmed.2023.08.003 PMID: 36775251

Reygaert, W. C. (2018). An overview of the antimicrobial resistance mechanisms of bacteria. *AIMS Microbiology*, *4*(3), 482–501. DOI: 10.3934/microbiol.2018.3.482 PMID: 31294229

Rima, M., Rima, M., Fajloun, Z., Sabatier, J.-M., Bechinger, B., & Naas, T. (2021). Antimicrobial peptides: A potent alternative to antibiotics. *Antibiotics (Basel, Switzerland)*, *10*(9), 1095. Advance online publication. DOI: 10.3390/antibiotics10091095 PMID: 34572678

Saha, M., & Sarkar, A. (2021). Review on multiple facets of drug resistance: A rising challenge in the 21st century. *Journal of Xenobiotics*, *11*(4), 4. Advance online publication. DOI: 10.3390/jox11040013 PMID: 34940513

Schlegel, H. G., & Zaborosch, C. (1993). *General microbiology*. Cambridge University Press.

Schwarz, S., Kehrenberg, C., Doublet, B., & Cloeckaert, A. (2016). Lincosamides, streptogramins, phenicols, and pleuromutilins: Mode of action and mechanisms of resistance. *Cold Spring Harbor Perspectives in Medicine*, *6*(11), a027037. Advance online publication. DOI: 10.1101/cshperspect.a027037 PMID: 27549310

Schwiertz, A., Taras, D., Schäfer, K., Beijer, S., Bos, N. A., Donus, C., & Hardt, P. D. (2010). Microbiota and SCFA in lean and overweight healthy subjects. *Obesity (Silver Spring, Md.)*, *18*(1), 190–195. DOI: 10.1038/oby.2009.167 PMID: 19498350

Sengupta, S., Chattopadhyay, M., & Grossart, H.-P. (2013). The multifaceted roles of antibiotics and antibiotic resistance in nature. *Frontiers in Microbiology*, *4*, 47. Advance online publication. DOI: 10.3389/fmicb.2013.00047 PMID: 23487476

Sheard, D. E., O'Brien-Simpson, N. M., Wade, J. D., & Separovic, F. (2019). Combating bacterial resistance by combination of antibiotics with antimicrobial peptides. *Pure and Applied Chemistry*, *91*(2), 199–209. DOI: 10.1515/pac-2018-0707

Simons, A., Alhanout, K., & Duval, R. E. (2020). Bacteriocins, antimicrobial peptides from bacterial origin: Overview of their biology and their impact against multidrug-resistant bacteria. *Microorganisms*, *8*(5), 639. Advance online publication. DOI: 10.3390/microorganisms8050639 PMID: 32349409

Stokholm, J., Sevelsted, A., Bønnelykke, K., & Bisgaard, H. (2014). Maternal propensity for infections and risk of childhood asthma: A registry-based cohort study. *The Lancet. Respiratory Medicine*, *2*(8), 631–637. DOI: 10.1016/S2213-2600(14)70152-3 PMID: 25066330

Thong, B. Y.-H. (2010). Update on the management of antibiotic allergy. *Allergy, Asthma & Immunology Research*, *2*(2), 77–86. DOI: 10.4168/aair.2010.2.2.77 PMID: 20358021

Tuomanen, E. I., Austrian, R., & Masure, H. R. (1995). Pathogenesis of pneumococcal infection. *The New England Journal of Medicine*, *332*(19), 1280–1284. DOI: 10.1056/NEJM199505113321907 PMID: 7708073

Wang, F., Zhou, H., Olademehin, O. P., Kim, S. J., & Tao, P. (2018). Insights into key interactions between vancomycin and bacterial cell wall structures. *ACS Omega*, *3*(1), 37–45. DOI: 10.1021/acsomega.7b01483 PMID: 29399648

Wong, W. S. W., Lee, M. W. Y., Dudley, E. G., & Kovac, J. (2020). Prenatal and peripartum exposure to antibiotics and cesarean section delivery are associated with differences in diversity and composition of the infant meconium microbiome. *Microorganisms*, *8*(2), 179. Advance online publication. DOI: 10.3390/microorganisms8020179 PMID: 32012716

Yin, J., Wang, L., Jin, Y., He, Q., Li, W., Wang, J., Wang, Y., & Sun, L. (2020). Mechanisms of bactericidal action and resistance of polymyxins for Gram-positive bacteria. *Applied Microbiology and Biotechnology*, *104*(9), 3771–3780. DOI: 10.1007/s00253-020-10525-y PMID: 32157424

Zanfardino, M., Pane, K., Mirabelli, P., Salvatore, M., & Franzese, M. (2019). TCGA-TCIA impact on radiogenomics cancer research: A systematic review. *International Journal of Molecular Sciences*, *20*(23), 6033. Advance online publication. DOI: 10.3390/ijms20236033 PMID: 31795520

Zhu, Y., Huang, W. E., & Yang, Q. (2022). Clinical perspective of antimicrobial resistance in bacteria. *Infection and Drug Resistance*, *15*, 735–746. DOI: 10.2147/IDR.S345574 PMID: 35264857

Zwittink, R. D., Renes, I. B., van Lingen, R. A., van Zoeren-Grobben, D., Konstanti, P., Norbruis, O. F., Martin, R., Knol, J., & Belzer, C. (2018). Association between duration of intravenous antibiotic administration and early-life microbiota development in late-preterm infants. *European Journal of Clinical Microbiology & Infectious Diseases*, *37*(3), 475–483. DOI: 10.1007/s10096-018-3193-y PMID: 29368074

# Chapter 4
# Influenza Virus

**Nadia A. Mohammed**
https://orcid.org/0009-0005-7705-8563
*Cairo Univercity, Egypt*

**Yasmine Ashraf**
*Cairo Univercity, Egypt*

**Ganna Ameen**
*Cairo Univercity, Egypt*

**Fatima M. Abbas**
*Cairo Univercity, Egypt*

**Nada Abdo**
*Cairo Univercity, Egypt*

## ABSTRACT

*Influenza, generally known as flu, is a viral respiratory disease. It can cause symptoms like fever, cough, sore throat, body aches, and fatigue. Researching treatments for influenza is important to develop effective antiviral medications and vaccines to prevent its spread and reduce its impact on public health. Influenza is typically a self-limiting illness, and most people recover during a week or two without any complications. It's worth noting that while influenza can cause significant illness and even death, it is distinct from the common cold, which is caused by different viruses and typically produces milder symptoms. This chapter provides Epidemiology, symptoms, prevention, advancements and future directions of Influenza.*

DOI: 10.4018/979-8-3693-1990-1.ch004

## INTRODUCTION

Influenza is a severe viral infection that predominantly affects the respiratory system. Influenza viruses belong to the Orthomyxoviridae family, characterized by a segmented, negative sense, single-stranded RNA. There are different types of Influenza viruses, but Influenza A and B Viruses are the sole shapes of Influenza viruses that cause illness in humans. Influenza A viruses are grouped based on the presence of particular surface proteins, namely hemagglutinin (H) and neuraminidase (N). These surface proteins undergo frequent changes, leading to the emergence of new strains and the need for updated vaccines. The influenza virus is responsible for causing significant illness in millions of individuals every year. Around 5 to 15 percent of the global population gets infected with influenza viruses every year, leading to approximately 950,000 hospitalizations and 300,000 to 650,000 deaths, (Vogel & Manicassamy, 2020) (De Jong et al., 2020) (Nagashima & Mousa, 2021).

## EPIDEMIOLOGY OF INFLUENZA

Influenza affects all age groups, with pregnant women, young children, elderly, and chronic medical conditions more susceptible. World Health Organization reports four influenza-related events since 2021, (Centers for Diease Control, 2021). The swine flu, caused by the A(H1N1) pdm09 virus, caused 284,000 deaths in 214 countries between 2009 and 2010. Younger people were disproportionately affected due to older populations' immunity. The virus is now circulating as a seasonal flu virus and is included in a vaccine for the Northern Hemisphere in 2021 and 2022, (Centers for Diease Control, 2021). Seasonal influenza, a prevalent respiratory infection in both the Northern and Southern Hemispheres, can cause respiratory infections year-round in tropical and subtropical regions, causing death for susceptible individuals. Annual seasonal influenza epidemics, varying in strain, can infect 20% of the global population, cause 290,000-650,000 deaths, strain healthcare systems, and decrease worker productivity, causing significant economic impact, (Centers for Diease Control, 2021). Influenza cases worldwide have decreased due to non-pharmacological measures like handwashing and social distancing, with 35.2% type A and 64.8% type B cases detected in March 2021, (Centers for Diease Control, 2021).

## SYMPTOMS OF INFLUENZA

Influenza symptoms vary in severity and are unique to each individual. Severity is influenced by age and the presence of other chronic conditions. Typical signs and symptoms of influenza that are common: abrupt or unplanned beginning, chills and a chronic, dry cough that may or may not cause chest pain discomfort in general weariness or lethargy, diaphoresis, A sudden-onset fever that could last for three to four days, a frontal or retroorbital headache, Pain in the arms, legs, and back, sometimes referred to as myalgia, rhinorrhoea, or nasal congestion (Joints) suffering swelling in the throat, Sneezing, Weakness; additionally This virus does not induce vomiting and diarrhea in young children or old individuals who are already vulnerable. Instead, it causes diarrhea, nausea, and vomiting, which can give rise to viral pneumonia or secondary bacterial pneumonia, (Lung.org, 2018) (Keilman, 2019) (World Health Organization, 2021).

## PREVENTION AND CONTROL MEASURES

As maintained by the Centres for Disease Control and Prevention (CDC), flu vaccination lessens the risk of flu illness by 40% to 60% among the overall community during seasons when most circulating flu viruses are well-matched to those used to make flu vaccines, (CDC, 2023).

A 2022 study showed that flu vaccination abates children's risk of severe life-threatening influenza by 75%, (CDC, 2022).

During the 2018-2019 flu season, flu vaccination lowered flu-related hospitalization by 41% and flu-related emergency department visits by half among children (aged 6 months to 17 years old), (CDC, 2022).

The CDC has been working with researchers at universities and hospitals since the 2003-2004 flu season to estimate how well flu vaccines work through observational studies using laboratory-confirmed flu as the outcome, (Yamayoshi & Kawaoka, 2019).

## Vaccine Composition and Strains Covered

Vaccines are intended to guard against influenza viruses; according to research, they are likely to spread and infect people over the next season. Every year, the ingredients in influenza vaccines are examined and changed as necessary to match the viruses that are currently in circulation, (Young *et al.,* 2018).

Some of the research projects undertaken to increase the efficacy of influenza vaccines include the development of high-yielding influenza A and B virus vaccine viruses, artificial generation of influenza vaccine viruses for quick response to pandemics, and generating and characterizing influenza A viruses in altered polymerase fidelity—consequently, the ingredients in influenza vaccinations. Therefore, the composition of influenza vaccines is reviewed per year and updated as needed to match circulating influenza viruses. The vaccine seed viruses are determined more than 6 months before each epidemic season, and occasionally, there may be an antigenic mismatch between vaccine candidates and circulating strains. Researchers are working to make influenza vaccines more effective through various methods, including the development of high-yield influenza A and B virus vaccine viruses, synthetic generation of influenza vaccine viruses for rapid response to pandemics, and generation and characterization of influenza A viruses with altered polymerase fidelity, (Young *et al.,* 2018) (Trombetta & Montomoli, 2016).

## Vaccine Effectiveness and Duration of Protection

Worldwide, inactivated vaccinations are the greatest often used method because of their great safety and comparatively inexpensive cost of manufacture. Beginning at 6–12 months of age, inactivated vaccines must be administered annually due to the short duration of the immunity they impart, (Yamayoshi & Kawaoka, 2019). A vaccine's effectiveness is determined by how well it protects against an infection. To assess vaccine immunogenicity, however, surrogates have been employed, such as virus-specific cytotoxic T lymphocyte (CTL) levels and hemagglutinin-inhibition (HI) antibody titers in sera, (Young *et al.*, 2018). Serum HI antibody Because a serum HI antibody titer of > 1:40 is associated with a significant reduction in influenza incidence, titer induction is used as a measure of vaccine efficacy in clinical studies, (Young *et al.*, 2018). Therefore, the duration of protection provided by the influenza vaccine is limited, and annual vaccinations are needed to maintain immunity. The vaccine's effectiveness is evaluated based on the level of protection it provides against infection, and serum HI antibody titer induction is used as an indication of vaccine efficacy in clinical trials, (Young *et al.*, 2018) (Miller *et al.,* 2013).

## Recommendations for Different Age Groups and High-Risk Populations

Influenza vaccinations are recommended by the (CDC) for individuals of any age. However, it highly encourages vaccination for individuals at a relatively high risk of getting infected with influenza, such as infants, the elderly, pregnant women, and those who suffer from chronic medical conditions. Specifically, inactivated and live attenuated vaccines are available for infants, with the former being suitable for individuals over 6 months of age and the latter for those over 2 years of age. Additionally, the elderly population, known to have a weaker immune response to vaccination, can benefit from adjuvant strategies developed to improve vaccination efficacy in this demographic. Therefore, the CDC's recommendations emphasize the importance of vaccination for all age groups, with particular emphasis on high-risk populations and tailored vaccination strategies for specific age groups, (Young *et al.,* 2018) (Miller *et al.,* 2013) (Rote, 2019).

## Non-Pharmaceutical Interventions

NPIs, or non-pharmaceutical interventions, are a crucial tactic in the management of influenza outbreaks. NPIs include things like respiratory protocol, social distance, hand cleanliness, and closing schools, (Young *et al.,* 2018).

Performing good hand hygiene, which includes washing your hands by using soap and water and using alcohol-based hand sanitizers, is an easy way to stop the flu from spreading. Practicing good respiratory hygiene, including covering the nose and mouth when sneezing or coughing, can also help stop the influenza from spreading. In addition, methods of social distancing that involve remaining at home while ill and avoiding close contact with sick people work well to stop the spread of influenza. Although closing schools can help stop the spread of the flu, there are several drawbacks to consider, including disruptions to education and financial losses. For this reason, they should only be used in conjunction with different non-pharmaceutical measures. Thus, preventing influenza outbreaks through non-pharmaceutical measures, including hand washing, respiratory protocol, social distancing, and closing schools, is crucial. Good hand hygiene and respiratory etiquette are two easy and efficient ways to stop the influenza virus from spreading. School closures are a possibility, but they should be carefully evaluated and carried out in tandem with other NPIs. Social separation tactics are additionally useful, (Young *et al.,* 2018).

## ADVANCEMENTS AND FUTURE DIRECTIONS

### Universal Influenza Vaccines

To get vaccinated annually, it is advised to be protected from seasonal influenza viruses owing to the substantial burden of influenza virus infection on public health. The effectiveness of seasonal vaccinations might vary significantly from year to year despite intense new variation tracking and comprehensive vaccine strain selection. Regardless of vaccination history, this frequently reduces population protection, (Vogel & Manicassamy, 2020).

### Strategies for Developing Vaccines Targeting Conserved Regions

Since there are many different influenza virus subtypes, creating universal vaccinations for the disease is still the best course of action, (Sun, Luo, & Li, 2020). Conventional influenza vaccinations aim to produce neutralizing antibodies against highly variable yet immunodominant hemagglutinin (HA) antigens. Focusing on conserved antigens and eliciting cross-reactive T-cell responses are two newly discovered strategies for developing influenza vaccines that result in more broadly protective and durable immunity. This field of study is rapidly growing, (Ostrowsky *et al.,* 2020) (De Jong *et al.,* 2020).

For example, the viral surface protein HA is made up of three protomers of the HA1 and HA2 subunits, which are created after the cleavage of the HA0 precursor protein. The stem domain, which is made up of parts from both HA1 and HA2, allows the viral membrane to fuse with the host endosomal membrane by conformational changes in the HA, (De Jong *et al.,* 2020) (Nagashima & Mousa, 2021). This is followed by the release of viral RNA into the host cytoplasm. Additional conserved areas can be found in HA as well, such as some residues in the stem domain and the receptor binding pocket. Neutralizing antibodies directed against them may provide cross-protection because these areas are conserved across strains or even subtypes. These conserved sections might be the subject of a potentially effective, all-encompassing vaccination, (De Jong *et al.,* 2020).

### Current Progress and Challenges in Universal Vaccine Development

The development of novel techniques for universal influenza vaccines has advanced significantly, but choosing the top candidates for human trials is a difficult process for a number of reasons:

1) Novel influenza vaccines are not consistently evaluated in preclinical studies. The assortment of vaccine platforms and targets is also to blame for this.
2) There are no recognized correlates of immunity for influenza-related broadly cross-reactive immunological responses. The standardization of assays measuring non-HA-head immune responses is insufficient.
3) There is a shortage of funds for the creation of universal vaccines, (Madsen & Cox, 2020).

## Novel Antiviral Therapies

In order to battle upcoming pandemic outbreaks and ongoing seasonal cycles of influenza, new antiviral medicines are required. The advent of drug-resistant influenza virus variants emphasizes this requirement, (Shin & Seong, 2018).

### New Classes of Antiviral Drugs Under Investigation

In case a virus resistant to a certain agent or class begins to proliferate, the growing diversity of antiviral classes should allow for an adequate public health response. Baloxavir marboxil, a brand-new antiviral, has been authorized for use in the United States to treat influenza in those who are at a high risk of experiencing complications from the illness. No antivirals have been licensed expressly for the indication of severe influenza or hospitalized influenza, with the exception of intravenous zanamivir in nations of the European Union, (Beigel & Hayden, 2020).

The most recent antiviral to be licensed is baloxavir marboxil (brand name: Xofluza), which blocks the transcription of viral mRNA by targeting the endonuclease activity of the viral PA polymerase subunit. The pharmacology of this novel medication, which enables efficient treatment of influenza A or B virus infection with just one dose, is its most encouraging feature. Greater viral load reductions were seen in a clinical experiment, (O'Hanlon & Shaw, 2019).

### Mechanisms of Action and Potential Benefits

There are different mechanisms of action according to the antiviral drug used. Certain drugs stop the spread of viruses by blocking the A/M2 proton channel, which the influenza A virus uses to communicate with itself (Amantadine). However, this limits its usage only for influenza A type, (Świerczyńska, Mirowska-Guzel, & Pindelska, 2022).

Other medications besides Neuraminidase Inhibitors (NAIs), the largest class of medications and currently the most prescribed and utilized medications for treating human influenza. Based on the example of Zanamivir, their mechanism of action involves the prevention of viral replication both in vitro and in vivo, (Świerczyńska, Mirowska-Guzel, & Pindelska, 2022).

Cap-dependent endonuclease Inhibitors are a New Group of Anti-Influenza Drugs as Baloxavir Marboxil. After being taken orally, the small molecule prodrug baloxavir marboxil is hydrolyzed to produce the active form of baloxavir acid in the liver, blood, and intestinal epithelial cells. By specifically attaching to the PA protein, active baloxavir prevents the influenza virus's RNA polymerase complex from replicating. The PA protein, which is in charge of snatching the host cell mRNA cap and is a crucial step in starting the process of vRNA transcription, is specifically bound by baloxaviric acid to prevent the synthesis of viral mRNA, (O'Hanlon & Shaw, 2019) (Świerczyńska, Mirowska-Guzel, & Pindelska, 2022).

## Improved Diagnostics

### Rapid Diagnostic Tests for Influenza Detection

Rapid Diagnostic tests (RDTs) for respiratory viruses may help with early diagnosis, direct patient management, and stop transmission through at-home testing. One type of RDT is the "Flu@home" test kit. Patients used their flu@home kit according to instructions on a mobile application and indicated what lines they saw on the RDT if they reported experiencing a cough along with aches, fever, chills, and/or sweats, (Kotnik *et al.,* 2022).

Due to their label-free mechanism, quartz crystal microbalance (QCM) systems have become a reliable biosensing platform, enabling the detection and quantification of a variety of biomolecules. For the early diagnosis of infections and the routine monitoring of illness progression, QCM-based biosensors are appealing due to their high sensitivity and quick detection times, which may be utilized to detect various viruses like influenza and COVID-19, (Lim *et al.*, 2020).

### Advancements in Molecular and Point-of-Care Testing Methods

One of respiratory viruses tests is called Rapid point-of-care testing (POCT), may enhance clinical care by lowering the need for antibiotics, reducing hospital stays, enhancing the detection and treatment of influenza, and rationalizing the use of isolation facilities; however, The use of it instead of regular clinical therapy is not supported by enough data. Rapid molecular testing technologies for respiratory viruses possess the capability to function as point-of-care (POC) assays, with diagnostic accuracies that are approximately equivalent to those of laboratory PCR. Rapid, sensitive, and dependable point-of-care (POC) molecular assays have been developed recently, which expedites the procedure from sample collection to result, (Brendish et al., 2017) (Rahamat-Langendoen et al., 2019).

Nathan and his colleagues – after a pragmatic, open-label, randomised controlled trial – have found that in comparison to laboratory PCR, the detection rate of viruses was enhanced by routine molecular POCT technique in adults presenting to secondary care with severe respiratory disease; however, this strategy did not affect the percentage of patients receiving antibiotic treatment or the overall duration of antibiotic use. It did result in a higher percentage of patients taking single doses and short (48 h) regimens of antibiotics without any evidence of hazard, (Brendish *et al.*, 2017).

## CONCLUSION

Influenza is a respiratory illness caused by influenza viruses. It poses a significant global health burden, leading to substantial morbidity and mortality each year. It affects individuals of all ages, with certain populations, like older people, young children, and those with weakened immune systems. Prevention plays a crucial role in controlling the outbreak of influenza. Vaccination is the most effective method of prevention and is recommended annually. By getting vaccinated, individuals can reduce their risk of contracting the flu and minimize its impact on their health and the community.

## REFERENCES


Beigel, J. H., & Hayden, F. G. (2020). Influenza therapeutics in clinical practice—Challenges and recent advances. *Cold Spring Harbor Perspectives in Medicine, 11*(4), a038463. Advance online publication. DOI: 10.1101/cshperspect.a038463 PMID: 32041763

Brendish, N. J., Malachira, A. K., Armstrong, L., Houghton, R., Aitken, S., Nyimbili, E., & Clark, T. W. (2017). Routine molecular point-of-care testing for respiratory viruses in adults presenting to hospital with acute respiratory illness (ResPOC): A pragmatic, open-label, randomised controlled trial. *The Lancet. Respiratory Medicine*, *5*(5), 401–411.

De Jong, N. M. C., Aartse, A., Van Gils, M. J., & Eggink, D. (2020). Development of broadly reactive influenza vaccines by targeting the conserved regions of the hemagglutinin stem and head domains. *Expert Review of Vaccines*, *19*(6), 563–577. DOI: 10.1080/14760584.2020.1777861 PMID: 32510256

Keilman, L. J. (2019). Seasonal Influenza (Flu). *The Nursing Clinics of North America*, *54*(2), 227–243. DOI: 10.1016/j.cnur.2019.02.009 PMID: 31027663

Kotnik, J. H., Cooper, S., Smedinghoff, S., Gade, P., Scherer, K., Maier, M., Juusola, J., Ramirez, E., Naraghi-Arani, P., Lyon, V., Lutz, B., & Thompson, M. (2022). Flu@home: The comparative accuracy of an at-home influenza rapid diagnostic test using a prepositioned test kit, mobile app, mail-in reference sample, and symptom-based testing trigger. *Journal of Clinical Microbiology*, *60*(3), e02070-21. Advance online publication. DOI: 10.1128/jcm.02070-21 PMID: 35107302

Lim, H. J., Saha, T., Tey, B. T., Tan, W. S., & Ooi, C. W. (2020). Quartz Crystal Microbalance-based biosensors as rapid diagnostic devices for infectious diseases. *Biosensors & Bioelectronics*, *168*, 112513. DOI: 10.1016/j.bios.2020.112513 PMID: 32889395

Madsen, A., & Cox, R. J. (2020). Prospects and challenges in the development of Universal Influenza Vaccines. *Vaccines*, *8*(3), 361. DOI: 10.3390/vaccines8030361 PMID: 32640619

Miller, E., Andrews, N., Stellitano, L., Stowe, J., Winstone, A. M., Shneerson, J., & Verity, C. (2013). Risk of narcolepsy in children and young people receiving AS03 adjuvanted pandemic A/H1N1 2009 influenza vaccine: Retrospective analysis. *BMJ (Clinical Research Ed.)*, *346*(feb26 2), f794. DOI: 10.1136/bmj.f794 PMID: 23444425

Nagashima, K. A., & Mousa, J. J. (2021). Next-generation influenza HA immunogens and adjuvants in pursuit of a broadly protective vaccine. *Viruses, 13*(4), 546. DOI: 10.3390/v13040546 PMID: 33805245

O'Hanlon, R., & Shaw, M. L. (2019). Baloxavir Marboxil: The new influenza drug on the market. *Current Opinion in Virology, 35*, 14–18. DOI: 10.1016/j.coviro.2019.01.006 PMID: 30852344

Ostrowsky, J., Arpey, M., Moore, K., Osterholm, M., Friede, M., Gordon, J., Higgins, D., Molto-Lopez, J., Seals, J., & Bresee, J. (2020). Tracking progress in Universal Influenza Vaccine Development. *Current Opinion in Virology, 40*, 28–36. DOI: 10.1016/j.coviro.2020.02.003 PMID: 32279026

Pragmatic, A. (2017, May). open-label, Randomised Controlled Trial. [PubMed<]. *The Lancet. Respiratory Medicine, 5*(5), 401–411. DOI: 10.1016/S2213-2600(17)30120-0

Rahamat-Langendoen, J., Groenewoud, H., Kuijpers, J., Melchers, W. J. G., & van der Wilt, G. J. (2019). Impact of molecular point-of-care testing on Clinical Management and in-hospital costs of patients suspected of influenza or RSV infection: A modeling study. *Journal of Medical Virology, 91*(8), 1408–1414. DOI: 10.1002/jmv.25479 PMID: 30950066

Rote, N. S. (2019). Infection. In McCance, K. L., & Huether, S. E. (Eds.), *Pathophysiology: the Biologic basis for disease in adults and children* (8th ed., pp. 289–322). Elsev-Ier.

Shin, W.-J., & Seong, B. L. (2018). Novel antiviral drug discovery strategies to tackle drug-resistant mutants of influenza virus strains. *Expert Opinion on Drug Discovery, 14*(2), 153–168. DOI: 10.1080/17460441.2019.1560261 PMID: 30585088

Sun, W., Luo, T., Liu, W., & Li, J. (2020). Progress in the development of Universal Influenza Vaccines. *Viruses, 12*(9), 1033. DOI: 10.3390/v12091033 PMID: 32957468

Świerczyńska, M., Mirowska-Guzel, D. M., & Pindelska, E. (2022). Antiviral drugs in influenza. *International Journal of Environmental Research and Public Health, 19*(5), 3018. DOI: 10.3390/ijerph19053018 PMID: 35270708

Trombetta, C. M., & Montomoli, E. (2016). Influenza immunology evaluation and correlates of protection: A focus on vaccines. *Expert Review of Vaccines, 15*(8), 967–976. DOI: 10.1586/14760584.2016.1164046 PMID: 26954563

Vogel, O. A., & Manicassamy, B. (2020). Broadly protective strategies against influenza viruses: Universal Vaccines and therapeutics. *Frontiers in Microbiology, 11*, 135. Advance online publication. DOI: 10.3389/fmicb.2020.00135 PMID: 32117155

World Health Organization. (2021,August 31) Available from: http://www.who.int

Yamayoshi, S., & Kawaoka, Y. (2019). Current and future influenza vaccines. *Nature Medicine*, *25*(2), 212–220. DOI: 10.1038/s41591-018-0340-z PMID: 30692696

Young, B., Sadarangani, S., Jiang, L., Wilder-Smith, A., & Chen, M. I. (2018). Duration of influenza vaccine effectiveness: A systematic review, meta-analysis, and meta-regression of test-negative design case-control studies. *The Journal of Infectious Diseases*, *217*(5), 731–741. DOI: 10.1093/infdis/jix632 PMID: 29220496

# Chapter 5 Parainfluenza, Adenoviruses, and RS-Viruses

**Abdulrahman Adel**
*Faculty of Science, Cairo University, Egypt*

**Nadia A. Mohammed**
https://orcid.org/0009-0005-7705-8563
*Faculty of Science, Cairo University, Egypt*

**Ahlam Ahmed**
https://orcid.org/0009-0005-5376-0067
*Faculty of Science, Cairo University, Egypt*

**Zeinab Abd ElTawab**
*Faculty of Science, Cairo University, Egypt*

**Manar Hamed**
*Faculty of Science, Cairo University, Egypt*

## ABSTRACT

*Adenoviruses, respiratory syncytial viruses, and parainfluenza viruses are among the major causes of respiratory infections, which are a serious global health concern. This thorough analysis examines the virology, clinical presentation, and epidemiology of these viruses, emphasizing the effects they have on a range of demographics, including young children, the elderly, and people with weakened immune systems. In order to address the changing landscape of respiratory viral infections, emphasis is given on recent developments in diagnostics, antiviral treatments, and vaccine development. Through an understanding of the unique characteristics and shared*

DOI: 10.4018/979-8-3693-1990-1.ch005

*traits of these viruses, this chapter hopes to support ongoing efforts to reduce the global burden of respiratory disorders.*

## INTRODUCTION

The Paramyxoviridae family of enveloped RNA viruses included parainfluenza viruses. They are divided into four major serotypes, namely HPIV1 to HPIV4, and are identified by their single-stranded RNA genomes. Notably, HPIV4 is further subdivided into the HPIV4a and HPIV4b genera. While HPIV2 and HPIV4 are classified as belonging to the Rubulavirus genus, HPIV1 and HPIV3 belong to the Respirovirus genus Pleomorphism is a characteristic of parainfluenza virus virions, ranging in diameter from 150 to 200 m. The nucleocapsid protein (NP), phosphoprotein (P), matrix protein (M), fusion glycoprotein (F), hemagglutinin neuraminidase (HN) glycoprotein, and RNA polymerase (L) are all encoded by a single negative-sense RNA strand found within these virions, (Branche & Falsey, 2016).

Adenoviruses are double-stranded, non-enveloped deoxyribonucleic acid (DNA) viruses that are linked to a variety of clinical disorders in humans, (Branche & Falsey, 2016) (Ison & Hayden, 2016). Thus far, seven (A–G) species have been identified from which 67 immunologically diverse adenovirus serotypes have been further classified into accordance with hemagglutinin characteristics, DNA homology, carcinogenic potential in rodents, and clinical disease, (Ison & Hayden, 2016).

Biologically, RSV is a member of the Paramyxoviridae virus family, which is distinguished by a single-stranded RNA genome that is roughly 15 kB long. Nearly ten genes and eleven protein entities, including those involved in the fusion (F) and attachment (G) of the virus, are found in this genome. These proteins are also useful as antigenic targets in the creation of medications and vaccines. RSV is divided into two subgroups (A and B) as a result of the relative antigenic differences among these proteins, particularly glycoproteins. Physically, the RSV can take on spherical or long filamentous shapes, (Malik *et al.,* 2023).

## PARAINFLUENZA VIRUS

Human parainfluenza viruses (HPIVs) are a group of RNA viruses that can cause respiratory illnesses. HPIVs are the second most common cause of respiratory illness-related hospitalizations in children under 5 years old, after respiratory syncytial virus (RSV). HPIVs exhibit seasonal circulation patterns, with HPIV-1 and HPIV-2 peaking in fall, HPIV-3 peaking in spring and early summer, and HPIV-4 having less well-defined seasonal patterns, (Schmidt & Varga, 2021) (Bhorat, Fong, & Corey, 2020).

## Symptoms

Symptoms of parainfluenza viruses often present with respiratory symptoms such as fever, runny nose, cough, sneezing, and sore throat, which are similar to the common cold, (Centers for Disease Control and Prevention, n.d.).

Other symptoms may include ear pain, irritability, and decreased appetite (Centers for Disease Control and Prevention, n.d.).

HPIVs can cause serious illness in children, such as, (Centers for Disease Control and Prevention, n.d.):

- croup: (viral Infection characterized by harsh, barking cough and difficulty breathing due to swelling around the vocal cords)
- bronchitis (main air passage infection)
- Bronchiolitis (smallest air passages infection in the lungs)
- Pneumonia (infection and inflammation of the lungs, causing chest pain and shortness of breath)

More serious symptoms may include barking cough, stridor (noisy or high-pitched sound with breathing), and wheezing(, (Centers for Disease Control and Prevention, n.d.).

## Diagnosis

Diagnosis of PIVs infection includes a combination of clinical evaluation and laboratory testing, some of commonly used methods for Diagnosis of PIVs include:

- Clinical presentation: The most common symptoms such as cough, sore throat and vomiting may raise susceptible infection of PIVs, (Hsieh, Chen, & Hsu, 2017).
- Laboratory testing (Centers for Disease Control and Prevention, n.d.).
- viral detection genome by PCR

Viral culture as PIVs can be grown in cell culture from respiratory specimens.

## Treatment

The treatment of PIV is primarily supportive, as there are no specific antiviral medications for PIV infection. However, to abate symptoms you can:

- Take acetaminophen, ibuprofen, and other over-the-counter medications for pain and fever (Caution: children should not taking aspirin.) (Centers for Disease Control and Prevention, n.d.).
- Use a room humidifier or take a hot shower to help ease a sore throat and cough, (Centers for Disease Control and Prevention, n.d.).
- Drink plenty of liquids, stay home, and rest, (Centers for Disease Control and Prevention, n.d.).

## Novel Research Strategies

Limiting the spread of parainfluenza virus infections depends on a combination of preventive measures and novel research strategies. Such as:

Vaccine Development: Several vaccine candidates are being investigated, including live attenuated, inactivated, and subunit vaccines, (Higgins, Trujillo, & Keech, 2019). However, no licensed vaccine specifically targeting parainfluenza viruses is available.

Public Health Interventions: Novel research strategies involve evaluating the effectiveness of public health interventions to limit the spread of parainfluenza viruses, such as hand hygiene, respiratory etiquette, mask-wearing, social distancing, and environmental disinfection. Research can help refine guidelines and policies for infection control practices in healthcare settings, schools, and community settings, (Centers for Disease Control and Prevention, 2021).

# ADENOVIRUS

## Epidemiology

The frequency of infection with HAdV was 2.8%. Throughout the whole year, HAdV was prevalent, increasing in the winter and early spring; a reduced number of HAdV infections were linked to higher average monthly temperatures ($p = 0.013$). Males made up the majority of HAdV hospitalized patients ($p = 0.003$). HAdV infection is age-related, as children from the ages of 1 to 5 constitute 30.8% of the outpatients.

Morbidity and death are caused by HAdV infection of the respiratory system, as people with heart disease and weakened immunity are the most at risk of death. Of all those infected with the HAdV, 3% die, and one of the common factors among those infected is the presence of an underlying condition such as heart disease or immunosuppression, (Pscheidt *et al.*, 2021).

The molecular epidemiology of HAdV shows that nine genotypes are found in HAdV cases. Although the F41 HAdV strain predominated, 10% of patients also had HAdV-A31, (Tang *et al.*, 2022).

## Transmission and Prevalence

Transmission of the HAdV infection can spread sporadically and epidemically, (Florescu & Schaenman, 2019). Adenoviruses are mostly spread through direct contact and fomites, such as respiratory droplets. Regular self-inoculation also takes place when someone touches their mouth, nose, or eyes after coming into contact with contaminated fomite (such a doorknob). When people spend extended periods of time in closed environments like psychiatric institutions, boarding schools, dormitories for college students, orphanages, public swimming pools, job-training centers, infant nurseries, long-term care facilities, and military barracks, (Bonville, n.d.).

## Symptoms

The symptoms of acute adenoviral pharyngitis include fever, a painful throat, widespread exudative tonsillitis, and, oftentimes, cervical adenopathy. The following symptoms are also present: cough, headache, myalgia, chills, and malaise. Abdominal pain is a common complaint in infants and preschoolers, and nasal congestion and discharge are more noticeable, (Pscheidt *et al.*, 2021).

## Diagnosis

The incubation period for adenoviruses ranges from 2 to 14 days, with an average of 5 to 8 days, (Bonville, n.d.). We can diagnose the disease by a histopathologic analysis of biopsy. To differentiate between infection and rejection, immunohistochemical staining for adenovirus may be helpful. When appropriate, PCR-based testing of respiratory secretions should be done to detect adenovirus.

## Treatment

The most effective antiviral medication for the treatment of adenovirus infections is cidofovir. (the ideal dose is not known), (Florescu & Schaenman, 2019). For prevention, it is recommended to take precautions with direct contact and droplets from the nose and mouth during treatment in hospitals, specifically for people with weak immunity.

## Risk Factors

From the previous discussion, we conclude that the risk factors are: Age, The degree of immunosuppression, use of adenovirus sero-mismatch, and lack of hygiene.

## RSV

Respiratory syncytial virus (RSV) is one of the most important viral pathogens causing respiratory tract infection in infants and can cause mild to severe illness in people of all ages but especially dangerous for infants (Shang, Tan, & Ma, 2021) young children, and older adults commonly called lifetaker disease in children who are few months old, (Suresh, 2023).

## Pathogensis

RSV is mainly transmitted from person to person through saliva or mucus droplets. Human Respiratory Syncytial Virus (RSV) from the family pneumoviridae, under the order Mononegavirales, is a single continuous. strand of negative sense RNA, (Shang, Tan, & Ma, 2021).

## Symptoms

Most common symptoms of RSV infection begin approximately 3 to 7 days after infection with RSV and include coughs, sneezes, stuffy nose, dyspenia, robust bronchiolar airway infection and inflammation, (Suresh, 2023).

the cough progress into a fever develop severe bronchiolar airway infection and apnea which is a common symptom these symptoms may develped into asthma, bronchiolitis and pneomonia in severe cases

In the developing world, this disease leads to a high number of deaths, causing approximately 200,000 young children to lose their lives every year worldwide. In tropical regions, RSV thrives more in hotter climates and is further intensified during the rainy season, on the other hand, respiratory syncytial virus (RSV) infections are typically influenced by seasonal changes and variations in different regions. In temperate areas such as Europe, RSV outbreaks occur mainly during the cold winter months

## Diagnosis

The weak sensitivity of viral culture and antigen cause respiratory syncytial virus (RSV) during acute infection is difficult, therefore several methods are used as, Cell culture is the most sensitive method for testing RSV infection. This involves growing RSV obtained from a nasal aspirate or nasopharyngeal swab in a laboratory culture. The virus is then identified by its ability to infect cells and cause characteristic changes. Although cell culture is considered the best method for diagnosing RSV, it can take several days to obtain results. Another test called enzyme-linked immunosorbent assay (ELISA) is used to detect RSV antibodies in the blood. RSV-specific IgM antibodies, which are produced early in the course of RSV infection, can be detected in the blood for several weeks and indicate recent infection. On the other hand, RSV-specific IgG antibodies, produced later during RSV infection, can be detected in the blood for many years and indicate past infection with RSV, (Gröndahl e*t al*., 2005)

Alternative techniques, such as real-time PCR(RT-PCR) methods, enable the measurement of viral genetic material in clinical samples. However, drawbacks of these nucleic acid-based tests include their expensive nature and lack of widespread standardization, (Falsey, Formica, & Walsh, 2002).

## Strategies to Limit the Spread

- Vaccination by developing and promoting vaccines against RSV can help limit the spread of the virus, especially among high-risk populations such as infants and the elderly
- Antiviral medications: Researching and developing new antiviral medications specifically targeting RSV can help reduce the spread of the virus and improve treatment outcomes
- Improved infection control measures: Implementing strict infection control measures in healthcare settings, such as proper hand hygiene, isolation protocols, and environmental cleaning, can help prevent RSV transmission among patients and healthcare workers
- Research on immune-boosting therapies: Investigating immune-boosting therapies that can enhance the body's ability to fight off RSV infection may provide novel strategies to limit the spread of the virus

- Targeted interventions for high-risk populations: Developing targeted interventions for high-risk populations, such as premature infants or individuals with underlying health conditions, can help reduce their susceptibility to RSV infection and limit its spread within these vulnerable groups

## CONCLUSIONS

In conclusion, major respiratory pathogens that can cause a variety of respiratory infections, especially in young and immunocompromised people, include parainfluenza viruses, adenoviruses, and respiratory syncytial viruses. Comprehending the unique attributes of every virus is crucial for precise diagnosis and efficient handling. The necessity of maintaining constant watchfulness in combating chronic respiratory illnesses and enhancing public health outcomes is highlighted by ongoing research and developments in preventative strategies, such as vaccination.

## REFERENCES


Bhorat, A. E., Fong, Y., & Corey, L. (2020). A phase 1, open-label, single-arm study to evaluate the safety and immunogenicity of a trivalent influenza vaccine in adults 18 to <50 years of age in South Africa. *Journal of Clinical Virology*, *124*, 104262. DOI: 10.1016/j.jcv.2020.104262

Bonville, C. (n.d.). Respiratory syncytial virus. In Domachowske, J. (Ed.), *Vaccines* (pp. 89–97).

Branche, A. R., & Falsey, A. R. (2016). Parainfluenza virus infection. *Seminars in Respiratory and Critical Care Medicine*, *37*(4), 538–554. DOI: 10.1055/s-0036-1584798 PMID: 27486735

Centers for Disease Control and Prevention. (2021). *Preventing the spread of respiratory viruses*. https://www.cdc.gov/flu/prevent/preventing.htm

Centers for Disease Control and Prevention. (n.d.). *Symptoms of parainfluenza viruses*. https://www.cdc.gov/parainfluenza/symptoms.html

Centers for Disease Control and Prevention. (n.d.). *Laboratory information for parainfluenza viruses*. https://www.cdc.gov/parainfluenza/hcp/lab.htm

Centers for Disease Control and Prevention. (n.d.). *Prevention and treatment of parainfluenza viruses*. https://www.cdc.gov/parainfluenza/prevention-treatment.html

Falsey, A. R., Formica, M. A., & Walsh, E. E. (2002). Diagnosis of respiratory syncytial virus infection: Comparison of reverse transcription-PCR to viral culture and serology in adults with respiratory illness. *Journal of Clinical Microbiology*, *40*(3), 817–820. DOI: 10.1128/JCM.40.3.817-820.2002 PMID: 11880399

Florescu, D. F., & Schaenman, J. M. (2019). Adenovirus in solid organ transplant recipients: Guidelines from the American Society of Transplantation Infectious Diseases Community of Practice. *Clinical Transplantation*, *33*(9), e13527. DOI: 10.1111/ctr.13527 PMID: 30859626

Gröndahl, B., Puppe, W., Weigl, J., & Schmitt, H.-J. (2005). Comparison of the BD Directigen Flu A+B Kit and the Abbott TestPack Influenza A/B for rapid detection of influenza viruses. *Clinical Microbiology and Infection*, *11*(2), 120–124. DOI: 10.1111/j.1469-0691.2004.01047.x PMID: 16153263

Higgins, D., Trujillo, C., & Keech, C. (2019). Progress in the development of parainfluenza virus vaccines. *Viruses*, *11*(12), 1122. DOI: 10.3390/v11121122 PMID: 31817188

Hsieh, Y.-C., Chen, H.-Y., & Hsu, H.-C. (2017). Molecular epidemiology of human adenovirus infections in Taiwan, 2013–2014. *Journal of Microbiology, Immunology, and Infection*, *50*(6), 784–790. DOI: 10.1016/j.jmii.2017.03.005

Ison, M. G., & Hayden, R. T. (2016). Adenovirus. *Microbiology Spectrum*, *4*(4), 4.4.41. Advance online publication. DOI: 10.1128/microbiolspec.DMIH2-0020-2015 PMID: 27726766

Malik, S., Ahmad, T., Muhammad, K., & Waheed, Y. (2023). Respiratory syncytial virus infection: Treatments and clinical management. *Vaccines*, *11*(2), 491. DOI: 10.3390/vaccines11020491 PMID: 36851368

Pscheidt, V. M., Gregianini, T. S., Martins, L. G., & Veiga, A. B. (2021). Epidemiology of human adenovirus associated with respiratory infection in southern Brazil. *Reviews in Medical Virology*, *31*(4), e2189. DOI: 10.1002/rmv.2189 PMID: 33156553

Schmidt, M. E., & Varga, S. M. (2021). Cytokines and CD8 T cell effector mechanisms during respiratory syncytial virus infection. *Clinical Infectious Diseases*, *73*(3), e773–e779. DOI: 10.1093/cid/ciaa149 PMID: 33569576

Shang, Z., Tan, S., & Ma, D. (2021). Respiratory syncytial virus: From pathogenesis to potential therapeutic strategies. *International Journal of Biological Sciences*, *17*(14), 3903–3918. DOI: 10.7150/ijbs.64762 PMID: 34671221

Suresh, S. (2023). The medical significance, epidemiology, pathogenesis, detection, and management of respiratory syncytial virus. *Preprints*. DOI: 10.20944/preprints202307.1733.v1

Tang, X., Yue, H., Zhong, X., & Xu, H. (2022). Molecular epidemiology of human adenovirus, astrovirus, and sapovirus among outpatient children with acute diarrhea in Chongqing, China, 2017–2019. *Frontiers in Pediatrics*, *10*, 826604. DOI: 10.3389/fped.2022.826600 PMID: 35311045

# Chapter 6
# Measles

**Katrine Faysal Ibrahim**
*Lebanese University, Lebanon*

**Jimmy Joseph Dagher**
*Holy Spirit University of Kaslik, Lebanon*

**Rasha Mustafa Harb**
*University of Balamand, Lebanon*

**Hussein Khalil Hmadi**
https://orcid.org/0009-0008-2901-535X
*Lebanese University, Lebanon*

## ABSTRACT

*Measles or rubeola is a highly contagious disease, that is often overlooked, keeps possessing global challenges due to its stability outside the body for long periods of time and complications especially in younger kids. Due to its high transmissibility over 90% of people get infected after being exposed to a potential measles risk. It usually spreads through respiratory droplets, aerosol particles and human contact. The measles virus initiates infection by the attachment to SLAM or CD150 receptors which is a lymphoid surface receptor involved in immune cell activation, then it is transmitted to epithelial cells through the use of CD46. Manifestations of measles are often associated with high fevers, rashes and koplik spots. Currently numerous diagnostic approaches are being employed to detect measles, some of them being serologic techniques that work on detecting IgM or IgG antibodies. Although no cure has been found to treat measles, few strategies have been developed in order to combat symptoms such as the use of vitamin A and vaccinations.*

DOI: 10.4018/979-8-3693-1990-1.ch006

## INTRODUCTION

Measles is a fierce disease, mostly attributed as the rash illness causing extreme cases of complications and death. It is considered as the most viral disease of the world due to its high contiguity and long life stance outside the body. Measles outbreaks have decreased tremendously throughout the decades, however global outbreaks are still present especially in low income countries, (Awotiwon *et al.*, 2017). In developing countries children less than 5 years, will have already acquired the disease and it is associated with deaths associated with respiratory, gastrointestinal, nutritional and neurological complications. There is no direct link between nutrition and measles mortality, although rates in developing countries prove the other otherwise where it has suggested that undernourished kids had higher rates of complications, (Toole *et al.*, 1989).

## DEFINITION

Measles or rubeola is a highly contagious exanthematous and enanthematous disease, caused by a viral agent that's transmitted mainly through the respiratory tract secretions, (Walter & Malani, 2022). Up to 90% of unvaccinated individuals get diagnosed with measles after being exposed to an infected person. The virus has a 2 hour viability on surfaces and has the capacity of spreading throughout unfiltered air, (Keller *et al.,* 2019). Annually speaking, a staggering number of approximately 10 million people are infected with over 100,000 mortalities, (Crecelius & Burnett, 2020).

## EPIDEMIOLOGY AND PREVALENCE IN DEVELOPING AND DEVELOPED NATIONS AND RISK FACTORS

Measles epidemiology varies by region and is mainly tightly linked with the immunization levels attained in each country. It was responsible for the death of 2.6 million people around the globe before immunization was introduced. Although vaccination in this era was implemented, 134,000 deaths were recorded by the World Health Organization in 2015, (Coughlin *et al.,* 2017). The global annual incidence of measles declined by 83% from 2000 to 2017, (Strebel & Orenstein, 2019).

Measles is very contagious, 90% of people exposed to measles will attract the disease, (Centers for Disease Control and Prevention, 2012). It is a disease that must be reported when found, one case could lead to approximately 18 more cases. This virus exclusively affects humans and has no other animal reservoir. It is spread generally through respiratory droplets, aerosols particles, and human-to-human close contact, (Furuse & Oshitani, 2017).

Measles mostly affects young children. Pregnant women and children both have a higher risk of infection if not vaccinated. As for infants, born from an immunized mother, are at lower risk of contracting the disease due to antibodies transfer. However, as these antibodies wear off, they become vulnerable (10). Concerning pregnant women who contract measles during their pregnancy, they are at a higher risk of premature delivery, miscarriage or low birth infants, (Perry & Halsey, 2004). People who have immunocompromised diseases such as HIV, leukemia or are on immunosuppressive drugs are also more susceptible to severe complications. As for environmental factors, overcrowded living conditions and poor hygiene can boost the rapid spread of this virus, (Moss, 2017). In addition, people without access to vaccination due to limited access to healthcare or low immunization coverage are particularly the most vulnerable, (Bester, 2016). The booming of international travel played a role in transmission of measles from regions with ongoing epidemics to other regions where it was previously eradicated. Vitamin A deficiency could be another risk factor as it could exacerbate the severity of the disease, (Moss, 2017).

## PATHOGENESIS

Measles virus is naturally found in humans, and there are no identified animal reservoirs for the virus, (Naim, 2015). Despite the existence of effective live vaccines, measles still causes 4% of fatalities among children under the age of 5 years old worldwide, (Bryce *et al.*, 2005). The pathogenesis of measles involves several stages, including transmission, entry into the host, spread within the host, and the resulting clinical manifestations. Measles is primarily transmitted through respiratory droplets when an infected person coughs or sneezes, infecting the respiratory epithelium and/or the circulating immune cells in the upper respiratory passages. The virus infects the host by attaching to specific receptors: SLAM or CD150(signaling lymphocyte activation molecule) a lymphoid surface receptor involved in immune cell activation. Following an initial infection of immune cells, MeV is transmitted to epithelial cells by using the ubiquitously expressed CD46 (membrane cofactor protein) present on epithelial cells, and a third potential receptor, which enables measles virus infection even in the absence of the above receptors, (Naim, 2015). The Measles virus (MeV) genome encodes crucial components, including the M protein, H and F envelope glycoproteins, P and L proteins, and the N protein. The P gene region contains two overlapping open reading frames that produce non-structural proteins, V and C, involved in suppressing the host immune response. While dispensable for in vitro virus replication, V and C are essential during natural infections within the host, highlighting their significant roles in the viral life cycle. Upon entering a host cell, Measles virus (MeV), like other Paramyxoviridae, initiates genome transcription in the cytoplasm. This process is facilitated by the RNA-dependent RNA polymerase (RdRp) associated with the viral genome. The RdRp is responsible for transcribing the viral genetic material, enabling the virus to hijack the host cell's machinery for its replication and propagation, (Delpeut *et al.*, 2012). The initial infection and replication of the Measles virus (MV) in respiratory tract epithelial cells, followed by spreading to regional lymphoid organs. Infected monocytes were thought to disseminate the virus during the viremic phase. However, the widely acknowledged receptor for MV, CD150, is not expressed in epithelial cells or circulating monocytes. Measles virus (MV) exhibits a pronounced tropism for lymphoid and myeloid tissues, utilizing dendritic cells (DCs) as potential carriers to reach their primary targets in lymphoid organs. Extensive replication within T- and B-lymphocytes expressing CD150 leads to the widespread spread of the Measles virus throughout the body. The virus has a specific inclination for infecting memory lymphocytes, resulting in the depletion of immunologic memory and contributing to measles-associated immunosuppression, (de Swart, 2008).

## SYMPTOMS AND SIGNS

Despite the 2017 declaration of measles elimination in the UK, ongoing vaccination efforts and vigilance are crucial as the disease still poses a threat, underscoring the need to maintain high immunity levels in the population. Measles ranks among the highly contagious viral illnesses disseminated through airborne droplet transmission or direct exposure to respiratory secretions from infected individuals. The incubation period for measles may vary between 7 and 21 days from the time of exposure to the onset of symptoms but is usually 10 days. The onset of measles is characterized by a 2–4-day prodromal phase, during which individuals commonly experience coryzal symptoms such as a runny or stuffy nose, accompanied by cough and conjunctivitis (inflammation of the eyes). A prominent feature of this initial phase is a high fever, often reaching or exceeding 39°C. Notably, the fever tends to escalate during the prodromal period and reaches its peak around the time when the characteristic rash is about to appear. The rash, a hallmark of measles, emerges after the prodromal illness, typically starting on the face and subsequently spreading to other parts of the body, lasting 3–7 days. This sequence of symptoms underscores the distinct stages of measles progression, with the prodromal phase serving as a precursor to the appearance of the characteristic rash. Koplik spots, small white lesions in the mouth, may appear around the time of the measles rash, but they are not a reliable marker for diagnosis since they are not consistently present in all cases, and measles can still be present without them. If someone is suspected of having measles or it is being considered as a possible cause of their symptoms, healthcare providers should be informed, even if not all typical symptoms are present at that time. Measles cases are contagious from four days before to four days after the onset of the characteristic rash. While measles is typically a self-limiting condition, certain populations, including immunocompromised individuals, infants under one year, and pregnant women, are at risk of serious complications such as viral pneumonitis, otitis media (ear infection), and encephalitis (inflammation of the brain), (Moten *et al.,* 2018). Measles primarily targets the respiratory system by infecting the mucous membranes of the throat and lungs, leading to severe symptoms such as Pneumonia, a potentially life-threatening complication of measles, arises when the virus weakens the immune system, making individuals more susceptible to bacterial infections in the lungs, emphasizing the systemic impact of the disease beyond its initial respiratory manifestations, (Schoini *et al.,* 2019). These complications underscore the importance of monitoring and providing appropriate care for vulnerable groups during measles infections. Measles can impact individuals of all ages, and a notable percentage of cases occur in adults, with those aged 15–25 being especially vulnerable in the UK, (Moten *et al.,* 2018).

## DIAGNOSIS

Diagnostic measures could be based on manifestations presented by the patient through recognizing the unique symptoms accompanying measles such as a maculopapular rash lasting 3+ days, cough, Coryza or conjunctivitis and koplik's spots that descend from head to trunk and out to the extremities, (World Health Organization, 2007).

Laboratory testing is further needed in order to confirm suspicions, the WHO recommends the testing of a serum sample used to diagnose acute measles infection and an additional urine sample or a nasopharyngeal sample used to determine the virus genotype. The initial diagnostic measures required a serum sample that was collected during the first week after the first onset rash outbreak, and a follow-up sample. However, due to the high transmissibility of measles this technique was not effective so logistically easier methods were developed such as:

1) IgM EIA testing, can be done using a single collection of the serum and has a staggering 83%-89% sensitivity including a 95%-100% specificity. This technique is used to diagnose acute measles infection for up to 4 weeks after premier rash onset.

2) IgG EIA is recognized by its convenience as a home-made kit, it presents substantial improvements over any other diagnostic measure due to its rapidity, sensitivity and specificity, (Bellini & Helfand, 2003).

Currently many diagnostic methods are being implemented to detect measles, some of them being serologic techniques that work on detecting IgM or IgG antibodies. However, using acute and convalescent-phase specimens to indicate the rise of IgG antibodies is considered as a disadvantage. The most sensitive laboratory test proven was an antibody-capture EIA configuration used for the detection of IgM specific to measles, and it has been known for the reduction of false positives caused by the rheumatoid factor, (Helfand *et al.,* 1997).

## TREATMENT

So far, no anti-viral treatment has been recognized for measles, however vitamin A supplementation has been proved to reduce measles mortality and tackle complications. Two doses of vitamin A, ranging between 200,000 IU 1+ years old and 100,000 for infants has been proven to reduce mortality by at least 62%, (Bester, 2016). Nigeria, such as the Ijebu area, has witnessed a great outbreak of measles between children so in order to combat this spread residents have opted for medicinal plants as a cure. Twenty-three plant species have been claimed to possess curative properties for measles, and the most important plant is said to belong to the cucurbitaceae family, (Sonibare, Moody, & Adesanya, 2009). The only confirmed strategy in measles prevention is full vaccination against the virus. In developed countries measles vaccine is recommended in 2 doses at the ages 12-15 months and 4-6 years, (Bester, 2016).

## CHALLENGES OF EACH INFECTION IN THESE NATIONS AND LACK OF KNOWLEDGE IN ANTIBIOTICS, NO VACCINATION,....

The persistence of measles not only varies between nations and within communities due to many factors that vary from the access to healthcare to socioeconomic status of the patients to the general knowledge on the importance of vaccination.

Countries are facing varying problems in their efforts to eradicate measles. In Italy, wide immunity gaps and nosocomial transmission are major challenges to measles elimination, (Filia *et al.,* 2017). China is facing great obstacles in its efforts to eradicate measles as the percentages of cases in children and adults have been on the rise, (Wang *et al.,* 2019).

Furthermore, the persistence of measles in low-income, high birth rate countries reflects the difficulties in achieving high vaccine coverage in areas with limited public health infrastructure, (Ferrari *et al.,* 2008). For example, frequent measles outbreaks in low-income countries are a reflection of the difficulties in attaining and sustaining high vaccination rates in the face of inadequate public health infrastructure, (Bharti *et al.,* 2011). Moreover, community's involvement in undervaccinated populations, delays in diagnosis, notification, and adequate case isolation, and a lack of reliable data on vaccine coverage in demographic subgroups are also major obstacles to the efficient control of measles outbreaks, (Mulchandani *et al.,* 2021). Furthermore, the endemic spread of the measles is a challenge facing many countries and nations despite the significant advancements made, (Muscat *et al.,* 2015). Measles coverage rates have decreased in developed nations due to vaccine reluctance, which has led to continuing epidemics, (Sabahelzain *et al.*, 2019). Alongside the obstacles mentioned above, there are known logistical obstacles, such as getting to epidemic areas in some nations and problems with vaccination acceptability, (Thompson & Tebbens, 2014). In order to stop uncontrolled measles outbreaks, vaccination coverage, immunity clustering, and contact investigations are essential, (Liu *et al.,* 2015). Different strategies should be used to address vaccine reluctance and boost the adoption of the measles vaccination due to the intricacy of the interaction between supply-side and demand-side factors and measles vaccine hesitancy, (Sabahelzain *et al.,* 2022).

Alongside the lack of vaccination, living in rural areas and the effect of socio-economic status on the spread of measles, multiple studies have shown that measles outbreak due to war and conflict is a serious public health problem. Research has demonstrated that wars and conflicts can cause disruptions to immunization efforts, resulting in lower vaccination rates and subsequent outbreaks. Measles can spread easily in large populations of unvaccinated children due to the disruption of the vaccination programs before, during, and after wars, (Takahashi *et al.,* 2015). A great consideration is the vulnerability of regional health systems and large-scale population displacement that occur after wartime situations may also lead to a reduction in the overall rate of vaccination, hence intensifying the danger of measles outbreaks, (Mugoša *et al.,* 2021).

The consequences of impeding vaccination due to war have been brought to light in a number of conflict-affected areas, including Yemen and Syria, where the spread of diseases that could have been prevented, like measles, has been linked to a lack of preventative services and a delay in responding to the situation, (Mehtar *et al.*, 2021). Moreover, data collected from specific geographical locations of infected cases also show that the use of weapons during wars has been linked to the resurgence of infectious illnesses, such as measles, (Mousavi & Anjomshoa, 2020). The effect of war on the spread of measles is exacerbated when populations are unsettled during humanitarian crises, raising the possibility of vaccine-preventable diseases, including measles, spreading among vulnerable populations like refugees and internally displaced people, (Lam *et al.,* 2016).

## NOVEL RESEARCH STRATEGIES TO LIMIT THE SPREAD

A number of strategies have been suggested and put into practice in an effort to stop the measles from spreading. These include the formation of an outbreak control committee, the isolation of cases, the exclusion and quarantining of individuals who do not exhibit immunity, the vaccination of susceptible individuals, the use of immunoglobulin for high-risk individuals, and the maintenance of laboratory proficiency for measles confirmation, (Gastañaduy *et al.,* 2018). There has also been talk of using a ring vaccination strategy to boost immunity and catch-up unvaccinated individuals as soon as the virus is detected, which could effectively stop the spread of the measles, (Javelle *et al.,* 2019). Moreover, it has been discovered that the widespread participation in epidemic response vaccination campaigns greatly slows the measles virus's transmission and offers inpatients a hazard-free buffer, (Fu *et al.,* 2019). Additionally, despite the fact that the measles virus is still spreading throughout the world, it has been highlighted that the best way to prevent and eradicate the disease is to administer two doses of the vaccination, (Seto *et al.,* 2023). Furthermore, it has been determined that an improved monitoring system which includes viral genotyping is a crucial instrument for assessing approaches to contain and eradicate the measles, (Curtale *et al.,* 2010). In low and middle-income nations, contact tracing has been investigated as a potential strategy to stop the transmission of measles during epidemics, (Mbiynjo, Lynch, & Huws, 2021). Additionally, in an effort to stop the measles from spreading, several tactics have been suggested and put into practice. These include forming an outbreak control committee, keeping laboratory proficiency for measles confirmation, isolating cases of the disease, excluding and quarantining people without proof of immunity, immunizing susceptible people, using immunoglobulin to prevent measles in exposed susceptible high-risk individuals, and immunizing susceptible people, (Gastañaduy *et al.,* 2018). In order to control acute cases of measles, stop outbreaks from spreading, and guarantee vaccination rates, health care providers are essential, (Bester, 2016). Additionally, minimizing secondary measles transmission can be achieved through developing and adhering to standards for the management of patients who present to hospitals with fever and rash, (Pillsbury *et al.,* 2016). The risk of nosocomial measles transmission can also be reduced by putting infection prevention and control procedures into place, making sure healthcare personnel are immunized, and only admitting severe cases of the disease to hospitals, (Donadel *et al.,* 2021).

## CONCLUSION

Although no specific implementations have been proven to eradicate measles disease, the WHO efforts in tackling measles have decreased the spread incidence by 83% in the past 17 years. A variety of tactics needed to be used in developing countries including immunization, contact tracing, improved surveillance systems and epidemic response immunization programs should be considered in stopping measles spread. These tactics should be molded and customized to suit particular demographics ranging from developing to developed countries in order to combat child mortality caused by this transmissible diseases.

## REFERENCES


Awotiwon, A. A., Oduwole, O., Sinha, A., & Okwundu, C. I. (2017). Zinc supplementation for the treatment of measles in children. *Cochrane Database of Systematic Reviews*, *2017*(6), 6. DOI: 10.1002/14651858.CD011177.pub3 PMID: 28631310

Bellini, W. J., & Helfand, R. F. (2003). The challenges and strategies for laboratory diagnosis of measles in an international setting. *The Journal of Infectious Diseases*, *187*(s1, Supplement_1), S283–S290. DOI: 10.1086/368040 PMID: 12721927

Bester, J. (2016). Measles and measles vaccination. *JAMA Pediatrics*, *170*(12), 1209. DOI: 10.1001/jamapediatrics.2016.1787 PMID: 27695849

Bester, J. C. (2016). Measles and Measles Vaccination: A Review. *JAMA Pediatrics*, *170*(12), 1209–1215. DOI: 10.1001/jamapediatrics.2016.1787 PMID: 27695849

Bester, J. C. (2016). Measles and measles vaccination: A review. *JAMA Pediatrics*, *170*(12), 1209–1215. DOI: 10.1001/jamapediatrics.2016.1787 PMID: 27695849

Bharti, N., Tatem, A., Ferrari, M., Grais, R., Djibo, A., & Grenfell, B. (2011). Explaining seasonal fluctuations of measles in niger using nighttime lights imagery. *Science*, *334*(6061), 1424–1427. DOI: 10.1126/science.1210554 PMID: 22158822

Bryce, J., Boschi-Pinto, C., Shibuya, K., & Black, R. E. (2005). WHO estimates of the causes of death in children. *Lancet*, *365*(9465), 1147–1152. DOI: 10.1016/S0140-6736(05)71877-8 PMID: 15794969

Centers for Disease Control and Prevention. Epidemiology and Prevention of Vaccine-Preventable Diseases. 12th ed, second printing. Atkinson W, Wolfe C, Hamborsky J, eds. Washington, DC: Public Health Foundation, 2012.

Coughlin, M. M., Beck, A. S., Bankamp, B., & Rota, P. A. (2017). Perspective on Global Measles Epidemiology and Control and the Role of Novel Vaccination Strategies. *Viruses*, *9*(1), 11. DOI: 10.3390/v9010011 PMID: 28106841

. Crecelius, E. M., & Burnett, M. W. (2020). Measles (Rubeola): An Update. *Journal of special operations medicine: a peer reviewed journal for SOF medical professionals, 20*(2), 136–138. DOI: 10.55460/3NFC-341T

Curtale, F., Perrelli, F., Mantovani, J., Atti, M., Filia, A., Nicoletti, L., & Lallo, D. (2010). Description of two measles outbreaks in the lazio region, italy (2006-2007). importance of pockets of low vaccine coverage in sustaining the infection. *BMC Infectious Diseases*, *10*(1), 62. Advance online publication. DOI: 10.1186/1471-2334-10-62 PMID: 20219143 de Swart, R. L. (2008). The pathogenesis of measles revisited. *The Pediatric Infectious Disease Journal, 27*(10), S84–S88. DOI: 10.1097/INF.0b013e31816857fe PMID: 18820585

Delpeut, S., Noyce, R. S., Siu, R. W., & Richardson, C. D. (2012). Host factors and measles virus replication. *Current Opinion in Virology, 2*(6), 773–783. DOI: 10.1016/j.coviro.2012.10.008 PMID: 23146309

Donadel, M., Stănescu, A., Pistol, A., Stewart, B., Butu, C., Janković, D., Paunescu, B., & Zimmerman, L. (2021). Risk factors for measles deaths among children during a nationwide measles outbreak – romania, 2016–2018. *BMC Infectious Diseases, 21*(1), 279. Advance online publication. DOI: 10.1186/s12879-021-05966-3 PMID: 33740895

Ferrari, M., Grais, R., Bharti, N., Conlan, A., Bjørnstad, O., Wolfson, L., Guerin, P. J., Djibo, A., & Grenfell, B. (2008). The dynamics of measles in sub-saharan africa. *Nature, 451*(7179), 679–684. DOI: 10.1038/nature06509 PMID: 18256664

Filia, A., Bella, A., Manso, M., Baggieri, M., Magurano, F., & Rota, M. (2017). Ongoing outbreak with well over 4,000 measles cases in italy from january to end august 2017 – what is making elimination so difficult? *Eurosurveillance, 22*(37). Advance online publication. DOI: 10.2807/1560-7917.ES.2017.22.37.30614 PMID: 28933342

Fu, J., Chu, J., Wang, J., Cai, R., Cheng, W., Lifei, S., & Xing, Y. (2019). A hospital-associated measles outbreak in health workers in beijing: Implications for measles elimination in china, 2018. *International Journal of Infectious Diseases, 78*, 85–92. DOI: 10.1016/j.ijid.2018.10.023 PMID: 30391419

Furuse, Y., & Oshitani, H. (2017). Global Transmission Dynamics of Measles in the Measles Elimination Era. *Viruses, 9*(4), 82. DOI: 10.3390/v9040082 PMID: 28420160

Gastañaduy, P., Banerjee, E., DeBolt, C., Bravo-Alcántara, P., Samad, S., Pastor, D., Rota, P. A., Patel, M., Crowcroft, N. S., & Durrheim, D. (2018). Public health responses during measles outbreaks in elimination settings: Strategies and challenges. *Human Vaccines & Immunotherapeutics, 14*(9), 2222–2238. DOI: 10.1080/21645515.2018.1474310 PMID: 29932850

Gastañaduy, P., Banerjee, E., DeBolt, C., Bravo-Alcántara, P., Samad, S., Pastor, D., Rota, P. A., Patel, M., Crowcroft, N. S., & Durrheim, D. (2018). Public health responses during measles outbreaks in elimination settings: Strategies and challenges. *Human Vaccines & Immunotherapeutics, 14*(9), 2222–2238. DOI: 10.1080/21645515.2018.1474310 PMID: 29932850

Helfand, R. F., Heath, J. L., Anderson, L. J., Maes, E. F., Guris, D., & Bellini, W. J. (1997). Diagnosis of measles with an IgM capture EIA: The optimal timing of specimen collection after rash onset. *The Journal of Infectious Diseases*, *175*(1), 195–199. DOI: 10.1093/infdis/175.1.195 PMID: 8985220

Javelle, E., Colson, P., Parola, P., & Raoult, D. (2019). Measles, the need for a paradigm shift. *European Journal of Epidemiology*, *34*(10), 897–915. DOI: 10.1007/s10654-019-00569-4 PMID: 31624970

Keller, J. M., Dela Cruz, C. S., Pasnick, S., Gross, J. E., Carlos, W. G., Maves, R., & Jamil, S. (2019). Measles. *American Journal of Respiratory and Critical Care Medicine*, *200*(1), 1–P2. DOI: 10.1164/rccm.2001P1 PMID: 31259630

Lam, E., Diaz, M., Maina, A., & Brennan, M. (2016). Displaced populations due to humanitarian emergencies and its impact on global eradication and elimination of vaccine-preventable diseases. *Conflict and Health*, *10*(1), 27. Advance online publication. DOI: 10.1186/s13031-016-0094-5 PMID: 27956938

Liu, F., Enanoria, W., Zipprich, J., Blumberg, S., Harriman, K., Ackley, S., Wheaton, W. D., Allpress, J. L., & Porco, T. (2015). The role of vaccination coverage, individual behaviors, and the public health response in the control of measles epidemics: An agent-based simulation for california. *BMC Public Health*, *15*(1), 447. Advance online publication. DOI: 10.1186/s12889-015-1766-6 PMID: 25928152

Mehtar, S., Almhawish, N., Shobak, K., Reingold, A., Guha-Sapir, D., & Haar, R. (2021). Measles in conflict-affected northern syria: Results from an ongoing outbreak surveillance program. *Conflict and Health*, *15*(1), 95. Advance online publication. DOI: 10.1186/s13031-021-00430-0 PMID: 34933672

Moss, W. J. (2017). Measles. *Lancet*, *390*(10111), 2490–2502. DOI: 10.1016/S0140-6736(17)31463-0 PMID: 28673424

Moten, M., Phillips, A., Saliba, V., Harding, N., & Sibal, B. (2018). Measles: Is it still a threat? *The British Journal of General Practice*, *68*(674), 404–405. DOI: 10.3399/bjgp18X697961 PMID: 29970395

Mousavi, S., & Anjomshoa, M. (2020). Covid-19 in yemen: A crisis within crises. *International Journal for Equity in Health*, *19*(1), 120. Advance online publication. DOI: 10.1186/s12939-020-01231-2 PMID: 32652995

Mugoša, B., Ceccarelli, G., Begic, S., Vujošević, D., Zekovic, Ž., Ciccozzi, M., & Vratnica, Z. (2021). Measles outbreak, montenegro january–july 2018: Lessons learned. *Journal of Medical Virology*, *94*(2), 514–520. DOI: 10.1002/jmv.27377 PMID: 34617629

Mulchandani, R., Sibal, B., Phillips, A., Suleman, S., Banerjee, A., Teagle, R., Foulkes, S., Spence, K., & Edeghere, O. (2021). A large outbreak of measles in the west midlands, england, 2017–2018: Descriptive epidemiology, control measures and lessons learnt. *Epidemiology and Infection*, *149*, e114. Advance online publication. DOI: 10.1017/S0950268821000868 PMID: 33866992

Muscat, M., Mamou, M., Shefer, A., Jankovic, D., Deshevoy, S., & Butler, R. (2015). Situación del sarampión y la rubéola en la región europea de la oms. *Revista Española de Salud Pública*, *89*(4), 345–351. DOI: 10.4321/S1135-57272015000400002 PMID: 26580789

Naim, H. Y. (2015). Measles virus. *Human Vaccines & Immunotherapeutics*, *11*(1), 21–26. DOI: 10.4161/hv.34298 PMID: 25483511

Perry, R. T., & Halsey, N. A. (2004). The clinical significance of measles: A review. *The Journal of Infectious Diseases*, *189*(Supplement_1), S4–S16. DOI: 10.1086/377712 PMID: 15106083

Pillsbury, A., Chiew, M., Bag, S., Hope, K., Norton, S., Conaty, S., Sheppeard, V., & McIntyre, P. (2016). The changing epidemiology of measles in an era of elimination: Lessons from health-care-setting transmissions of measles during an outbreak in new south wales, australia, 2012. *Western Pacific Surveillance and Response Journal : WPSAR*, *7*(4), 12–20. DOI: 10.5365/wpsar.2016.7.1.010 PMID: 28246577

Sabahelzain, M., Moukhyer, M., Borne, B., & Bosma, H. (2022). Vaccine hesitancy among parents and its association with the uptake of measles vaccine in urban settings in khartoum state, sudan. *Vaccines*, *10*(2), 205. DOI: 10.3390/vaccines10020205 PMID: 35214664

Sabahelzain, M., Moukhyer, M., Dubé, E., Hardan, A., Borne, B., & Bosma, H. (2019). Towards a further understanding of measles vaccine hesitancy in khartoum state, sudan: A qualitative study. *PLoS One*, *14*(6), e0213882. DOI: 10.1371/journal.pone.0213882 PMID: 31220092

Schoini, P., Karampitsakos, T., Avdikou, M., Athanasopoulou, A., Tsoukalas, G., & Tzouvelekis, A. (2019). Measles pneumonitis. *Advances in Respiratory Medicine*, *87*(1), 63–67. DOI: 10.5603/ARM.a2019.0010 PMID: 30830960

Seto, J., Aoki, Y., Komabayashi, K., Yamada, K., Ishikawa, H., Ichikawa, T., Ahiko, T., & Mizuta, K. (2023). Measles outbreak response activity in japan, and a discussion for a possible strategy of outbreak response using cycle threshold values of real-time reverse transcription pcr for measles virus in measles elimination settings. *Viruses*, *15*(1), 171. DOI: 10.3390/v15010171 PMID: 36680212

Sonibare, M. A., Moody, J. O., & Adesanya, E. O. (2009). Use of medicinal plants for the treatment of measles in Nigeria. *Journal of Ethnopharmacology, 122*(2), 268–272. DOI: 10.1016/j.jep.2009.01.004 PMID: 19168120

Strebel, P. M., & Orenstein, W. A. (2019). Measles. *The New England Journal of Medicine, 381*(4), 349–357. DOI: 10.1056/NEJMcp1905181 PMID: 31184814

Takahashi, S., Metcalf, C., Ferrari, M., Moss, W., Truelove, S., Tatem, A., Grenfell, B. T., & Lessler, J. (2015). Reduced vaccination and the risk of measles and other childhood infections post-ebola. *Science, 347*(6227), 1240–1242. DOI: 10.1126/science.aaa3438 PMID: 25766232

Thompson, K., & Tebbens, R. (2014). Framework for optimal global vaccine stockpile design for vaccine-preventable diseases: Application to measles and cholera vaccines as contrasting examples. *Risk Analysis, 36*(7), 1487–1509. DOI: 10.1111/risa.12265 PMID: 25109229

Toole, M. J., Steketee, R. W., Waldman, R. J., & Nieburg, P. (1989). Measles prevention and control in emergency settings. *Bulletin of the World Health Organization, 67*(4), 381. PMID: 2805216

Walter, K., & Malani, P. N. (2022). What Is Measles? *Journal of the American Medical Association, 328*(23), 2370. DOI: 10.1001/jama.2022.21363 PMID: 36374512

Wang, H., Zhang, Y., Mao, N., Zhu, Z., Cui, A., Xu, S., Song, J., Chen, M., Fang, X., Li, C., Feng, D., Zhou, S., Wang, S., Shi, J., Ji, Y., Cao, L., Ren, L., Gao, L., & Xu, W. (2019). Molecular characterization of measles viruses in china: Circulation dynamics of the endemic h1 genotype from 2011 to 2017. *PLoS One, 14*(6), e0218782. DOI: 10.1371/journal.pone.0218782 PMID: 31220172

World Health Organization. (2007). *Manual for the laboratory diagnosis of measles and rubella virus infection* (No. WHO/IVB/07.01). World Health Organization.

Yu, C. P., Chen, B. C., Chou, Y. C., Hsieh, C. J., & Lin, F. H. (2022, October 28). Epidemiological features and risk factors for measles and rubella in Taiwan during 2011 to 2020. *Medicine, 101*(43), e31254. DOI: 10.1097/MD.0000000000031254 PMID: 36316902

# Chapter 7
# Rubella

**Layal Bassam Msheik**
*Faculty of Medical Sciences, Lebanese University, Beirut, Lebanon*

**Zeinab Kazan**
https://orcid.org/0009-0002-9138-1154
*Faculty of Medical Sciences, Lebanese University, Beirut, Lebanon*

**Ahmad Afyouni**
*Faculty of Medical Sciences, Lebanese University, Beirut, Lebanon*

**Ahmad Saifan**
*Faculty of Medical Sciences, Lebanese University, Beirut, Lebanon*

**Mohammad Barakat**
https://orcid.org/0000-0001-7254-083X
*Faculty of Medical Sciences, Lebanese University, Beirut, Lebanon*

## ABSTRACT

*This chapter provides a comprehensive exploration of rubella, encompassing its definition, epidemiology, risk factors, pathogenesis, signs and symptoms, as well as diagnosis and treatment modalities. It delves into the challenges posed by rubella in both developed and developing countries, addressing issues such as misinformation, high birthrates, and healthcare infrastructure constraints. Furthermore, the abstract outlines potential solutions to these challenges, emphasizing the importance of strengthening immunization programs, improving healthcare infrastructure, and implementing targeted educational initiatives. The holistic approach presented here aims to contribute to a deeper understanding of rubella and offers insights into effective strategies for minimizing its impact on global health.*

DOI: 10.4018/979-8-3693-1990-1.ch007

## INTRODUCTION

Rubella is a contagious viral infection caused by the rubella virus. It is also known as German measles. The virus is a member of the Togaviridae family and belongs to the genus Rubivirus. Rubella is usually a mild sickness, especially in children, but it can be dangerous if received by a pregnant woman since it can cause congenital rubella syndrome (CRS) in the developing fetus (Camejo Leonor & Mendez, 2023). Rubella may be found all over the world. Pandemics occur every 10 to 30 years, whereas epidemics occur every 6 to 9 years. The most recent worldwide epidemic occurred between 1962 and 1964 (Rodriguez, 2003). It is usually transferred from person to person by respiratory droplets produced by infected individuals when they cough or sneeze. Direct contact with respiratory secretions or touching surfaces or items infected with the virus and then contacting the face can potentially transmit the infection. It is very contagious, and people are most infectious when they have the rash, but transmission can happen before symptoms appear. Symptoms include a rash that begins on the face and spreads across the body, a low-grade fever, and enlarged lymph nodes. Transient arthralgia or arthritis is prevalent, especially among rubella-infected women (Meissner & Hamer, 2017). A clinical examination of symptoms is combined with a medical history review, which includes probable viral exposure. Serological assays identify particular antibodies (IgM and IgG) to suggest recent or prior infection. In addition, viral culture from respiratory samples may be used to detect the rubella virus (Camejo Leonor & Mendez, 2023; Meissner & Hamer, 2017). The measles, mumps, and rubella (MMR) vaccination has an excellent safety record and is very effective. MMR vaccination has resulted in the abolition of endemic measles, rubella, and congenital rubella syndrome in the United States. The greatest hurdles to worldwide measles and rubella management and eradication are low global vaccine coverage and rising skepticism (Bankamp, Hickman, Icenogle, & Rota, 2019). This chapter will look at a general overview of rubella. The challenges that both industrialized and developing countries confront will be explored. Additionally, possible remedies, particularly in developing nations, will be highlighted.

## DISCUSSION

### Definition

German scientists initially identified rubella as an illness in the middle of the 18th century, referring to it as Rötheln (Plotkin, Reef, Cooper, & Alford, 2011). The single-stranded RNA virus known as the rubella virus is a member of the

Togaviridae family's genus Rubivirus. It falls under the category of enveloped viruses having positive-sense RNA genomes. The virus is spherical and measures between 40 to 80 nanometers in diameter. The primary cause of German measles, also known as rubella, is the rubella virus, which is mostly spread by respiratory droplets. The respiratory epithelium is where it replicates and infects. Its capacity to cross the placenta during pregnancy plays a crucial role in the development of congenital rubella syndrome (CRS) in the fetus (Camejo Leonor & Mendez, 2023; Plotkin et al., 2011).

## Epidemiology

Before the advent of vaccines, rubella was a viral illness that impacted children and young adults on a global scale. The introduction of rubella vaccination strategies has significantly diminished the incidence of rubella cases in numerous countries. Notably, in the World Health Organization Region of the Americas (0 cases in 2023) (Tiller et al., 2023), endemic transmission of rubella has been successfully halted since 2009, marking a significant achievement in the control of the disease (Lambert, Strebel, Orenstein, Icenogle, & Poland, 2015). Based on monthly submissions of provisional rubella data by member states to the World Health Organization, the Africa region recorded a total of 3640 cases in 2023, with Ethiopia and Nigeria collectively accounting for 42% of these cases. In the East Mediterranean region, there were 2459 reported cases in 2023, and Yemen alone represented 49% of that total. Europe reported 317 cases, with the majority (69%) in Poland and 17% in Turkey. The south-east Asia region documented 2001 cases, while the west Pacific region reported 911 cases. Notably, the nations with the highest incidence rates per million were Guinea-Bissau (73.14), Yemen (45.76), and the Central African Republic (22.05) (Tiller et al., 2023).

## Risk Factors

Partial vaccination programs in specific regions stand out as prominent risk factors for rubella outbreaks (Rodriguez, 2003). An incomplete vaccination campaign in Japan targeting young females and neglecting the vaccination of males had the population suspectable to an outbreak (Minakami, Kubo, & Unno, 2014). A case control study carried out during a rubella outbreak in Zimbabwe highlighted several risk factors, including exposure to a classmate or household contact and having more than three children in a household (Makoni, Chemhuru, Bangure, Gombe, & Tshimanga, 2015) . Another case control study conducted in Ethiopia identified additional risk factors such as crowded and poorly-ventilated living conditions, along with not receiving vitamin A in the last 6 months (Leung, Hon, & Leong, 2019) .

These findings underscore the importance of comprehensive vaccination strategies and addressing environmental factors to mitigate the risk of rubella transmission.

## Pathophysiology

Droplets from an infected person's respiratory system can colonise the upper respiratory tract and spread the rubella virus. The virus then initiates the first stage of replication in the nasopharyngeal cells and lymphoid tissue of the nasopharynx and upper respiratory tract after entering the cells by receptor-mediated endocytosis (Camejo Leonor & Mendez, 2023). Viraemia happens five to seven days after inoculation and affects the skin, lymph nodes, and placenta in pregnant women (Winter & Moss, 2022). Remember that before the infection manifests clinically, infected people are infectious. Maternal immunity protects against intrauterine rubella infection in pregnant women; but, in vulnerable women, the virus can infect the placenta and then cross it to infect the fetus's vascular system causing rubella in fetus (Camejo Leonor & Mendez, 2023; Winter & Moss, 2022).

*Table 1. Overview of the crucial stages in the pathophysiology of Rubella*

| **Transmission** | **Droplets from an infected person's respiratory system** |
|---|---|
| Replication Cite | nasopharyngeal cells and lymphoid tissue of the nasopharynx and upper respiratory tract |
| Spread | Viraemia happens five to seven days after inoculation |
| Target Organs | skin, lymph nodes, and placenta in pregnant women |

## Signs and Symptoms

Postnatally acquired rubella takes 14 to 21 days to incubate. About 25 to 50% of patients are asymptomatic (subclinical infection), and the maximum time a patient can spread the rubella to others is seven days prior to and seven days following the rash's emergence (Winter & Moss, 2022). Usually occurring one to five days before to the rash, the symptoms include low-grade fever, anorexia, nausea, malaise, lethargy, coryza, cough, headaches, non-exudative conjunctivitis, sore throat, myalgia, and painful lymph nodes (Camejo Leonor & Mendez, 2023; Winter & Moss, 2022). Retroauricular, suboccipital and posterior cervical lymph nodes are usually involved in the lymphadenopathy, and they frequently become more noticeable as the rash appears (Meissner & Hamer, 2017; Winter & Moss, 2022). While uncommon in young children, the symptoms are prevalent in adults (Winter & Moss, 2022). Rubella is known for a particular type of rash called a spotty maculopapular rash that begins on the face, spreads caudally to the trunk and limbs, and also becomes generalized in less than a day (Best & Enders, 2006; Camejo Leonor & Mendez, 2023). The rash often fades in the same pattern it began with and can be rather itchy (Winter & Moss, 2022).

## Diagnosis

### Serology

Antigenic consistency has been demonstrated across rubella virus (RV) strains all over the world, indicating that serological assays based on antigens from one strain can successfully identify antibodies produced in response to any circulating RV strain (Mushahwar, 2006). Blood tests that are often used seek to detect certain antibodies, such as immunoglobulin M (IgM) and immunoglobulin G (IgG). IgG antibodies are indicative of a previous infection or immunization, whereas IgM antibodies are indicative of a current rubella infection (Mushahwar, 2006; Shukla & Maraqa, 2023). Furthermore, both rubella infection and reinfection can be verified by observing a four-fold or more rise in rubella-specific IgG titers when comparing acute and convalescent sera. Additionally, recent primary rubella infections can be confirmed through the detection of rubella-specific low-avidity IgG (Camejo Leonor & Mendez, 2023).

### Polymerase Chain Reaction (PCR)

Numerous reverse transcription-polymerase chain reaction (RT-PCR) assays for the identification of rubella virus (RV) RNA have been documented in scientific literature. Currently, there are no commercially available RT-PCR assays for RV RNA. The most suitable biological samples for conducting RV RT-PCR analysis include blood, nasopharyngeal aspirates, throat swabs, urine, as well as three types of fetal tissues—chorionic villi, amniotic fluid, and umbilical cord blood (Shukla & Maraqa, 2023). The elevated GC content in the rubella virus (RV) genome has presented challenges in establishing a dependable reverse transcription-polymerase chain reaction (RT-PCR) method. Consequently, various protocols have been rigorously validated to identify the most effective approach tailored for diverse purposes (Mushahwar, 2006).

### Treatment

Considering that rubella is a mild, benign, and self-limiting infection, therapy is primarily symptomatic in the absence of pregnancy (Best & Enders, 2006). Whenever treating severe arthralgia or arthritis, non-steroidal anti-inflammatory medications are used (Winter & Moss, 2022). On the contrary, the gestational age at infection determines the course of treatment for an expecting mother who has an infection (Mushahwar, 2006). Due to the increased chance of fetal deformity before 18 weeks of gestation, discussions on pregnancy termination have to be started in accordance with local laws (Mahmood, Gerriets, & Tadi, 2023). Immunoglobulin administered intramuscularly or intravenously should be given to vulnerable women who have known early pregnancy rubella exposure and for whom pregnancy termination is not an option (Winter & Moss, 2022).

On the other hand, congenital rubella syndrome and rubella infection can be avoided by immunizing all children and vaccinating those who are more susceptible to the virus with a rubella vaccine (Sodha & Dietz, 2015).

### Challenges

Ensuring effective healthcare involves the operation of well-equipped health centers with convenient service hours, maximizing opportunities to vaccinate children during health visits, expanding outreach to overcome site limitations, maintaining a continuous vaccine supply and proper cold chain storage, reporting accurate vaccination data, implementing national immunization plans and localized microplans, fostering community demand for vaccines, and ensuring competent management and supervision at all program levels with dedicated healthcare professionals (Priyadharshini & Jasmine, 2019).

## Challenges in Developing Countries

### Misinformation

Promoting widespread acceptance of vaccination also calls for a multidisciplinary approach aimed at tackling misinformation and correcting false perceptions of vaccination risks (Sodha & Dietz, 2015). However, according to Priyadharshini et al. a significant number of parents declined rubella vaccination for their children primarily due to concerns and misunderstandings about potential adverse effects, coupled with a lack of awareness regarding the benefits of vaccines. The hesitancy was fueled by various rumors circulating during the vaccination campaign, contributing to widespread fear of negative outcomes (Peters et al., 2008).

## Weak Healthcare Systems

Administering the MMR vaccine necessitates a collaborative, interprofessional approach that involves various members of the healthcare team. This team typically comprises clinicians such as Medical Doctors (MDs), Doctors of Osteopathic Medicine (DOs), Nurse Practitioners (NPs), Physician Assistants (PAs), as well as nurses and pharmacists. The effective and proper administration of the MMR vaccine is contingent on the patient population and the specific clinical context, highlighting the importance of coordination and expertise from a diverse range of healthcare professionals (Sodha & Dietz, 2015). While there have been advancements in enhancing healthcare access in developing nations, significant portions of their populations still face restricted entry. The impoverished individuals in these countries bear a disproportionate share of the disease burden, yet they typically encounter greater obstacles to healthcare access. This limitation is evident in various aspects, including geographic accessibility, availability, financial accessibility, acceptability, and the quality of care (Lessler & Metcalf, 2013).

## High Birthrates

Furthermore, Epidemiological theory and real-world observations indicate that the average age of infection for a vaccine-preventable disease, providing lifelong immunity, is mainly influenced by factors such as the population birthrate, the extent of vaccine coverage, and the transmissibility of the disease (Nargund, 2009). In developing nations, children are crucial for labor and providing care for aging parents, contributing to higher fertility rates. Limited access to contraceptives and lower levels of female education are key factors influencing the increased fertility rates in these countries (Allerberger, 2017).

# Challenges in Developed Countries

Global measles and rubella management confronts problems due to inadequate vaccine coverage and growing skepticism. Despite the eradication of native rubella and CRS in the Americas, the majority of US mothers of CRS cases are born in nations that do not currently have structured rubella immunization programs (Bankamp et al., 2019).

While in Europe, measles and rubella might be completely eradicated if 100% of people receive vaccinations. Although vaccination is generally recognized in most European countries, vaccine-preventable illnesses may spread more extensively if advised vaccinations are not administered with diligence. Under-vaccinated people and groups may be hidden by national vaccination coverage figures, increasing the risk of transmission. Moreover, healthcare personnel who are not vaccinated put their sensitive patient population in danger in an irresponsible manner (Hviid, Hansen, Frisch, & Melbye, 2019). A significant reason why parents choose not to vaccinate their children or are worried about vaccinations is the notion that vaccines cause autism. However, the research did not support the idea that an increased risk of autism results from receiving the MMR vaccination (Hübschen et al., 2017).

Another challenge relies upon rubella diagnostic essays which is further complicated by the potential for false-positive IgM results brought on by cross-reactive antibodies from other infections, interference from rheumatoid factor, or antibodies from pregnant women's serum that cross-react with the membrane component of the whole virus preparation. Furthermore, for prompt actions in elimination settings, public health professionals must get feedback quickly. However, the examination of isolated cases and transmission networks is more intricate, time-consuming, and expensive. That emphasizes the need for more effective and efficient rubella control methods (Fabiani et al., 2017).

The growth of international migration in the past decade has significantly impacted public health, making migrants more vulnerable to infectious diseases. Despite being generally healthy, they often face socioeconomic disadvantages, cultural differences, and limited access to health-preventative programs. Immigrant women have lower rates of rubella vaccination. Informal and cultural barriers further exacerbate these issues (O'Connor et al., 2017).

Although there has been a decrease in measles and rubella infections in the World Health Organization's (WHO) European Region, adolescents and young adults with poor vaccination histories have been the main target of outbreaks. The region has difficulties providing immunization services and conducting surveillance. Large outbreaks happen in a few countries each year, whereas the majority of nations record few cases. Rubella surveillance is still challenging since fewer nations have developed systems. In addition to additional initiatives and routine vaccine strengthening, very sensitive surveillance backed by an approved laboratory network is required to accomplish regional eradication (Kesson, 2012).

## Novel Strategies to Limit the Spread

### Elimination and Eradication Policies

Rubella virus is a potential contender for worldwide eradication, since humans are the only known host, there are safe and highly efficient vaccinations available, as well as precise diagnostic and molecular testing (Andrus & de Quadros, 2013).

The Global Measles and Rubella Strategy Plan was introduced by the main partners of the Measles and Rubella Initiative to eradicate measles, rubella, and congenital rubella syndrome. This will be accomplished through maintaining high levels of population immunity, reaching ≥95% vaccination coverage, monitoring disease with efficient surveillance programs, preparing for potential outbreaks, fostering public confidence, and conducting research to support efficient operations and enhance vaccination and diagnostic tools (Lambert et al., 2015).

### Vaccination Optimization

Live attenuated rubella virus vaccination has proven to be effective in preventing infection, epidemics, and congenital rubella syndrome—one of the most dangerous side effects. Because it is a combination vaccination, it is quite affordable in both industrialized and developing nations, the latter of which have profited from financial initiatives to incorporate the vaccine into routine vaccination programs (Lambert et al., 2015). The primary vaccination strategy is the routine program, which aims to increase coverage to the greatest extent. Then, additional mass immunization campaigns are made available (Parkman, 1996).

To completely understand the behavior of cell-based rubella receptors, more study is necessary. This will open the door to advancements in the development of vaccines, diagnostic tools, and possible treatment possibilities. Furthermore, technological advancements such as a vaccination that doesn't require cold chain or highly skilled healthcare personnel to give it would be a huge benefit and a top priority. A non-live viral vaccination that is available to all patients and populations would also be advantageous (Lambert et al., 2015). The genome of the rubella virus is stable and conserved, and the antigenic reactions of different strains are comparable (Lambert et al., 2015; Terracciano, Amadori, Pettinicchio, Zaratti, & Franco, 2020). Nonetheless, the immune response to rubella is regulated by polymorphisms or genetic variations across individuals, which is the source of the variation in immunological response amongst people. Comprehending the immunogenetics of rubella can facilitate the creation of innovative vaccine candidates, enhance the detection of possible adverse effects through screening techniques, and boost protection across a diverse population (Lambert et al., 2015).

## Enhanced Surveillance Programs

By identifying high-risk groups and stepping up vaccination campaigns in these risky areas, surveillance aims to achieve equity in the interventions by defining trends in disease burden and enabling appropriate action or adjustments to be made in response to inevitable outbreaks or to limit the extensive spread of disease. For this to operate well, a sufficient investment in infrastructure and human resources is needed. Well-trained personnel in case detection, investigation, and response are part of human resources. Infrastructure, on the other hand, necessitates a well-regulated and coordinated interaction between reporting sites and the vast national, regional, and subnational network of laboratories that will accept and process specimens for genetic and immunologic testing (Parkman, 1996). A top-notch surveillance system relies heavily on the laboratory, not just for etiology confirmation and diagnosis but also for diagnosis. In actuality, laboratory studies can provide information regarding vaccination success or failure and seroprevalence in the general population and high-risk groups (Santibanez et al., 2017). Moreover, molecular surveillance plays a critical role in tracking the spread of wild-type viruses within an area, locating probable viral spread sites, and detecting persistent transmission networks. Documenting the eradication process, tracking developments, and providing proof to halt the spread of endemic viruses are crucial. The WHO GMRLN provides technical assistance, instruction, training, knowledge exchange, and quality control initiatives in addition to coordinating laboratory-based surveillance. A molecular External Quality Assessment Programm was then initiated by the WHO and CDC to assess GMRLN laboratories' performance. This indicates that real-time data submission from national reference laboratories is encouraged to aid in the analysis of global viral transmission chains. So, no matter what the circumstances, the national molecular surveillance system needs to be operational and ready to respond quickly (Giambi et al., 2015).

## Social Network Analysis

Two primary issues were identified in the primary risk category of reproductive-age women: vulnerability and limited knowledge. Adequate health promotion initiatives might be used to counter them (Santibanez et al., 2017). Rubella-susceptible women must be screened for the disease before conception by examining vaccination records or testing for rubella-specific IgG antibodies. They should also be administered vaccinations as soon as possible, including post-partum and post-abortion shots. Additionally, public education programs are required to raise awareness of the possibility of contracting rubella during pregnancy. Areas with high incidence rates require special care. Moreover, to actively look for seronegative women, it may be helpful for laboratories to systematically report to vaccination services any negative rubella antibody findings (Bechini et al., 2012). Even in nations where rubella has been eliminated, immigrant women, who comprise the population with greater fertility and are a vulnerable and sometimes disregarded demographic, pose a danger of transmission (Santibanez et al., 2017; Song et al., 2012). Targeted advertising and early visits to the healthcare system are essential to increasing vaccine coverage since they guarantee that the initial interaction with susceptible persons is favorable (Santibanez et al., 2017).

Knowing that women have been the primary focus of the conventional rubella vaccination method [34], males have emerged as a substantial reservoir of vulnerable people. Thus, male adults should receive extra immunizations to prevent the spread of endemic rubella (Santibanez et al., 2017).

A delay in vaccination acceptance or rejection, known as vaccine hesitancy, is frequently associated with socioeconomic status, education level, race, and ethnicity (Peters et al., 2008; Song et al., 2012). The CDC suggests identifying populations with low vaccination rates, engaging families via provider-parent dialogues, and dispelling myths and false information to lessen reluctance. Public health partners should use surveillance tools and vaccine coverage monitoring systems to identify under-vaccinated communities and use science-based strategies to promote vaccination. Healthcare providers should also have the resources to initiate early conversations with expectant women (Nguyen et al., 2022).

## CONCLUSION

In conclusion, this chapter has shown the problems that rubella poses in both developed and underdeveloped nations. Despite advances, concerns such as inadequate vaccination access, disinformation, and healthcare infrastructure limits remain. Solutions include expanding vaccination programs, enhancing healthcare facilities, and launching targeted educational campaigns. A concerted effort is required to reduce the worldwide danger of rubella and ensure the health of communities at all stages of development.

## REFERENCES


Allerberger, F. (2017). Eliminating measles and rubella in Europe. *Clinical Microbiology and Infection*, *23*(8), 502–503. DOI: 10.1016/j.cmi.2017.04.008 PMID: 28412385

Andrus, J. K., & de Quadros, C. A. (2013). Perspectives on the role of surveillance in eliminating rubella and congenital rubella syndrome in the Americas. *Expert Review of Vaccines*, *12*(9), 989–993. DOI: 10.1586/14760584.2013.841435 PMID: 24053393

Bankamp, B., Hickman, C., Icenogle, J. P., & Rota, P. A. (2019). Successes and challenges for preventing measles, mumps and rubella by vaccination. *Current Opinion in Virology*, *34*, 110–116. DOI: 10.1016/j.coviro.2019.01.002 PMID: 30852425

Bechini, A., Boccalini, S., Tiscione, E., Pesavento, G., Mannelli, F., Peruzzi, M., Rapi, S., Mercurio, S., & Bonanni, P. (2012). Progress towards measles and rubella elimination in Tuscany, Italy: The role of population seroepidemiological profile. *European Journal of Public Health*, *22*(1), 133–139. DOI: 10.1093/eurpub/ckq134 PMID: 20880991

Best, J. M., & Enders, G. (2006). Laboratory Diagnosis of Rubella and Congenital Rubella. In Banatvala, J., & Peckham, C. (Eds.), *Perspectives in Medical Virology* (Vol. 15, pp. 39–77). Elsevier.

Camejo Leonor, M., & Mendez, M. D. (2023). Rubella *StatPearls*. Treasure Island (FL) with ineligible companies. Disclosure: Magda Mendez declares no relevant financial relationships with ineligible companies.: StatPearls Publishing

Fabiani, M., Ferrante, G., Minardi, V., Giambi, C., Riccardo, F., Declich, S., & Masocco, M. (2017). Comparison of rubella immunization rates in immigrant and Italian women of childbearing age: Results from the Italian behavioral surveillance system PASSI (2011-2015). *PLoS One*, *12*(10), e0178122. DOI: 10.1371/journal.pone.0178122 PMID: 28968403

Giambi, C., Filia, A., Rota, M. C., Del Manso, M., Declich, S., Nacca, G., & Bella, A. (2015). Congenital rubella still a public health problem in Italy: Analysis of national surveillance data from 2005 to 2013. *Eurosurveillance*, *20*(16). Advance online publication. DOI: 10.2807/1560-7917.ES2015.20.16.21103 PMID: 25953272

Hübschen, J. M., Bork, S. M., Brown, K. E., Mankertz, A., Santibanez, S., Ben Mamou, M., Mulders, M. N., & Muller, C. P. (2017). Challenges of measles and rubella laboratory diagnostic in the era of elimination. *Clinical Microbiology and Infection*, *23*(8), 511–515. DOI: 10.1016/j.cmi.2017.04.009 PMID: 28412379

Hviid, A., Hansen, J. V., Frisch, M., & Melbye, M. (2019). Measles, Mumps, Rubella Vaccination and Autism: A Nationwide Cohort Study. *Annals of Internal Medicine*, *170*(8), 513–520. DOI: 10.7326/M18-2101 PMID: 30831578

Kesson, A. M. (2012). 12 - Rubella. In Jong, E. C., & Stevens, D. L. (Eds.), *Netter's Infectious Diseases* (pp. 51–54). W.B. Saunders. DOI: 10.1016/B978-1-4377-0126-5.00012-4

Lambert, N., Strebel, P., Orenstein, W., Icenogle, J., & Poland, G. A. (2015). Rubella. *Lancet*, *385*(9984), 2297–2307. DOI: 10.1016/S0140-6736(14)60539-0 PMID: 25576992

Lessler, J., & Metcalf, C. J. (2013). Balancing evidence and uncertainty when considering rubella vaccine introduction. *PLoS One*, *8*(7), e67639. DOI: 10.1371/journal.pone.0067639 PMID: 23861777

Leung, A. K. C., Hon, K. L., & Leong, K. F. (2019). Rubella (German measles) revisited. *Hong Kong Medical Journal*, *25*(2), 134–141. DOI: 10.12809/hkmj187785 PMID: 30967519

Mahmood, R., Gerriets, V., & Tadi, P. (2023). Rubella Vaccine *StatPearls*. Treasure Island (FL) ineligible companies. Disclosure: Valerie Gerriets declares no relevant financial relationships with ineligible companies. Disclosure: Prasanna Tadi declares no relevant financial relationships with ineligible companies.: StatPearls Publishing Copyright © 2023, StatPearls Publishing LLC.

Makoni, A. C., Chemhuru, M., Bangure, D., Gombe, N. T., & Tshimanga, M. (2015). Rubella outbreak investigation, Gokwe North District, Midlands province, Zimbabwe, 2014 - a case control study. *The Pan African Medical Journal*, *22*, 60. DOI: 10.11604/pamj.2015.22.60.5939 PMID: 26834913

Meissner, H. C., & Hamer, D. H. (2017). Rubella. In Quah, S. R. (Ed.), *International Encyclopedia of Public Health* (2nd ed., pp. 410–413). Academic Press. DOI: 10.1016/B978-0-12-803678-5.00392-1

Minakami, H., Kubo, T., & Unno, N. (2014). Causes of a nationwide rubella outbreak in Japan, 2012-2013. *The Journal of Infection*, *68*(1), 99–101. DOI: 10.1016/j.jinf.2013.09.002 PMID: 24029626

Mushahwar, I. K. (2006). Rubella Virus: Molecular Composition, Pathogenesis, Diagnosis, and Control. In Mushahwar, I. K. (Ed.), *Perspectives in Medical Virology* (Vol. 13, pp. 211–221). Elsevier.

Nargund, G. (2009). Declining birth rate in Developed Countries: A radical policy re-think is required. *Facts, Views & Vision in ObGyn*, *1*(3), 191–193. PMID: 25489464

Nguyen, K. H., Srivastav, A., Lindley, M. C., Fisher, A., Kim, D., Greby, S. M., Lee, J., & Singleton, J. A. (2022). Parental Vaccine Hesitancy and Association With Childhood Diphtheria, Tetanus Toxoid, and Acellular Pertussis; Measles, Mumps, and Rubella; Rotavirus; and Combined 7-Series Vaccination. *American Journal of Preventive Medicine*, *62*(3), 367–376. DOI: 10.1016/j.amepre.2021.08.015 PMID: 35190101

O'Connor, P., Jankovic, D., Muscat, M., Ben-Mamou, M., Reef, S., Papania, M., Singh, S., Kaloumenos, T., Butler, R., & Datta, S. (2017). Measles and rubella elimination in the WHO Region for Europe: Progress and challenges. *Clinical Microbiology and Infection*, *23*(8), 504–510. DOI: 10.1016/j.cmi.2017.01.003 PMID: 28111293

Parkman, P. D. (1996). Togaviruses: Rubella Virus. In S. Baron (Ed.), *Medical Microbiology*. Galveston (TX): University of Texas Medical Branch at Galveston Copyright © 1996, The University of Texas Medical Branch at Galveston.

Peters, D. H., Garg, A., Bloom, G., Walker, D. G., Brieger, W. R., & Rahman, M. H. (2008). Poverty and access to health care in developing countries. *Annals of the New York Academy of Sciences*, *1136*(1), 161–171. DOI: 10.1196/annals.1425.011 PMID: 17954679

Plotkin, S. A., Reef, S. E., Cooper, L. Z., & Alford, C. A. (2011). CHAPTER 28 - Rubella. In Remington, J. S., Klein, J. O., Wilson, C. B., Nizet, V., & Maldonado, Y. A. (Eds.), *Infectious Diseases of the Fetus and Newborn* (7th ed., pp. 861–898). W.B. Saunders. DOI: 10.1016/B978-1-4160-6400-8.00028-6

Priyadharshini, & Jasmine, A. (2019). Coverage survey of Measles-Rubella mass vaccination campaign in a rural area in Tamil Nadu. *J Family Med Prim Care, 8*(6), 1884-1888. DOI: 10.4103/jfmpc.jfmpc_319_19

Rodriguez, D. L. (2003). Rubella. In Samuels, M. A., & Feske, S. K. (Eds.), *Office Practice of Neurology* (2nd ed., pp. 493–495). Churchill Livingstone. DOI: 10.1016/B0-44-306557-8/50076-9

Santibanez, S., Hübschen, J. M., Ben Mamou, M. C., Muscat, M., Brown, K. E., Myers, R., Donoso Mantke, O., Zeichhardt, H., Brockmann, D., Shulga, S. V., Muller, C. P., O'Connor, P. M., Mulders, M. N., & Mankertz, A. (2017). Molecular surveillance of measles and rubella in the WHO European Region: New challenges in the elimination phase. *Clinical Microbiology and Infection*, *23*(8), 516–523. DOI: 10.1016/j.cmi.2017.06.030 PMID: 28712666

Shukla, S., & Maraqa, N. F. (2023). Congenital Rubella *StatPearls*. Treasure Island (FL) ineligible companies. Disclosure: Nizar Maraqa declares no relevant financial relationships with ineligible companies.: StatPearls Publishing Copyright © 2023, StatPearls Publishing LLC.

Sodha, S. V., & Dietz, V. (2015). Strengthening routine immunization systems to improve global vaccination coverage. *British Medical Bulletin*, *113*(1), 5–14. DOI: 10.1093/bmb/ldv001 PMID: 25649959

Song, N., Gao, Z., Wood, J. G., Hueston, L., Gilbert, G. L., MacIntyre, C. R., Quinn, H. E., Menzies, R., & McIntyre, P. (2012). Current epidemiology of rubella and congenital rubella syndrome in Australia: Progress towards elimination. *Vaccine*, *30*(27), 4073–4078. DOI: 10.1016/j.vaccine.2012.04.025 PMID: 22554644

Terracciano, E., Amadori, F., Pettinicchio, V., Zaratti, L., & Franco, E. (2020). Strategies for elimination of rubella in pregnancy and of congenital rubella syndrome in high and upper-middle income countries. *Journal of Preventive Medicine and Hygiene*, *61*(1), E98–e108. DOI: 10.15167/2421-4248/jpmh2020.61.1.1310 PMID: 32490275

Tiller, E. C., Masters, N. B., Raines, K. L., Mathis, A. D., Crooke, S. N., Zwickl, R. C., French, G. K., Alexy, E. R., Koch, E. M., Tucker, N. E., Wilson, E. M., Krauss, T. S., Leasure, E., Budd, J., Billing, L. M., Dewart, C., Tarter, K., Dickerson, K., Iyer, R., & Roberts, M. W. (2023). Notes from the Field: Measles Outbreak - Central Ohio, 2022-2023. *MMWR. Morbidity and Mortality Weekly Report*, *72*(31), 847–849. DOI: 10.15585/mmwr.mm7231a3 PMID: 37535476

Winter, A. K., & Moss, W. J. (2022). Rubella. *Lancet*, *399*(10332), 1336–1346. DOI: 10.1016/S0140-6736(21)02691-X PMID: 35367004

# Chapter 8
# Poliomyelitis: A Global Perspective on the Challenges and Progress in Developing and Developed Countries


**Rahma Mahmoud Saad**
https://orcid.org/0009-0005-1259-3944
*Faculty Of Medicine, Modern University For Technology And Information-MTI, Cairo, Egypt*

**Ahmed Tharwat Al-Namrouti**
https://orcid.org/0009-0006-1588-2597
*Faculty of Medicine, Galala University, Suez, Egypt*

**Esraa Y. Salem**
*Faculty of Medicine, Modern University for Technology and Information (MTI), Cairo, Egypt*

**Karim S. Shata**
*Faculty of Medicine, Cairo University, Cairo, Egypt*

**Shahd Gamal Abdelsamad**
https://orcid.org/0009-0000-8322-0153
*Faculty of Medicine, Ain Shams University, Cairo, Egypt*

**safaa AlMawas**
https://orcid.org/0000-0001-5785-3950
*Faculty of Medicine, Mansoura University, Mansoura, Egypt*


## ABSTRACT


*Poliomyelitis, also known as polio, is a highly contagious disease that affects children under the age of five, mostly transmitted through the fecal-oral route by contaminated water and food. It is caused by three different types of wild polioviruses (WPV), a non-enveloped, single-stranded RNA virus, and can cause a range of symptoms and signs, from a mild flu-like illness to acute flaccid paralysis in severe cases. People have been plagued by this illness for many generations, which has resulted in global epidemics and high rates of morbidity and mortality. Nonetheless, vaccinations like*



DOI: 10.4018/979-8-3693-1990-1.ch008

*the live Sabin vaccine and the inactivated Salk vaccine, which were developed in the 20th century, have been crucial in both lowering the disease's occurrence and eliminating it. Numerous challenges have been faced in the fight to eradicate polio, such as outbreaks of vaccine-derived poliovirus (VDPV) and resistance. Despite all these challenges, there is still a worldwide responsibility and constant cooperation to work toward a world free of polio.*

## INTRODUCTION

Erwin Popper and Karl Landsteiner identified the poliovirus (PV) in 1908 as a positive-sense, non-enveloped, single-stranded RNA virus that is smaller than bacteria (Mohammed et al., 2021; Mohanty et al., 2023). This virus was the first animal virus to have both a reverse genetic technique and its entire genome sequence deciphered (Quarleri, 2023). The virus is a member of Enterovirus Group C from the Picornaviridae family. Humans are the only hosts for the three wild poliovirus types (WPV-1, -2, and -3), which cause poliomyelitis. Of them, WPV-1 is the primary source of the majority of global outbreaks, but WPV-2 and WPV-3 only create sporadic clusters (Mohanty et al., 2023; Quarleri, 2023).

Poliomyelitis is a debilitating and potentially fatal viral disease that frequently begins in children under the age of five and can result in lifelong paralysis in about 1% of affected people (paralytic polio) (Martini & Orsini, 2022). The Greek terms "polio" (grey) and "myelon" (marrow), which denote the most dreaded condition, are the source of the phrase "poliomyelitis" (Quarleri, 2023). The socioeconomic standing of the impacted communities dictates the pattern of disease spread. Fecal-oral transmission is the most common mode of infection in low-income countries; oral-to-oral transmission via saliva and oropharyngeal secretions is the mode of transmission in high-income countries. Replication occurs in the intestines, from which it might spread to the nervous system and cause paralysis (Al-Tawfiq et al., 2023; Martini & Orsini, 2022).

In addition to the lack of a conclusive treatment for polio, post-polio syndrome (PPS) may develop 25–30 years after the initial paralysis. PPS's primary symptoms include joint and muscular pain, abnormal fatigability, and new or worsening muscle weakness (Chu et al., 2016; Martini & Orsini, 2022). Since the only effective treatment for polio is prevention, two trivalent vaccinations were developed: the live Sabin vaccine (OPV) in 1961 and the inactivated Salk vaccine (IPV) in 1955, following the virus's discovery by electron microscopy in 1950. These vaccinations gave children lifetime protection against poliomyelitis, profoundly altered the epidemiology of the disease, and markedly reduced the number of cases (Al-Tawfiq et al., 2023; Martini & Orsini, 2022; Mohammed et al., 2021).

Eradicating polio is a critical global health priority due to its profound impact on public health and the potential for significant social and economic benefits. With the aim of eradicating polio by the year 2000, the World Health Organization (WHO) launched the Global Polio Eradication Initiative (GPEI) in 1988. GPEI was incredibly effective; by 2012, there had been a 99% reduction in the total number of polio cases reported (from 350 000 cases in 1988 to only 6 cases in 2021). Since then, only WPV1 infections have been reported worldwide due to the eradication of two polio virus serotypes: type 2 in 2015 (the last known case was in 1999) and type 3 in 2019 (the last recorded case was in 2012) (Al-Tawfiq et al., 2023). As of 2022 (5), the endemic transmission of WPV1 is still present in Afghanistan and Pakistan, despite these efforts to eradicate it (Mbani et al., 2023).

## DEFINITION

Poliovirus, which is a positive single-strand, non-enveloped RNA enterovirus virus causative agent of poliomyelitis commonly known as polio crippling and potentially fatal illness, The poliovirus has a diameter of roughly 25–30 nm (Wolbert, 2022). The 60 protomers that make up their outer coat are divided into four versions (VP1, VP2, VP3, and VP4). Additionally, the poliovirus has been identified as having three serotypes: 1, 2, and 3 placed in icosahedral symmetry (Bolaños-Martínez et al., 2022). The poliovirus has a very rapid replicated cycle and synthesis up to 10,000 virions per cell, which yields the ability to spread to other cells and/or new hosts (Burrill et al., 2013). The virus usually affects children six years of age or younger. The fecal-oral pathway primarily distributes it and spreads through person-to-person contact; naturally, humans are the only reservoir (Kaslow et al., 2014).

## EPIDEMIOLOGY AND PREVALENCE AMONG COUNTRIES

The disease did not begin epidemically; rather, it was identified by the ancient Egyptians in the 13th century BC as a representation of an atrophied limp and crutch, and a few isolated occurrences of paralysis with severe feverish sickness were documented. By the late 19th century, the epidemics had spread to the United States and other European countries. Still, the epidemics began in the 1920s and lasted until the 1950s, only spreading to Europe, Canada, and the United States (Walter & Malani, 2022).

Furthermore, during the first half of the 20th century, "the prevaccine era," larger epidemics with a high mortality toll were caused by improved sanitation, which led to decreased exposure and an increase in the age of initial infection. Then, with the introduction of the inactivated polio vaccine (IPV) in 1955 and the oral polio vaccine (OPV) in 1961, the incidence of the disease significantly decreased from almost 21,000 paralytic cases recorded in 1952; just 2,525 cases were reported in 1960 and 61 cases in 1965, leading to a decrease and elimination of the circulation of WPV in the United States in 1979. In the United States, 162 cases of paralytic poliomyelitis were confirmed, with an average of 8 occurrences each year between 1980 and 1999, as WPV was the cause of 6 cases and vaccine-associated paralytic polio (VAPP) was responsible for the remaining 154 cases (Centers for Disease Control and Prevention, 2022). Moreover, the incidence of vaccine-derived polio virus (VDPV) is significantly greater globally than that of WPV; between 2016 and 2021, 40 nations reported 1,818 incident instances of VDPV circulation (Polio Factsheet, 2023).

More than 50,000 cases of polio worldwide were reported in 1980, and about 350,000 cases per year in 125 countries were confirmed in 1988, so the WHO launched the GPEI, aiming to eradicate the disease globally, and that resulted in reducing the number of cases to 649 in 2021. Figure 1 and Table 1 show the prevalence of polio in some developed and developing countries in 1988 and 2021 (Centers for Disease Control and Prevention, 2022; Dattani et al., 2023). However, with the success of GPEI to eradicate WPV2 in 2015 and WPV3 in 2019 and decrease the incidence worldwide, 4 countries (Pakistan, Afghanistan, Mozambique, and Malawi) still have new WPV1 cases (Polio Factsheet, 2023). By 2020, the WHO will have certified six world regions, not only countries, to be polio-free: Africa, the Americas, the Eastern Mediterranean, Europe, South-East Asia, and the Western Pacific (Dattani et al., 2023).

*Table 1. Prevalence of polio in selected countries in 1988 and 2021*

| | Year 1988 | Year 2021 |
|---|---|---|
| **Zambia** | 11.187 | 0 |
| **Yemen** | 10.624 | 0.623 |
| **United Arab Emirates** | 5.531 | 0 |
| **Syria** | 2.901 | 0 |
| **Sudan** | 4.929 | 0 |
| **South Africa** | 4.957 | 0 |
| **Senegal** | 2.54 | 0.989 |
| **Philippines** | 5.851 | 0 |
| **Pakistan** | 9.222 | 0.04 |
| **Nigeria** | 16.151 | 1.963 |

continued on following page

*Table 1. Continued*

| | Year 1988 | Year 2021 |
|---|---|---|
| **Niger** | 4.372 | 0.676 |
| **Mauritania** | 8.806 | 0 |
| **Mali** | 14.808 | 0 |
| **Malawi** | 1.274 | 0.051 |
| **Madagascar** | 3.835 | 0.457 |
| **Libya** | 2.369 | 0 |
| **Liberia** | 2.811 | 0.579 |
| **Kenya** | 76.195 | 0 |
| **Iraq** | 4.154 | 0 |
| **Indonesia** | 4.418 | 0 |
| **India** | 28.419 | 0 |
| **Guinea** | 42.624 | 0.445 |
| **Europe** | 0.057 | 0.045 |
| **Ethiopia** | 2.949 | 0.085 |
| **Egypt** | 10.3 | 0 |
| **China** | 0.586 | 0 |
| **Central African Republic** | 20.045 | 0 |
| **Canada** | 0.112 | 0 |
| **Cameroon** | 11.106 | 0.11 |
| **Cambodia** | 12.328 | 0 |
| **Bangladesh** | 5.5 | 0 |
| **Africa** | 7.612 | 0.392 |
| **Afghanistan** | 26.424 | 1.18 |

*Figure 1. Prevalence of polio in selected developed and developing countries in 1988 and 2021*

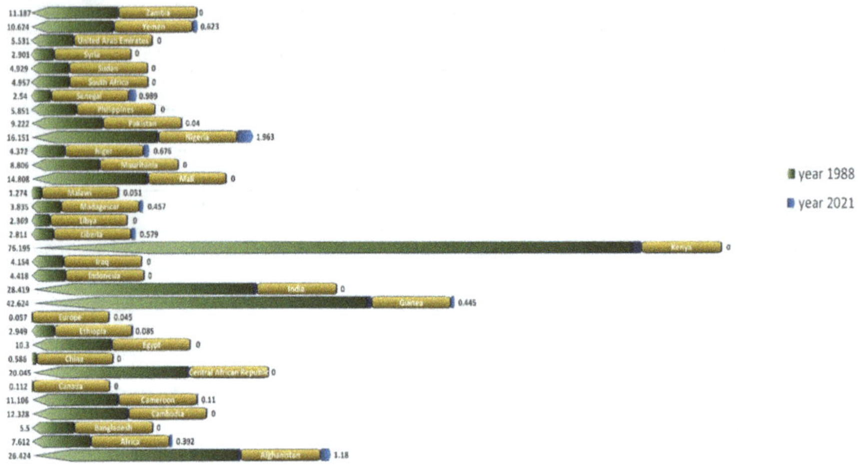


In 1988, Kenya, Guinea, India, Afghanistan, the Central African Republic, and Nigeria had the highest prevalence rates, recorded at 76.195, 42.624, 28.419, 26.424, 20.045, and 16.151, respectively. By 2021, these numbers had declined significantly, with Kenya, India, and the Central African Republic reporting zero cases, while Guinea, Afghanistan, and Nigeria recorded reduced prevalence rates of 0.445, 1.18, and 1.963, respectively.

## RISK FACTORS

Numerous environmental, demographic, and socioeconomic factors influence the frequency of poliomyelitis in both developed and developing countries, with a high prevalence of infectious diseases in developing countries. Several variables contribute to the spread of the polio virus, including (Bhardwaj, 2016; Noori et al., 2017; O'Reilly et al., 2017):

- population density
- sanitation (such as in low-income countries with inadequate hygiene)
- waste-water management
- public health services
- habitats, and climate conditions
- reduced immunity within these countries
- increase in migration from countries where wild poliomyelitis is common

- limited access to vaccines, and a decline in the number of vaccinated children because of refusal, violence, fear, and missed children.
- Malnutrition, insufficient breastfeeding, and diarrheal illnesses may also lessen the effectiveness of OPV
- increasing the risk of vaccine-derived polio epidemics.
- Patients with impaired immune systems are more likely to contract type 2 polio, while healthy individuals are more likely to contract type 3 polio.
- Reducing maternal antibodies may exacerbate the lack of protection against polioviruses, according to some epidemiologists.

However, there is no proof that the transmission of polio is influenced by genes, ethnicity, sex, or gender. In countries with large populations and low vaccination rates, polio persistence is desirable.

## PATHOGENESIS

The polio virus is from the Picornaviradae family, an enterovirus subgroup. It has three different serotypes (Centers for Disease Control and Prevention, 2021). The human is the only reservoir and natural host of PV (polio virus) (Blondel et al., 2005). The virus principally spreads by the fecal-oral pathway or by pharyngeal droplets (Marzia & Ali, 2024), or even oral-to-oral spread (Wolbert, 2022) commonly by unhygienic patients. It enters through the mouth and multiplies in the oropharynx and gastrointestinal tract, especially tonsils and Peyer's patches in the small intestine (Nathanson, 2008), The virus proceeds to the draining lymph nodes, where it proliferates and enters the circulation through the thoracic duct and efferent lymphatic vessels (Blondel et al., 2005). The virus can be transmitted in feces for several weeks post-infection, even in individuals who lack symptoms or just mild ones. It is often accessible in nasopharyngeal secretions for one to two weeks (Centers for Disease Control and Prevention, 2021). PV particles bind to and are endocytosed by human intestinal M cells, indicating that PV penetration of the intestinal epithelial barrier occurs in human M cells. Immune cells are potential candidates for PV transport to mesenteric lymph nodes because M cells can directly deliver virions to underlying mucosa-associated lymphoid tissue as the PV's capacity for replication in blood mononuclear phagocytic cells (Blonde et al., 2005). It's released from the apical surfaces of intestinal epithelial cells into the gut lumen and from lymphoid tissues into the blood (Blondel et al., 2005). The circulating virus invades the CNS probably through the blood-brain barrier, it primarily targets motor neurons in the spinal cord and brain stem in the central nervous system (CNS), and it most likely spreads from cell to cell (Mehndiratta et al., 2014). Paralysis is caused by the destruction of motor neurons as a result of PV replication (Mehndiratta et al., 2014). The striking feature of paralytic poliomyelitis is its localization to lower motor neurons, which results in a flaccid paralysis that frequently affects one or both legs. First-order sensory neurons are not completely destroyed, nor are sensory function significantly compromised. Similarly, there is not much involvement from the brain, with the exception of the brain stem's lower motor neurons (Nathanson, 2008).

## SYMPTOMS AND SIGNS

The signs and symptoms of polio can vary greatly, from flu-like symptoms to quadriplegia and even respiratory failure, may be suspected in cases of viral prodrome. Thankfully, most poliovirus infections (about 70%) do not cause symptoms. About 25% experience symptoms like the flu for two to five days. These symptoms can include fever, headache, pharyngitis, stiff neck, and exhaustion, as well as gastrointestinal problems including nausea, vomiting, and abdominal pain. About 1 in 200 poliovirus-infected people experience asymmetrical muscular weakness or paralysis, which typically appears one to three weeks after the infection. 1% to 5% of infected individuals develop meningitis (Walter & Malani, 2022).

There are various stages of poliomyelitis that might manifest especially in adults, including the acute, recovery, and residual paralysis stages as the following:

- The acute phase consists of minor associated illnesses characterized by flu-like symptoms, which are followed by large associated illnesses, which include all types of CNS diseases caused by either the poliovirus alone or in combination. This stage typically lasts two to three weeks, although it can last up to two months. The persistence of the acute stage is obvious in the residual muscle soreness (Ranade, 2022).
- The acute symptoms and muscle soreness subside during the convalescent or recovery stage, which can extend up to two years following the start of the disease, and paralyzed muscles heal with partial recovery of muscle strength, but permanent weakness is unavoidable due to anterior horn cell necrosis. Transverse myelitis, on the other hand, is less common and manifests as partial leg paralysis, urine retention, and sensory manifestations (Ranade, 2022).
- The disease enters the residual-paralysis stage two years after it first appears. At this point, muscle power does not recover. Muscle power equivalency is a common cause of deformities (Ranade, 2022).

Acute paralysis patients experience a continuous state of paralysis. In contrast to acute flaccid myelitis (AFM), which is caused by other viruses that have a higher propensity for the upper limb, severe muscle spasms and aches are the first signs of infection if it reaches the spinal cord. This is followed by an asymmetrical flaccid paralysis, with the lower limb being more susceptible (Wolbert & Higginbotham, 2021). However, tens of years after the initial infection, between thirty and forty percent of polio patients are expected to develop post-polio syndrome (Wolbert, & Higginbotham, 2021).

There are three forms of paralytic polio that can affect adults; spinal poliomyelitis is the most prevalent, bulbar poliomyelitis (2%), and a mix of the two, bulbospinal poliomyelitis (about 19%). On the other hand, in children, polio may follow a biphasic course, starting with a prodromal phase, followed by a symptom-free interval of seven to ten days, and then the onset of asymmetrical limb paralysis. The defining feature is flaccid paralysis, accompanied by the progressive loss of deep tendon reflexes (Mehndiratta et al., 2014).

## POST-POLIOMYELITIS SYNDROME (PPS): A LATE COMPLICATION OF POLIO

PPS is a neurological disorder that affects polio survivors and is characterized by a range of symptoms, and it is considered the most severe complication of poliomyelitis. Additionally, even if the precise origin of the disease is still unknown, it is recognized that its pathophysiology is multifactorial. Also, there is little evidence to establish that immune-mediated illness or poliovirus reinfection is the cause of PPS. However, the late sequelae of poliomyelitis, including osteoporosis, tendinitis, arthritis, and muscle atrophy, may resemble or worsen PPS. Long-term compensation of orphaned muscle fibers, which can result from overusing muscles or from other muscle groups compensating for weaker polio-affected muscles, may cause surviving neurons to age prematurely. Several serious conditions can also result in joint pain, including aberrant biomechanics, muscle atrophy, leg length discrepancy, joint stiffness, and age-related changes. Neuropathic pain, primarily from nerve impingement or disc herniation, affects some survivors. In order to rule out other possible explanations for new symptoms and clinical worsening, relevant investigations are conducted based on the comprehensive clinical evaluation (Chu & Lam, 2019).

Diagnosing PPS is an exclusion-based method that does not include the use of specific tests. To rule out other potential reasons for fatigue and weakness, such as anemia, thyroid issues, or liver and renal failure, it could be as simple as blood tests. While nerve conduction or electromyography (EMG) cannot diagnose polio or post-polio, they can show how the disease affects a patient's muscles and rule out neuropathies and myopathies. Imaging tests such as MRIs, CT scans, and X-rays may be necessary. A muscle biopsy may also be useful, but it is not specific to PPS and can identify certain features, like current degeneration. A preliminary study suggests the potential of disease-specific proteins in the CSF of PPS patients as a diagnostic biomarker; however, more studies are required to verify its specificity (Lo & Robinson, 2018). Ultrasonography shows potential as a prognosis method rather than a diagnostic one, as it has been used recently to non-invasively distinguish between healthy formal polio patients and those with PPS (Mateos-Angulo et al., 2022).

The criteria of the European Federation of Neurological Societies (EFNS) are internationally recognized standards for diagnosis. These standards include (Chu & Zoubi, 2023):

- A verified history of acute paralytic polio with denervation signs on an electromyogram
- Partial or complete recovery followed by at least 15 years of stable neurologic function
- Abnormal muscle fatigability or gradual or sudden onset of progressive and persistent muscle weakness
- Symptoms that last for at least a year; and the exclusion of other neuromuscular, medical, and orthopedic conditions as possible causes.

Since conservative therapy is the primary method of managing PPS, interdisciplinary treatment is the best strategy for individuals with PPS. It has been shown that customized rehabilitation significantly increases physical effort and reduces discomfort. This type of treatment involves water therapy, endurance training, and muscle strengthening. Even though benzodiazepines, acetaminophen, and opioids are among the many medications used to treat post-polio muscle pain, their effectiveness is questionable. Amitriptyline is one of the tricyclic antidepressants (TCA) that works well for alleviating fatigue and pain. Properly fitted orthoses can improve biomechanical movement patterns and lower energy expenditure. Correcting postural irregularities can sometimes result in the prevention or reduction of biomechanical discomfort as well as the building of stronger muscles for standing, sitting, walking, and other activities (Chu & Lam, 2019).

## DIAGNOSIS

Poliomyelitis can be diagnosed using a combination of the patient's medical history, clinical examination, and investigative procedures. Together with the clinical findings during the examination, a prodromal stage's history can aid in the diagnosis of the condition (Wolbert & Higginbotham, 2021). Inquiring about past travel history may aid in diagnosis, as exposure to foreign locations where poliomyelitis is prevalent increases the likelihood of contracting the virus (Centers for Disease Control and Prevention, 2023). Polio is known to have been eradicated through vaccination; however, unusual occurrences of a vaccine-associated paralytic poliovirus have been reported (Centers for Disease Control and Prevention, 2022).

The most sensitive diagnostic test is the isolation of viruses on culture, typically from stool specimens. Though this is only possible in the first week, it is thought to be less dependable and less likely from blood or cerebrospinal fluid (CSF). It can also be isolated from a pharyngeal swab. It is more likely to be isolated if two stool samples are taken 24 hours apart and within the first 14 days of the illness starting (Marzia & Ali, 2024; Mehndiratta et al., 2014). Real-time reverse polymerase chain reaction (real-time PCR) intertypic differentiation can be helpful in distinguishing between vaccine-like and potentially wild strains. Partial genome sequencing is utilized to determine the virus genotype and most likely geographic origin. If vaccination history indicates missed vaccination, serology can support the diagnosis if done as early as possible by an acute serum specimen followed by a convalescent specimen 3 weeks later. It is unusual to detect poliovirus in CSF; however, lymphocytic pleocytosis is sometimes evidenced along with a slight increase in protein (Centers for Disease Control and Prevention, 2021).

## MANAGEMENT

Supportive therapy is useful in controlling symptoms and averting complications, even though there is no known cure or antiviral for poliomyelitis. Antipyretics, protection from respiratory infections, ventilation support if respiratory muscles are involved, hot packs for muscle spasms, immobilization of the affected limb, and the use of assistive devices to support weak joints and muscles are the mainstays of management during the acute and recovery stages (Wolbert et al., 2024).

Moreover, physical therapy and rehabilitation play a vital role in treatment of chronic cases, these includes: gait training, muscle strengthening exercises, exercises for range of motion, and usage of appropriate assistive devices (Marzia & Ali, 2024). In 1926, President Franklin Theodore Roosevelt established the first sophisticated rehabilitation clinic in the United States for polio sufferers (Mehndiratta et al., 2014).

Additionally, surgical techniques are frequently employed to avoid deformity and reduce disparities in limb length such as orthopedic and spinal surgeries for lengthening or transferring tendons and spinal fusion. Sadly, a large number of survivors have relied on iron lungs, assisted breathing, or wheelchairs throughout their lives (Rosenberg & Rovito, 2021; Marzia & Ali, 2024).

## PREVENTION

During the 20$^{th}$ century, the development of polio vaccinations marked the beginning of the disease's prevention, which varied in price, risks, and benefits. These immunizations significantly decreased the quantity of poliomyelitis cases, resulting in an adequate elimination of the illness (Thompson & Kalkowska, 2021).

### OPV, Or Oral Poliovirus Vaccines

OPV, sometimes known as Sabin, is a live-attenuated polio vaccine introduced in 1961. OPV is characterized by its easy administration, limitation of virus spread through induction of gut mucosal immunity, and cheapness, so it is most used in low- and middle-income nations. Four different types of OPV were identified, including: trivalent OPV (tOPV), monovalent OPV-1 (mOPV1), monovalent OPV-3 (mOPV3), and bivalent OPV (bOPV). tOPV was the recommended vaccine for routine immunization, eradicating poliovirus among these variants. After the complete eradication of WPV-2 in 1999, bOPV was introduced for the circulated WPV-1 and WPV-3 in endemic areas. The bOPV, mOPV1, and mOPV3 formulas have higher immunogenicity than tOPV (Ciapponi et al., 2019). However, vaccine-associated paralytic polio (VAPP) has a risk of developing in individuals immunized with OPV without previous exposure to poliovirus, and these OPV-related viruses may become circulating VDPVs (cVDPVs) that act like WPVs, causing outbreaks (Thompson & Kalkowska, 2021).

### IPV, or Inactivated Polio Vaccine

This one, called Salk, is a killed or inactivated vaccine derived from the three serotypes of WPV, which were first made available in 1955. Unlike OPV, IPV does not produce VAPP and is more expensive than it is; for this reason, in high-income countries (HICs), this vaccination is the preferred option for routine immunizations (Ciapponi et al., 2019). It comes in a trivalent form only, guards against paralysis, and offers humoral immunity that does not lessen the likelihood of gut infections (Thompson & Kalkowska, 2021).

*Table 2. Comparison between the two types of polio vaccines: IPV and OPV*

| Feature | OPV (Sabin) | IPV (Salk) |
|---|---|---|
| **Type of vaccine** | Live attenuated (weakened) virus | Inactivated (killed) virus |
| **Route of administration** | Oral drops | Injection (IM or SC) |
| **Number of doses** | 3 – 4 doses in primary series | |
| **Stability and storage** | Requires strict cold chain maintenance | Requires refrigeration but more stable than OPV |
| **Types** | 4 types: tOPV - mOPV1 - mOPV3 - bOPV | Only trivalent form |
| **Immunity provided** | Both systematic and intestinal immunity | Strong systemic (blood) immunity |
| **Prevention of transmission** | Very effective in reducing virus shedding | Less effective in stopping virus shedding |
| **Prevention of paralysis** | Very effective | |
| **Risk of VAPP** | High risk | No risk |
| **Cost** | Less expensive | More expensive |

## CHALLENGES OF INFECTION AMONG NATIONS

Worldwide success in eliminating polio has been attributed to the genetically stable character of the virus and efficacious immunization. According to the World Health Organization, two of the three wild poliovirus serotypes (WPV2 and 3) have been eliminated worldwide. Since 1988, the number of recorded global WPV cases has dropped by more than 99.9%, from 350,000 to 6 cases in 2021 (World Health Organization, 2019).

Even though the virus is almost completely eradicated, there are still a lot of challenges with immunization. Just one of the main obstacles is vaccine reluctance. Certain people are not sure whether to get vaccinated. because of low health literacy and knowledge regarding vaccinations and the hazards involved. Because immunizations have successfully reduced many previously frequent childhood infectious disorders, parents are now less familiar with these conditions. As a result, concerns have switched to perceived vaccine reactions which frequently involve childhood health issues and coincide with routine immunization regimens (Salmon et al., 2015). Polio epidemics have occurred in some places due to mistrust of immunizations or simple fear leading to low vaccination rates, which caused the polio outbreak in Malawi in 2022 (Chunda et al., 2022). A study conducted in Nigeria reported that the OPV refusal during the immunization campaign in 2011 was due to the low education level of the heads of households and lack of knowledge of vaccinations benefits (Mohammed et al., 2021). Therefore, dispelling myths about vaccines and their safety and educating communities have been the main goals of several public programs.

Poor sewage systems and contaminated water supplies are two of the main environmental risk factors. Due to its high contagious nature and the fact that the fecal-oral route is the main means of transmission in environments with inadequate hygiene and sanitation, polio mainly affects developing nations with inadequate sanitation; as a result, it is endemic in Pakistan and Afghanistan (Lee et al., 2023). Also, there were several obstacles in the battle against polio. Insufficient government, unstable geopolitics, insecurity, extremism, and difficulty reaching isolated regions (Shabbir et al., 2022). Similarly, in 2021, in Nigeria, they faced an infection caused by circulating vaccine-derived poliovirus (cVDPV) in areas with poor sanitation (Menon et al., 2024).

Wars provide fertile ground for infections and limit access to proper vaccination. It can be challenging to vaccinate children in war-torn and insecure areas, and health workers may become targets of violence, migration, and population shifts, such as the migration of Afghans to Pakistan (Ghosh, 2019). The success of immunization efforts is intimately linked to territory control, with GPEI urging for coordination with government forces (Taylor, 2023).

In Afghanistan, Taliban-controlled districts in Kandahar have been unreachable for years, and Afghan government attacks on health facilities have impaired immunization attempts. In Nigeria, Boko Haram insurgents prevent vaccination teams from reaching the populations they control (Taylor, 2023). In Aug 2024, the polio outbreak in Gaza, which includes the first case in 25 years in a 10-month-old baby, is a direct result of the ongoing conflict, which has damaged the region's healthcare and sanitation facilities (Devi, 2024). The conflict, which began in October 2023, has severely destroyed 70% of Gaza's water and sanitation infrastructure, denying nearly 1.6 million people access to clean water (Dardona et al., 2024; Menon et al., 2024). A situation where any infectious disease can spread quickly has been created by overcrowded shelters, some of which have just one restroom per 700 people and furthermore, hospital devastation has hampered immunization efforts, which further complicates containment (Dardona et al., 2024). Adding to the situation, polio has been found in sewage, which, combined with waste accumulation and overflowing sewage, has resulted in an increase in insect populations, further spreading disease (Menon et al., 2024). The ongoing conflict has also displaced 1.9 million people to temporary camps with extremely inadequate hygienic conditions (Dardona et al., 2024). Meanwhile, attacks on humanitarian workers and restrictions on medical assistance access have jeopardized polio response efforts and the United Nations claimed that approximately 300 aid workers and over 880 healthcare personnel have been killed, and Israeli authorities continued to deny humanitarian missions access (Mahase, 2024).

## POLIO IN THE COVID-19 ERA

The COVID-19 pandemic has drastically disrupted global polio eradication efforts and vaccine campaigns, putting years of progress at risk. In 2020, it resulted in a decrease in both national and GPEI immunization activities, as well as alterations in human contact patterns. These disruptions reduced vaccine coverage; however physical separation techniques lessened the impact by limiting poliovirus transmission (Thompson & Kalkowska, 2021; Uwishema et al., 2022).

If these disruptions are temporary and short-lived, the long-term impact on polio incidence may be minimal. However, the pandemic has had a huge economic impact, lowering productivity in many countries and possibly impacting funders' desire to continue prioritizing polio eradication. As resources are diverted to COVID-19 response actions, funding for polio vaccine programs may become difficult, jeopardizing eradication efforts (Thompson & Kalkowska, 2021).

Beyond the immediate disruptions, the global reduction of vaccine coverage, combined with increased international travel, has increased the likelihood of poliovirus spreading to formerly polio-free areas. This concern is highlighted by the discovery of WPV1 cases in Malawi (2021) and Mozambique (2022), as well as circulating vaccine-derived poliovirus type 2 (cVDPV2) cases in the United States, United Kingdom, Canada, and Israel in 2022 (Bandyopadhyay et al., 2024). These developments underline the continuous vulnerability of polio-free areas, as well as the crucial necessity for continued immunization efforts to avoid any setbacks in eradication progress.

On the other hand, a study by Yagovkina et al. (2022) evaluated the effect of bOPV on COVID-19 incidence. In a randomized, parallel group comparative study, 1115 healthy volunteers were allocated into 2 equal groups; one group received oral single dose of bOPV and the other group received placebo. Over a three-month period, the number of confirmed cases of COVID-19 was significantly low in the vaccinated group compared to placebo group. These findings suggested that immunization with bOPV could reduce the number of COVID-19 cases (Yagovkina et al., 2022).

## RESEARCH STRATEGIES TO LIMIT THE SPREAD

Community engagement has been critical to the Global Polio Eradication Initiative's (GPEI) success, with techniques such as awareness campaigns, education sessions, door-to-door messaging, and cross-border initiatives all helping to preserve vaccination compliance. Examples from Ethiopia and India demonstrate the importance of community-selected volunteers, schoolchildren, and religious influences in fostering trust and overcoming vaccine skepticism. Collaborations with local governments, prominent citizens, and groups such as Rotary Clubs have also aided outreach initiatives (Agrawal et al., 2023).

High-quality supplemental immunization activities (SIAs) and improved surveillance are two examples of the technical and financial support that GPEI offers to the polio epidemic response in collaboration with the Extended Program of Immunization (EPI), Ministries of Health (MOH), and WHO. Coordinated interventions and synchronized SIAs are advised for cross-border outbreaks (Shabana et al., 2024).

Faith-based organizations (FBOs) and public health agencies (PHAs) have teamed up to address vaccine reluctance in communities that face language hurdles, religious concerns, and medical mistrust. Multilingual toolkits, interaction with religious experts, and digital awareness campaigns have all been employed to increase vaccine confidence. Collaborative educational initiatives, such as outreach tactics and webinars, have aided in dispelling myths and promoting acceptance, especially among marginalized and vulnerable groups (Song et al., 2024).

A new approach to polio eradication has been launched by the Global Polio Eradication Initiative (GPEI). The objectives of this strategy are to take advantage of every chance to vaccinate children, foster a sense of collective ownership and accountability for the eradication campaign, and guarantee an urgency appropriate for the stage at which the polio outbreak is currently at. Three ambitious goals have been established by the GPEI to permanently stop the spread of the poliovirus in Pakistan and Afghanistan, stop outbreaks in non-endemic nations, and declare the globe polio-free by 2026. Additionally, the GPEI has created a thorough plan of action that will enable it to fulfil a pledge that pushes global support for the eradication of polio (World Health Organization, 2021).

Furthermore, the creation of a unique instrument to eliminate circulating vaccine-derived poliovirus type 2 (cVDPV2) has required the production of oral polio vaccine type 2 (nOPV2) (Bandyopadhyay & Zipursky, 2023). This vaccination is well tolerated by newborns, young children, and adults and has not exhibited any significant side effects. Also, it's the first vaccine to receive an Emergency Use Listing (EUL) recommendation from the WHO in 2020 (Macklin, 2023).

## CONCLUSION

Poliomyelitis continues to pose a substantial global health challenge, regardless of significant progress in its eradication efforts. This chapter has delved into the definition, epidemiology, and global prevalence of polio, emphasizing the risk factors that facilitate its transmission. We've covered the disease's pathogenesis, clinical signs, and long-term consequences of post-poliomyelitis syndrome (PPS). Advances in diagnosis, management, and prevention techniques, particularly the use of oral (OPV) and inactivated (IPV) polio vaccinations, have played critical roles in reducing disease burdens. However, issues such as vaccine-derived poliovirus outbreaks, discrepancies in immunization coverage, and the influence of the COVID-19 pandemic on eradication efforts continue to hinder progress.

In the battle against polio, ongoing research and innovative strategies are still essential. There is hope for polio eradication worldwide thanks to initiatives to strengthen surveillance systems, increase vaccine stability, and include polio vaccination into larger immunization campaigns. Achieving a world free of polio requires boosting international cooperation and dealing with political and practical obstacles.

As we approach eradication, governments, healthcare professionals, and policymakers need to be dedicated to immunization and public health programs. The elimination of polio will not only eradicate a crippling disease but will also serve as a model for fighting other contagious diseases across the world. The road ahead requires caution, innovation and unwavering global cooperation. With consistent effort, a polio-free future is achievable.

*Figure 2. Summary of the pathogenesis and clinical picture of polio.*

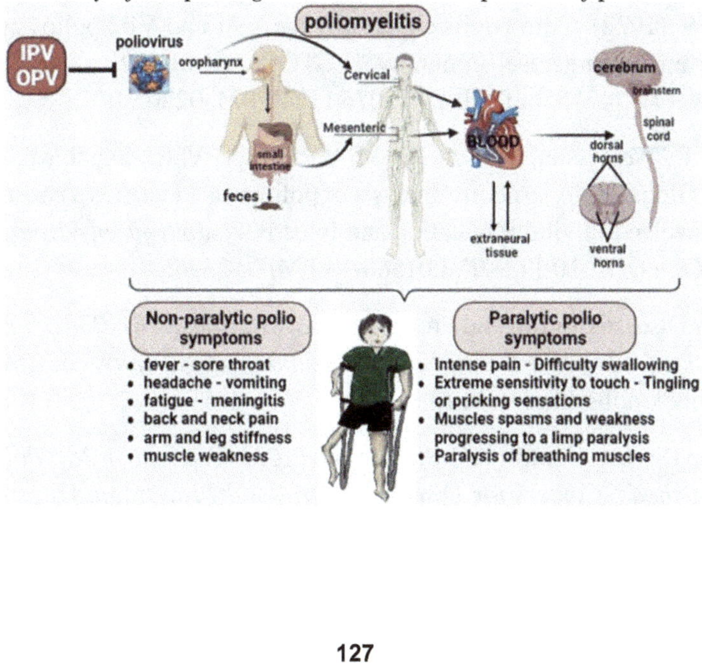

## REFERENCES


Agrawal, P., Neel, A., Deresse, A. S., Gerber, S., & Alonge, O. (2023). Facilitators and barriers to community engagement in the Global Polio Eradication Initiative–A mixed methods study. *PLOS Global Public Health*, *3*(4), e0001643. DOI: 10.1371/journal.pgph.0001643 PMID: 37027352

Al-Tawfiq, J. A., Kattan, R. F., Almoallem, S. A. S., Altawfiq, K. J., Mohsni, E., & Memish, Z. A. (2023). Worldwide poliomyelitis outbreaks: Should mass gathering organizers be concerned? *Journal of Travel Medicine*, *30*(1), taac128. DOI: 10.1093/jtm/taac128 PMID: 36331257

Bandyopadhyay, A. S., Burke, R. M., & Hawes, K. M. (2024). Polio Eradication: Status, Struggles and Strategies. *The Pediatric Infectious Disease Journal*, *43*(6), e207–e211. DOI: 10.1097/INF.0000000000004330 PMID: 38564755

Bandyopadhyay, A. S., & Zipursky, S. (2023). A novel tool to eradicate an ancient scourge: The novel oral polio vaccine type 2 story. *The Lancet. Infectious Diseases*, *23*(2), e67–e71. DOI: 10.1016/S1473-3099(22)00582-5 PMID: 36162417

Bhardwaj, S. (2016). The Epidemiology of Poliomyelitis Deconstructed. UC Merced Undergraduate Research Journal, 8(2).

Blondel, B., Colbere-Garapin, F., Couderc, T., Wirotius, A., & Guivel-Benhassine, F. (2005). Poliovirus, pathogenesis of poliomyelitis, and apoptosis. Role of apoptosis in infection, 25-56.

Bolaños-Martínez, O. C., Govea-Alonso, D. O., Fragoso, G., Sciutto, E., & Rosales-Mendoza, S. (2022). Carrot cells expressing the VP1 and VP2 poliovirus proteins effectively elicited mucosal immunity. [PCTOC]. *Plant Cell, Tissue and Organ Culture*, *148*(3), 545–556. DOI: 10.1007/s11240-021-02205-0

Burrill, C. P., Westesson, O., Schulte, M. B., Strings, V. R., Segal, M., & Andino, R. (2013). Global RNA structure analysis of poliovirus identifies a conserved RNA structure involved in viral replication and infectivity. *Journal of Virology*, *87*(21), 11670–11683. DOI: 10.1128/JVI.01560-13 PMID: 23966409

Centers for Disease Control and Prevention. *(2021, August 18). Pinkbook: Poliomyelitis. Centers for Disease Control and Prevention.* Https://www.cdc.gov/vaccines/pubs/pinkbook/polio.html. (n.d.).

Centers for Disease Control and Prevention. *(2021, September 28). Poliovirus diagnostic methods. Centers for Disease Control and Prevention.* Https://www.cdc.gov/polio/us/lab-testing/diagnostic.html. (n.d.).

Centers for Disease Control and Prevention. *(2022, August 3). Vaccine-associated paralytic polio. Centers for Disease Control and Prevention.* Https://www.cdc.gov/vaccines/vpd/polio/hcp/vaccine-associated-paralytic-polio-faq.html. (n.d.).

Centers for Disease Control and Prevention. *(2022) Chapter 18: Polio; epidemiology and prevention of vaccine-preventable, Available at:* Https://www.cdc.gov/vaccines/pubs/pinkbook/downloads/polio.pdf. (n.d.).

Centers for Disease Control and Prevention. *(2023, July 5). Polio: For travelers. Centers for Disease Control and Prevention.* Https://www.cdc.gov/polio/us/travelers.html. (n.d.).

Chu, E. C. P., & Lam, K. K. W. (2019). Post-poliomyelitis syndrome. *International Medical Case Reports Journal, 12*, 261–264. DOI: 10.2147/IMCRJ.S219481 PMID: 31496835

Chu, E. C.-P., & Zoubi, F. A. (2023). Post-polio syndrome presenting as isolated neck extensor myopathy: A case report. *AME Case Reports*, *7*(0), 0. Advance online publication. DOI: 10.21037/acr-22-76 PMID: 37122964

Chu, M., Yuan, W., Wu, S., Wang, Z., Mao, L., Tian, T., Lu, Y., Zhu, B., Yang, Y., Wang, B., Gao, H., Jiang, L., & Zhuang, X. (2016). Quantitative assessment of polymorphisms in H19 lncRNA and cancer risk: A meta-analysis of 13,392 cases and 18,893 controls. [CrossRef] [PubMed]. *Oncotarget*, *7*(48), 78631–78639. DOI: 10.18632/oncotarget.12530 PMID: 27732938

Chunda, P., Chisema, M. N., Mwale, A., Kambalame, D., Mapemba, D., & Muula, A. S. (2022). The 2022 Malawi Polio outbreak. *Malawi Medical Journal : the Journal of Medical Association of Malawi*, *34*(3), 223–224. DOI: 10.4314/mmj.v34i3.14 PMID: 36406100

Ciapponi, A., Bardach, A., Ares, L. R., Glujovsky, D., Cafferata, M. L., Cesaroni, S., & Bhatti, A. (2019). Sequential inactivated (IPV) and live oral (OPV) poliovirus vaccines for preventing poliomyelitis. [n.d.]. *Cochrane Database of Systematic Reviews*, *2019*(12), 12. DOI: 10.1002/14651858.CD011260.pub2 PMID: 31801180

Dardona, Z., Amane, M., & Boussaa, S. (2024). Polio in Gaza: Another disastrous outcome of the Gaza conflict, 2023-2024. *Asian Pacific Journal of Tropical Medicine*, *17*(9), 381–383. DOI: 10.4103/apjtm.apjtm_535_24

Dattani, S., Spooner, F., Ochmann, S., & Roser, M. *Polio. Our World Data [Internet]. 2023 Nov 10 [cited 2023 Nov 22]; Available from:* Https://ourworldindata.org/polio. (n.d.).

Devi, S. (2024). Calls for Gaza ceasefire to tackle poliovirus. *Lancet*, *404*(10455), 837. DOI: 10.1016/S0140-6736(24)01776-8 PMID: 39217989

Ghosh, A. (2019). Afghan migration and pakistan's policy response: Dynamics of continuity and change. Public Policy Research in the Global South: A Cross-Country Perspective, 215-230. (n.d.).

Kaslow, R. A., Stanberry, L. R., & Le Duc, J. W. (Eds.). (2014). *Viral infections of humans: epidemiology and control.* Springer.

Lee, S. E., Greene, S. A., Burns, C. C., Tallis, G., Wassilak, S. G., & Bolu, O. (2023). Progress Toward Poliomyelitis Eradication—Worldwide, January 2021–March 2023. *MMWR. Morbidity and Mortality Weekly Report*, *72*(19), 517–522. DOI: 10.15585/mmwr.mm7219a3 PMID: 37167156

Lo, J. K., & Robinson, L. R. (2018). Postpolio syndrome and the late effects of poliomyelitis. Part 1. Pathogenesis, biomechanical considerations, diagnosis, and investigations. *Muscle & Nerve*, *58*(6), 751–759. DOI: 10.1002/mus.26168 PMID: 29752819

Macklin, G. R., Peak, C., Eisenhawer, M., Kurji, F., Mach, O., Konz, J., Gast, C., Bachtiar, N. S., Bandyopadhyay, A. S., & Zipursky, S. (2023). Enabling accelerated vaccine roll-out for public health emergencies of international concern (PHEICs): Novel oral polio vaccine type 2 (nOPV2) experience. *Vaccine*, *41*, A122–A127. DOI: 10.1016/j.vaccine.2022.02.050 PMID: 35307230

Mahase, E. (2024). Gaza: Polio vaccination campaign gets underway as attacks on humanitarian aid continue. *BMJ (Clinical Research Ed.)*, *386*, q1918. DOI: 10.1136/bmj.q1918 PMID: 39271192

Martini, M., & Orsini, D. (2022). The fight against poliomyelitis through the history: Past, present and hopes for the future. Albert Sabin's missing Nobel and his "gift to all the world's children". *Vaccine*, *40*(47), 6802–6805. DOI: 10.1016/j.vaccine.2022.09.088 PMID: 36244880

Marzia, A., & Ali, L. (2024). A short review on poliomyelitis: Types, transmission, diagnosis, prevention, treatment. *Journal of Contemporary Pharmacy*, *8*(1), 1. DOI: 10.56770/jcp2024819

Mateos-Angulo, Á., Salazar-Agulló, J. A., Roldán-Jiménez, C., Trinidad-Fernández, M., & Cuesta-Vargas, A. I. (2022). Ultrasonography Assessment Based on Muscle Thickness and Echo Intensity in Post-Polio Patients. *Diagnostics (Basel)*, *12*(11), 2743. DOI: 10.3390/diagnostics12112743 PMID: 36359586

Mbani, C. J., Nekoua, M. P., Moukassa, D., & Hober, D. (2023). The Fight against Poliovirus Is Not Over. *Microorganisms, 11*(5), 1323. DOI: 10.3390/microorganisms11051323 PMID: 37317297

Mehndiratta, M. M., Mehndiratta, P., & Pande, R. (2014). Poliomyelitis: Historical Facts, Epidemiology, and Current Challenges in Eradication. *The Neurohospitalist, 4*(4), 223–229. DOI: 10.1177/1941874414533352 PMID: 25360208

Menon, T. P., Zinszer, K., & Abuzerr, S. (2024). Detection of polio virus in Gaza's sewage demands immediate action. *Frontiers in Public Health, 12*, 1474554. Advance online publication. DOI: 10.3389/fpubh.2024.1474554 PMID: 39691657

Mohammed, A., Tomori, O., & Nkengasong, J. N. (2021). Lessons from the elimination of poliomyelitis in Africa. *Nature Reviews. Immunology, 21*(12), 823–828. DOI: 10.1038/s41577-021-00640-w PMID: 34697501

Mohanty, A., Rohilla, R., Zaman, K., Hada, V., Dhakal, S., Shah, A., & Al-Tawfiq, J. A. (2023). Vaccine Derived Poliovirus (VDPV). *Le Infezioni in Medicina, 31*(2), 174. PMID: 37283637

Nathanson, N. (2008). The pathogenesis of poliomyelitis: What we don't know. *Advances in Virus Research, 71*, 1–50. DOI: 10.1016/S0065-3527(08)00001-8 PMID: 18585526

Noori, N., Drake, J. M., & Rohani, P. (2017). Comparative epidemiology of poliovirus transmission. *Scientific Reports, 7*(1), 17362. DOI: 10.1038/s41598-017-17749-5 PMID: 29234135

O'Reilly, K. M., Lamoureux, C., Molodecky, N. A., Lyons, H., Grassly, N. C., & Tallis, G. (2017). An assessment of the geographical risks of wild and vaccine-derived poliomyelitis outbreaks in Africa and Asia. *BMC Infectious Diseases, 17*(1), 1–14. DOI: 10.1186/s12879-017-2443-4 PMID: 28549485

*Polio eradication strategy 2022–2026: Delivering on a promise.* (n.d.). Retrieved November 30, 2023, from https://www.who.int/publications-detail-redirect/9789240031937

Polio Factsheet. *(2023, February 23). Health Protection Surveillance Centre.* Https://www.hpsc.ie/a-z/vaccinepreventable/polio/factsheet/. (n.d.).

*Poliomyelitis (polio). (2019, November 18).* Https://www.who.int/health-topics/poliomyelitis. (n.d.).

Quarleri, J. (2023). Poliomyelitis is a current challenge: Long-term sequelae and circulating vaccine-derived poliovirus. *GeroScience*, *45*(2), 707–717. DOI: 10.1007/s11357-022-00672-7 PMID: 36260265

Ranade, S. *A. (2022). Poliomyelitis clinical presentation. History and Physical Examination, Postpolio Syndrome, Complications.* Https://emedicine.medscape.com/article/1259213-clinical.

Rosenberg, D., & Rovito, C. (Eds.). *(2021). Post-Polio Syndrome: Background, Management and Treatment, An Issue of Physical Medicine and Rehabilitation Clinics of North America, E-Book (Vol. 32, No. 3). Elsevier Health Sciences.*

Salmon, D. A., Dudley, M. Z., Glanz, J. M., & Omer, S. B. (2015). Vaccine hesitancy: Causes, consequences, and a call to action. *Vaccine*, *33*, D66–D71. DOI: 10.1016/j.vaccine.2015.09.035 PMID: 26615171

Shabana, M. R., Salamony, A., Elleboudy, N. S., & Aboshanab, K. M. (2024). Vaccine-Derived Poliovirus: Epidemiology, Types, Global Response and Future Prospectives. *Archives of Pharmaceutical Sciences Ain Shams University*. DOI: 10.21608/aps.2024.268453.1159

Shabbir, H., Saeed, S., Farhan, M., Abbas, K., Rehman, M. E., Gul, F., & Basit, J. (2022). Poliomyelitis in Pakistan: Challenges to polio eradication and future prospects. *Annals of Medicine and Surgery (London)*, *80*, 104274. DOI: 10.1016/j.amsu.2022.104274 PMID: 36045811

Song, M. Y., Blake-Hepburn, D., Karbasi, A., Fadel, S. A., Allin, S., Ataullahjan, A., & Ruggiero, E. D. (2024). Public health partnerships with faith-based organizations to support vaccination uptake among minoritized communities: A scoping review. *PLOS Global Public Health*, *4*(6), e0002765. DOI: 10.1371/journal.pgph.0002765 PMID: 38837963

Taylor, S. (2023). Poliomyelitis and Child Paralysis. In *The Palgrave Encyclopedia of Global Security Studies* (pp. 1143–1147). Palgrave Macmillan., DOI: 10.1007/978-3-319-74319-6_550

*The effort to eradicate polio globally faces new challenges. (N.d.). UNICEF.* https://www.unicef.org/stories/the-effort-to-eradicate-polio-globally-faces-new-challenges.(n.d.).

Thompson, K. M., & Kalkowska, D. A. (2021). Potential future use, costs, and value of poliovirus vaccines. *Risk Analysis*, *41*(2), 349–363. DOI: 10.1111/risa.13557 PMID: 32645244

Thompson, K. M., & Kalkowska, D. A. (2021). An Updated Economic Analysis of the Global Polio Eradication Initiative. *Risk Analysis*, *41*(2), 393–406. DOI: 10.1111/risa.13665 PMID: 33590521

Uwishema, O., Elebesunu, E. E., Bouaddi, O., Kapoor, A., Akhtar, S., Effiong, F. B., Chaudhary, A., & Onyeaka, H. (2022). Poliomyelitis amidst the COVID-19 pandemic in Africa: Efforts, challenges and recommendations. *Clinical Epidemiology and Global Health*, *16*, 101073. DOI: 10.1016/j.cegh.2022.101073 PMID: 35664665

Walter, K., & Malani, P. N. (2022). What Is Polio? *Journal of the American Medical Association*, *328*(16), 1652–1652. DOI: 10.1001/jama.2022.17159 PMID: 36112391

Wolbert, J. G. *(2022). Poliomyelitis. StatPearls—NCBI Bookshelf.* Https://www.ncbi.nlm.nih.gov/books/NBK558944/?report=reader.

Wolbert, J. G., & Higginbotham, K. (n.d.). *(2021). Poliomyelitis.* StatPearls.

Wolbert, J. G., Rajnik, M., Swinkels, H. M., & Higginbotham, K. (2024). Poliomyelitis. In *StatPearls* [Internet]. StatPearls Publishing., https://www.ncbi.nlm.nih.gov/sites/books/NBK558944/

Yagovkina, N. V., Zheleznov, L. M., Subbotina, K. A., Tsaan, A. A., Kozlovskaya, L. I., Gordeychuk, I. V., Korduban, A. K., Ivin, Y. Y., Kovpak, A. A., Piniaeva, A. N., Shishova, A. A., Shustova, E. Y., Khapchaev, Y. K., Karganova, G. G., Siniugina, A. A., Pomaskina, T. V., Erovichenkov, A. A., Chumakov, K., & Ishmukhametov, A. A. (2022). Vaccination With Oral Polio Vaccine Reduces COVID-19 Incidence. *Frontiers in Immunology*, *13*, 907341. DOI: 10.3389/fimmu.2022.907341 PMID: 35711442

# Chapter 9
# Rabies

**Ala'a Fawaz**
*Lebanese University, Lebanon*

**Fatima Al Amin**
https://orcid.org/0009-0003-3453-9151
*Faculty of Medical Sciences, Lebanese University, Beirut, Lebanon*

**Fatima Ahmad Mroueh**
*Lebanese University, Beirut, Lebanon*

**Zeinab Karaki**
*Lebanese University, Beirut, Lebanon*

**Zahraa Awada**
*Lebanese University, Beirut, Lebanon*

**Jina Hasan**
*Lebanese University, Beirut, Lebanon*

## ABSTRACT

*Rabies is a fatal neurological infection caused by the Rabies Virus (RABV) and transmitted through wild animals and unvaccinated pets via saliva contact, especially through bites. The virus enters the CNS, and after a certain incubation period, it causes encephalitic or paralytic symptoms. Diagnosis relies on clinical evaluation and specialized assays, though no effective treatment exists once symptoms appear. Rabies has a variety of risk factors primarily including lack of post-exposure prophylaxis (PEP) and unvaccinated dogs. Transmission routes vary by virus strain and exposure type, affecting incubation periods. Symptoms of this infection include prodromal signs like pruritus and fever, with furious and paralytic forms defining the disease. Prevention involves vaccination—pre-exposure prophylaxis (PrEP) for high-risk individuals and postexposure prophylaxis (PEP) for suspected exposures. However, no effective treatment exists once symptoms manifest. Recent advancements in diagnostic tools and vaccine development aim to enhance detection and preventive strategies..*

DOI: 10.4018/979-8-3693-1990-1.ch009

## INTRODUCTION

Rabies is an acute neurological infection that affects both humans and animals. It is caused by the Rabies Virus (RABV), an enveloped virus with a single-stranded and negative-sense RNA genome and a type species of the Lyssavirus Genus within the Rhabdoviridae family, (Gup et al., 2019). It is mostly transmitted by wild animals such as bats, raccoons, skunks and foxes, and unvaccinated domesticated cats and dogs, (Liu & Cahill, 2020). It is spread through contact between infectious saliva and broken skin or mucous membranes, typically via bites, as well as through scratches or licks, (Fisher, Streicker, & Schnell, 2018). Its particles enter the CNS by budding from muscle cells into the synaptic cleft of neuromuscular junctions (NMJs), this is followed by retrograde axonal transport, replication and assembly in the neuronal cell body, until it is widely distributed in the CNS. The incubation period lasts weeks or longer, followed by a variety of prodromal symptoms. Encephalitic rabies, which is the most common presentation, is associated with episodes of generalised arousal or hyperexcitability and hydrophobia, in which spasms involve the contraction of inspiratory muscles with swallowing. Paralytic rabies, occurring less frequently, is characterised by progressive weakness in the lower motor neurons, (Jackson, 2018). Its diagnosis is usually clinical in the absence of available specific lab tests, (Chaudhary et al., 2021). However, recent advances have paved the way to the improvement or development of several diagnostic assays, including methods for rabies viral antigen and antibody detection and assays for viral nucleic acid detection and identification of specific biomarkers, (Mani & Madhusudana, 2013). Moreover, although the disease is rare, the prognosis is poor: No effective treatment that can save the life of a symptomatic rabies patients is currently available, (Davis, Rall, & Schnell, 2015). Efficacious rabies vaccines have been around for a long time and, combined with stray animal control measures, public health infrastructure, and good clinical evaluation of exposure, the risks posed by terrestrial animals can be minimized. However, effective treatment for the disease remains elusive. Safe and efficacious biologicals for active (vaccines) and passive (HRIG/ERIG) immunization are available, which are extremely valuable in prevention and control of this dreaded disease, (Mahadevan et al., 2016).

## EPIDEMIOLOGY

Rabies remains one of the deadliest infections known in humanity since antiquity with a case-fatality rate approaching 100%, (Mshelbwala et al., 2021). Rabies results in approximately 59,000 fatalities worldwide each year and accounts for a loss of around 3.7 million years of life due to associated diseases. Asia and Africa account for the majority of deaths, (Liu & Cahill, 2020). However, the estimated annual figure of almost 60,000 human rabies fatalities is probably an underestimate, (Fooks et al., 2014). Rabies in the US is rare and is now primarily transmitted through wild animal vectors such as bats, foxes, raccoons, and skunks. There have been two fatalities annually on average since 1980 in the US. Out of the 25 instances of human rabies documented in the US between 2000 and 2007, 20 were domestically acquired. Among those 20 cases, 17 were associated with bat rabies virus variants. The rate of rabies exposures is about 16 to 200 per 100,000 travelers. Approximately 16,000 to 39,000 patients are exposed to rabies and receive PEP annually in the U.S, (Liu & Cahill, 2020). Nevertheless, despite the historical and more recent success in controlling rabies, it continues to be a neglected illness in many developing nations, especially in Asia and Africa where the disease mostly affects the most impoverished segments of the society. As a disease of low priority, surveillance for rabies is woefully inadequate. In turn, the disease impact is not measured or appreciated, and evidence to support the increased spending required to control rabies in dogs remains absent. Given this cycle of neglect, it is not surprising that the best available estimates suggest that around 59,000 human deaths and 3.7 million disability-adjusted life years (DALYs) are lost each year due to canine rabies, and the cumulative cost of economic losses is estimated to be over 8.6 billion US$ every year. In a global context, the pattern of inequality is very marked, with the vast majority of the canine rabies burden falling on Africa and Asia, (Taylor & Nel, 2015).

## RISK FACTORS

Rabies virus is commonly transmitted by animal bites, such as dogs, bats, monkeys, and cats, (Saepudin et al., 2022). 95% of deaths by rabies in Africa and Asia is due to the lack of post-exposure prophylaxis (PEP) for animal-bites. Moreover, a major risk factor is the absence of dogs' vaccinations, that is because rabies vaccines are shown to provide herd immunity and cut off its transmission between the carrying species, (Ling et al., 2023). A study has demonstrated that rabies in humans is mostly found in those under 15 years of age (OR: 4.8, $p = 0.05$), with no previous PEP (OR: 16.7, $p = 0.01$), who didn't wash the bite with soap and water (OR: 17.1, $p = 0.00$), whose bite is in the head (OR: 11.6; $p = 0.00$) and causing a deep wound (OR: 6.1, $p = 0.02$), and where the dog is stray (OR: 13.6, $p = 0.00$) and unvaccinated (OR: 16.7, $p = 0.01$), (Salomão et al., 2017). Regarding the dogs, research has shown that rabies is more prevalent in male dogs (67.75%) than female dogs (32.25%). And 75.53% of the male dogs were uncastrated. Another study shows that dogs of unfenced houses (72.06%) were more susceptible to rabies than those of fenced houses (27.94%), (Roland et al., 2022).

## PATHOGENESIS

RABV is transmitted through different routes. The most typical one is through a bite exposing the skin. It might range from severe bites to insignificant scratches. Other modes of transmission include organ transplantation from an undetected rabies donor or aerosol transmission, (Fooks et al., 2017). The latter occurs via the direct olfactory pathway, (Jackson, 2018).

The chance of getting infected with the dog RABV variant is greatest after serious penetrating bites affecting the muscle. This is because the virus gains its motor entrance route by the nicotinic acetylcholine receptor (nAChR) at the neuromuscular junction. In contrast, the bat RABV variant can cause serious infection through tiny bites due to epidermal proliferation, as demonstrated in vitro. Some particularities of bat variants that have been demonstrated, including a higher prevalence of neuropathic pain, symptoms and signs of Horner syndrome, along with other atypical traits, imply a potential alternative pathway for transmission via sensory neurons, and this needs to be further studied and investigated, (Hemachudha et al., 2013).

Depending on the inoculation site, density of innervations, and virus concentration, the incubation period, which is the time from exposure to the virus to the onset of signs and symptoms, can range from two weeks to six years. Short incubation periods are caused by the larger number and shorter length of neurons, such as injuries to the hands, neck, face, and head, (Davis, Rall, & Schnell, 2015). On the other hand, low inoculum and natural RNA silencing mechanisms slow down viral replication, which results in longer periods, (Hemachudha et al., 2013).

After passing through the synapse, the neuroinvasion begins with centripetal proliferation. The virus is transmitted to the central nervous system via retrograde rapid axonal transmission. The rate of spread is roughly 250 mm every day. Concurrently, the central nervous system (CNS) experiences a centrifugal anterograde spread of RABV into multiple extra-neural organs such as the skin, hair follicles, heart, adrenal glands, tongue, and salivary glands, (Singh et al., 2017). The virus has already spread throughout the central nervous system and peripheral tissues by the time symptoms appear. The most extensively studied receptor in rabies neuronal invasion is the nAChR mentioned above beside additional host receptors or attachment factors, like integrin β1, mGLUT2R, the low-affinity nerve growth factor receptor (p75NTR), neural cell adhesion molecule (NCAM), and heparan sulfate, (Bastos et al., 2023).

In terms of immunity, the earlier the response, the better it is in targeting the virus. Since the CNS is a privileged organ, the immune system is less aggressive in its viral reaction to avoid brain parenchyma destruction. This aids the virus's establishment and spread in the CNS. Furthermore, the virus evades the immune system through its INF type 1 antagonist (phosphoprotein P), which inhibits interferon type 1 induction and slows further immunological responses, (Bastos et al., 2023).

## SIGNS AND SYMPTOMS

After a variable incubation period, rabies usually presents as a prodrome that is followed by an acute phase, which then progresses to coma and death, (Hemachudha et al., 2013). The incubation period of rabies is variable as mentioned earlier but generally averages 1-2 months, (hemachudha, Laothamatas, & Rupprecht, 2002).

The prodrome can start as pruritus, pain, and parathesia at the bite site, and the intense itching can sometimes lead to excoriation, (Bastos et al., 2023) (Hemachudha, Laothamatas, & Rupprecht, 2002). Fatigue, anorexia, headache, trouble sleeping, anxiety, and irritability are also non-specific symptoms that can be present. Moreover, fever occurs in all forms of rabies, (Jackson, 2016).

Rabies can present in 3 forms: furious, paralytic, and non-classic atypical rabies. Both furious and paralytic rabies are known as the classic form of the disease, (Hemachudha, Laothamatas, & Rupprecht, 2002).

### Furious Rabies

This form starts with hyperactivity, which can increase in intensity if stimulated by factors like thirst, light, or noise. Subsequently, the typical signs of furious rabies ensue, which include altered consciousness, phobic and inspiratory spasms, and autonomic disturbances, (Hemachudha, Laothamatas, & Rupprecht, 2002). These signs are often present in most furious rabies patients but may not show up simultaneously and are not apparent once the patient progresses to coma, (Hemachudha et al., 2013). The patient deteriorates and shows more agitation and irritability with time. Simply a breeze of air on the patient's face or chest or just offering a drink can cause phobic spasms, aerophobia, and hydrophobia to manifest, which are important signs. In addition, hypersalivation, temporary dilation or constriction of pupils, localized or generalized piloerection, hyperhidrosis, and spontaneous ejaculations can also be part of the clinical picture, (Hemachudha, Laothamatas, & Rupprecht, 2002).

### Paralytic Rabies

Unlike furious rabies, patients with this form maintain a normal consciousness and mental state at the beginning, (Jackson, 2016). The bitten limb is first affected by flaccid paralysis which progresses in an ascending fashion. It could be symmetric or asymmetric. Moreover, pain and muscle twitching arise along with sensory alterations, inability to voluntarily move the lower limbs or paraplegia, and sphincter disturbances. Hydrophobia is unusual and uncommon in contrast to furious rabies where it's a major sign. In the advanced diseased state, muscles involved in respiration and swallowing become paralyzed as well leading to death, (McKay & Wallis, 2005).

### Non-Classical Rabies

This form is typically noted in patients bitten by bats. The signs and symptoms include radicular and neuropathic pain, difficulties in motor and sensory functions, and problems with coordination like jerking or writhing, (Singh et al., 2017). Other problems that have been noted are ataxia, vertigo, or Horner's syndrome, as well as seizures and hallucinations, with the latter being rather common unlike the other forms, (Hemachudha, Laothamatas, & Rupprecht, 2002).

## DIAGNOSIS

First and foremost, a diagnosis of rabies can't be excluded in the absence of a bite history by a rabid animal, especially if the patient comes from endemic areas, (Hemachudha, Laothamatas, & Rupprecht, 2002). It should also be strongly suspected in any case of acute encephalitis of unknown cause, even more strongly if this case advances to a comatose state in 1-2 weeks, (Gadre et al., 2010).

MRI can be especially useful in differentiating rabies from other conditions with encephalitis; even though it varies between patients, there are still some typical signs, particularly when used in conjunction with other clinical features. Moreover, both classic forms have similar presentations on MRI. These include T2 hyper-intensities in the spinal cord, brainstem, thalamus, limbic system, and white matter, and are seen on images without contrast enhancement. Such changes are seen in stages preceding coma. As for changes to be expected in comatose patients, hyperintense signals can be noted throughout the brainstem and forebrain, (Hemachudha et al., 2013).

Laboratory tests may show normal results or increased white blood cell counts, with mononuclear cells being the most prominent, (Jackson, 2016) (Gadre et al., 2010). Protein may also be slightly increased in CSF studies, while glucose remains unchanged, (Jackson, 2016). Furthermore, identifying rabies specific antibodies in the CSF or blood of unvaccinated patients can be helpful in later stages, as the antibodies usually appear in the second week of infection and onwards, (Gadre et al., 2010). Other tests include the direct fluorescent antibody test (DFA) which can be used on tissues obtained from salivary glands, liver, spleen, pancreas, skin, or brain, (Gelbart, 2019). Tests on brain tissue are especially important in comatose patients who previously presented with encephalitis or paralysis, with DFA testing for the rabies virus antigen being a cheap but highly sensitive option, (Hemachudha, Laothamatas, & Rupprecht, 2002). DFA is also useful in detecting the viral antigen in skin biopsies from the posterior neck, but the biopsies should contain hair follicles, and it's best to obtain several sections, (Jackson, 2016). These skin biopsies or polymerase chain reaction (PCR) can confirm the diagnosis in early stages; PCR can be used on body fluids like saliva, urine, or CSF to detect viral RNA. Recently, a new diagnostic tool called mouse inoculation technique (MIT) is being used where mice are inoculated with saliva from patients, and their fresh tissues are subsequently examined by PCR for rabies virus RNA, (McKay & Wallis, 2005) (Gelbart, 2019).

It is imperative to differentiate paralytic rabies from Guillain-Barre syndrome (GBS), (Singh et al., 2017). Signs which orient toward a diagnosis of paralytic rabies include limb weakness accompanied by fever and bladder problems. Sensation is also typically preserved in paralytic rabies except at the wound site, which is not the case for GBS. Moreover, percussion myoedema can be used as a differentiating sign present in paralytic rabies. This sign is noted as a localized contraction of the muscle when percussed that lasts for a few seconds, and the best sites to be tested are the chest, deltoid, and thigh. The clinician must interpet this sign carefully since it can manifest in other disorders like hyponaterima, SIADH, hypothyroidism, among others, so other conditions must be excluded, (Hemachudha, Laothamatas, & Rupprecht, 2002).

## TREATMENT AND PROPHYLAXIS

Although there is no definitive treatment for rabies, the infection can be prevented through vaccination, (Gelbart, 2019). Rabies vaccines are inactivated virus vaccines inducing an immune response that triggers the differentiation of T cells (CD4+) to initiate the activation of B cells and their proliferation to plasma cells. Then, neutralizing antibodies are produced, and they persist for years, (Weant & Baker, 2013) (Ertl, 2018). The World Health Organization (WHO) prequalification has only approved the efficacy of 3 vaccines: the human diploid cell vaccine (HDCV), the purified chick embryo cell vaccine (PCECV), and the purified Vero cell vaccine (PVRV), (World Health Organization, 2018).

In the US, available cell-culture vaccines are Imovax Rabies (one of the HDCV) and RabAvert (from the PCECV family). RabAvert, based on embryonated eggs, is unsuitable for severe egg allergies, (Weant & Baker, 2013).

The vaccines are administered either intramuscularly (IM) into the deltoid region or the anterolateral area of the thigh in young children and infants or intradermally (ID) into the deltoid region, the anterolateral thigh or suprascapular regions, and it is not allowed to be given subcutaneously, intravascularly, or as a gluteal injection.

Since no preservatives are added to rabies vaccines, they should be stored at 2-8°C, never frozen, then used within six to eight hours. No evidence supports the superiority of one vaccine over another, (Weant & Baker, 2013) (Warrell, 2018) (World Health Organization, 2018).

## Pre-Exposure Prophylaxis (PrEP)

The vaccine can be given before exposure to rabies. This is called pre-exposure prophylaxis. Treating exposed individuals who have received pre-immunization is more straightforward, cost-effective, and safer than those who haven't been immunized. Three 0.5 mL or 1.0 mL intramuscular (IM) or 0.1 mL intradermal (ID) doses of rabies vaccine are given on days 0, 7, and any time between days 21 to 28. ID injection saves time and money due to the less doses needed, (World Health Organization, 2018) (Gherardin & Lau, 2007).

Only high-risk individuals are recommended to take the pre-exposure vaccine. This category of people includes veterinarians, spelunkers, certain laboratory workers handling live rabies and rabies-related viruses, and individuals whose professional or personal activities might lead to direct contact with bats or other mammals that may be infected with rabies such as raccoons, skunks, cats, and dogs, (Gelbart, 2019) (Weant & Baker, 2013) (Gherardin & Lau, 2007).

## Post-Exposure Prophylaxis (PEP)

After exposure to the virus, a post-exposure vaccine is either recommended or not according to the immunization status of the patient and the type of contact with the suspected rabid animal, (World Health Organization, 2018).

First, soap and water should be used to clean the wound whatever its type, with topical use of virucidal antiseptics like povidone iodine and ethanol, and it's better to keep the lesion without a cover. Then, the PEP administration is discussed, (Weant & Baker, 2013). The type of exposure is divided into 3 categories according to the WHO, (Scholand, Quiambao, & Rupprecht, 2022). The first category includes people who have contact with a rabid animal without having any skin lesions. This category doesn't need any PEP. The second category includes superficial wounds without bleeding, and the third category is formed of deep scratches with bleeding, exposures with contaminated mucosa, and bites from rabid animals. These 2 categories require PEP. The only difference is that rabies immune globulin (RIG) is sometimes added in the case of category 3, (World Health Organization, 2018) (Scholand, Quiambao, & Rupprecht, 2022). The PEP dose schedules are summarized in Table 1, (World Health Organization, 2018). RIG is given only in severe cases without previous vaccination. It should be administered concomitantly with the vaccine to provide passive immunity for 7 to 10 days until the body starts developing active immunity in response to the vaccine, (Warrell, 2018).

Overall, treatment involves wound care, RIG administration, and vaccination. Furthermore, the antiviral drugs ribavirin, ketamine, interferon alpha, and midazolam are recommended to treat rabies. Nimodipine was also added to relieve vasospasm, (Hemachudha et al., 2013).

Despite multiple attempted therapies, no treatment is effective after symptoms onset. Supportive care remains the only treatment option. Fatality is unavoidable once symptoms develop, (Weant & Baker, 2013) (Hemachudha et al., 2013) (Smith et al., 2019).

*Table 1. Post-exposure prophylaxis (PEP) by category of exposure*

| | Category I exposure | Category II exposure | Category III exposure |
|---|---|---|---|
| **Immunologically naive individuals of all age groups** | Washing of exposed skin surfaces. No PEP required. | Wound washing and immediate vaccination:<br>▪ 2-sites ID on days 0, 3 and 7 or<br>▪ 1-site IM on days 0, 3, 7 and between day 14–28 or<br>▪ 2-sites IM on days 0 and 1-site IM on days 7, 21(c)<br>RIG is not indicated. | Wound washing and immediate vaccination:<br>▪ 2-sites ID on days 0, 3 and 7 or<br>▪ 1-site IM on days 0, 3, 7 and between day 14–28 or<br>▪ 2-sites IM on days 0 and 1-site IM on days 7, 21<br>RIG administration is recommended. |
| **Previously immunized individuals of all age groups** | Washing of exposed skin surfaces. No PEP required. | Wound washing and immediate vaccination:<br>▪ 1-site ID on days 0 and 3 or<br>▪ 4-sites ID on day 0 or<br>▪ 1-site IM on days 0 and 3<br>RIG is not indicated. | Wound washing and immediate vaccination:<br>▪ 1-site ID on days 0 and 3 or<br>▪ 4-sites ID on day 0 or<br>▪ 1-site IM on days 0 and 3<br>RIG is not indicated. |

**ID:** intradermal injection; **IM:** intramuscular injection; **RIG:** rabies immunoglobulins
Source: (World Health Organization, 2018)

## PROGNOSIS

Human rabies has been an issue since the beginning of time. Although rabies can be effectively averted after a detected exposure, medical care after the clinical disease develops has nearly always been futile, leading to a deadly end, (Rupprecht & Salahuddin, 2019). However, rabies has the unique feature of being almost completely avoidable with timely and proper postexposure treatment. There are safe and effective biologicals available for both active (vaccinations) and passive (HRIG/ERIG) immunization, which are immensely important in the prevention and control of this dreadful disease, (Mahadevan et al., 2016). The detection of anti-rabies virus antibodies at the beginning of a patient's clinical history, which is anticipated to occur in less than 20% of all rabies patients, is considered to be an essential factor leading to a favorable result. Anti-rabies virus antibodies that neutralize the virus are a sign of an active immune system response that is required for viral clearance. Six rabies survivors were given the rabies vaccine before the commencement of their condition. This lends credence to the notion that an early immune response is connected with a favorable outcome. Furthermore, healing from rabies is based on an immunological response that includes viral clearance. To avoid the host immune response, pathogenic strains of the rabies virus use immunosubversive tactics; there is a virally-mediated suppression of the immune system with a diminished cellular-mediated immunity. Furthermore, removal of the virus from the brain is challenging since immune effectors do not permeate the blood-brain barrier or the brain well, (Rupprecht & Salahuddin, 2019). However, correct and fast wound cleansing and post-exposure immunization lower the risk of developing rabies from 50% to less than 5% before the virus enters the neurological system. Following head bites, the risk is greatest. Clothing placement, the extent of tissue injury, and prompt local therapy all influence the prognosis, (Dutta, 2014).

## NOVEL STUDIES

Advances in research are paramount for the discovery and improvement of diagnostic, preventive, therapeutic, and prophylactic techniques, as well as to keep guidelines up-to-date.

In 2017, the WHO created the Strategic Advisory Group of Experts (SAGE) which is responsible fer rabies vaccine and rabies immune globulin (RIG) recommendations. This group has been issuing important updates on human prophylaxis, but hasn't recommended any new treatment strategies for rabies yet, (Rupprecht & Salahuddin, 2019). It has recently updated its guidelines regarding rabies prophylaxis in 2018, which was based on evidence to improve the cost and feasibility and shorten regimens. WHO is now recommending shorter intramuscular PrEP approaches (only done over 3 days), which reduce cost by as much as 30%, or a two-site intradermal PrEP regimen done during a single month duration unlike the prior demand of a three-visit program. Such approaches have been supported by studies for their safety and similar effectiveness, (Pattanaik & Mani, 2019).

Evolutions in diagnostic tools put forward new techniques in hope of facilitating the detection of the disease. These include tests like the direct rapid immunohistochemical test (dRIT), which is a rapid test that can give results in less than an hour, and is characterized by being less costly and more practical with a very high sensitivity and specificity. Another test is the indirect rapid immunohistochemistry test (iRIT) which utilizes light microscopy to detect virus variants and is also cost-effective especially for the use on reservoir hosts. The rapid immunodiagnostic test (RIDT), an immunochromatographic technique, is also promising for animal screening. Other tests based on amplification, including nucleic acid sequence-based amplification (NASBA) and Loop-Mediated Isothermal Amplification (LAMP), are emerging as better options since they need constant temperatures unlike PCR, and thus can be speedy alternatives. There are also new alternatives in antibody detection such as ELISA-based methods and rapid neutralizing antibody detection tests (RAPINA). Moreover, quantitative proteomic analysis is being considered as an option to detect different rabies proteins which can serve as potential biomarkers in diagnosis, (Mani & Madhusudana, 2013) (Rohde & Rupprecht, 2020).

As for treatment strategies, there are increasing efforts to discover anti-viral treatments despite the fatal inevitable outcome of rabies. Drug classes like nucleoside inhibitors are showing promise in stopping viral replication, but the success remains limited to in vitro studies. An example is a drug called Favipiravir. Effectiveness in humans is greatly challenged, and proper animal models are yet to be available, which is leading researchers to consider using naturally occurring rabid animals for experiments, (Rohde & Rupprecht, 2020).

Regarding prevention, efforts have been oriented towards decreasing doses and opting for intra-dermal approaches, with less cumbersome regimens. Pre-exposure prophylaxis has also been a main focus for the past years, and work is being done to develop more effective vaccines. Recently, monoclonal antibodies (Mabs) have emerged as an alternative to RIG with potential applications in animal post-exposure prophylaxis. In addition, purified, more thermo-stable, and serum-free vaccines based on Vero cells are on their way to being licensed. Other techniques being researched include simian-based recombinant adenovirus vaccines as well as flavivirus based ones that express viral glycoproteins. Such recombinant vectors are important to achieve various combinations and an oral route of administration. This route is used on major reservoirs as part of efforts to limit spread, and intradermal PrEP rabies vaccines are being considered for animals that can't receive oral modalities, like hematophagous bats. Moreover, decreasing dog populations and controlling them has been considered, with surgical animal birth control (ABC) being an option, but it requires much logistical planning. All of this serves to achieve the aim of Global Elimination of Human Rabies Deaths (GEHRD) by 2030, which needs immense efforts and collaborative strategies between nations. The immense success of animal vaccination in eradicating rabies sources in developed countries is sufficient evidence to opt for advancing these strategies and working on more integrated and coordinated efforts, (Rupprecht & Salahuddin, 2019) (Rohde & Rupprecht, 2020).

## REFERENCES


Bastos, V., Pacheco, V., Rodrigues, É. D. L., Moraes, C. N. S., Nóbile, A. L., Fonseca, D. L. M., Souza, K. B. S., do Vale, F. Y. N., Filgueiras, I. S., Schimke, L. F., Giil, L. M., Moll, G., Cabral-Miranda, G., Ochs, H. D., Vasconcelos, P. F. da C., de M Bastos, V., Pacheco, V., Rodrigues, É. D. L., Moraes, C. N. S., Nóbile, A. L., Fonseca, D. L. M., Souza, K. B. S., do Vale, F. Y. N., Filgueiras, I. S., Schimke, L. F., Giil, L. M., Moll, G., Cabral-Miranda, G., Ochs, H. D., Vasconcelos, P. F. da C., de Melo, G. D., Bourhy, H., Casseb, L. M. N., & Cabral-Marques, O. (2023). Neuroimmunology of rabies: New insights into an ancient disease. Journal of Medical Virology, 95(10), e29042. [Online]. Available: ,DOI: 10.1002/jmv.29042

Chaudhary, S. C., Khandelwal, A., Tandon, R., & Sawlani, K. K. (2021). Rabies encephalitis. BMJ case reports, 14(4), e239249., [Online]. Available: .DOI: 10.1136/bcr-2020-239249

Davis, B. M., Rall, G. F., & Schnell, M. J. (2015). Everything You Always Wanted to Know About Rabies Virus (But Were Afraid to Ask). Annual review of virology, 2(1), 451–471., [Online]. Available: .DOI: 10.1146/annurev-virology-100114-055157

Dutta, Tarun Kumar. Rabies: An overview. International Journal of Advanced Medical and Health Research 1(2):p 39-44, Jul–Dec 2014., [Online]. Available: .DOI: 10.4103/2349-4220.147998

Ertl H. C. J. (2018). Human immune responses to traditional and novel rabies vaccines. Human immune responses to traditional and novel rabies vaccines. Revue scientifique et technique (International Office of Epizootics), 37(2), 649–656. [Online]. Available: DOI: 10.20506/rst.37.2.2830

Fisher, C. R., Streicker, D. G., & Schnell, M. J. (2018). The spread and evolution of rabies virus: conquering new frontiers. Nature reviews. Microbiology, 16(4), 241–255., [Online]. Available: .DOI: 10.1038/nrmicro.2018.11

Fooks, A. R., Banyard, A. C., Horton, D. L., Johnson, N., McElhinney, L. M., & Jackson, A. C. (2014). Current status of rabies and prospects for elimination. Lancet (London, England), 384(9951), 1389–1399., [Online]. Available: .DOI: 10.1016/S0140-6736(13)62707-5

Fooks, A. R., Cliquet, F., Finke, S., Freuling, C., Hemachudha, T., Mani, R. S., Müller, T., Nadin-Davis, S., Picard-Meyer, E., Wilde, H., & Banyard, A. C. (2017). Rabies. Nature Reviews Disease Primers, 3(1), 17091., [Online]. Available: .DOI: 10.1038/nrdp.2017.9

Gadre, G., Satishchandra, P., Mahadevan, A., Suja, M. S., Madhusudana, S. N., Sundaram, C., & Shankar, S. K. (2010). Rabies viral encephalitis: clinical determinants in diagnosis with special reference to paralytic form. Journal of neurology, neurosurgery, and psychiatry, 81(7), 812–820., [Online]. Available: DOI: 10.1136/jnnp.2009.185504

Gelbart D. (2019). Rabies. JAAPA: official journal of the American Academy of Physician Assistants, 32(10), 46–47., [Online]. Available: .DOI: 10.1097/01.JAA.0000580572.87216.17

Gherardin, A., & Lau, S. (2007). Intradermal rabies vaccine. The Medical journal of Australia, 187(1), 58–59., [Online]. Available: .DOI: 10.5694/j.1326-5377.2007.tb01128.x

Hemachudha, T., Laothamatas, J., & Rupprecht, C. E. (2002). Human rabies: a disease of complex neuropathogenetic mechanisms and diagnostic challenges. The Lancet. Neurology, 1(2), 101–109., [Online]. Available: .DOI: 10.1016/S1474-4422(02)00041-8

Hemachudha, T., Ugolini, G., Wacharapluesadee, S., Sungkarat, W., Shuangshoti, S., & Laothamatas, J. (2013). Human rabies: Neuropathogenesis, diagnosis, and management. The Lancet Neurology, 12(5), 498–513, [Online]. Available: .DOI: 10.1016/S1474-4422(13)70038-3

Jackson A. C. (2016). Human Rabies: a 2016 Update. Current infectious disease reports, 18(11), 38., [Online]. Available: .DOI: 10.1007/s11908-016-0540-y

Jackson A. C. (2018). Rabies: a medical perspective. Rabies: a medical perspective. Revue scientifique et technique (International Office of Epizootics), 37(2), 569–580., [Online]. Available: .DOI: 10.20506/rst.37.2.2825

Jane Ling, M. Y., Halim, A. F. N. A., Ahmad, D., Ramly, N., Hassan, M. R., Syed Abdul Rahim, S. S., Saffree Jeffree, M., Omar, A., & Hidrus, A. (2023). Rabies in Southeast Asia: a systematic review of its incidence, risk factors and mortality. BMJ open, 13(5), e066587, [Online]. Available: , [Online].DOI: 10.1136/bmjopen-2022-066587

Liu, C., & Cahill, J. D. (2020). Epidemiology of Rabies and Current US Vaccine Guidelines. Rhode Island medical journal (2013), 103(6), 51–53., [Online]. Available: https://pubmed.ncbi.nlm.nih.gov/32752569/

Mahadevan, A., Suja, M. S., Mani, R. S., & Shankar, S. K. (2016). Perspectives in Diagnosis and Treatment of Rabies Viral Encephalitis: InsightsfromPathogenesis. Neurotherapeutics: the journal of the American Society for Experimental NeuroTherapeutics, 13, (3), 477–492., [Online]. Available: DOI: 10.1007/s13311-016-0452-4

Mani, R. S., & Madhusudana, S. N. (2013). Laboratory diagnosis of human rabies: recent advances. TheScientificWorldJournal, 2013, 569712., [Online]. Available: .DOI: 10.1155/2013/569712

McKay, N., & Wallis, L. (2005). Rabies: a review of UK management. Emergency medicine journal: EMJ, 22(5), 316–321., [Online]. Available: .DOI: 10.1136/emj.2003.013805

Mshelbwala, P. P., Weese, J. S., Sanni-Adeniyi, O. A., Chakma, S., Okeme, S. S., Mamun, A. A., Rupprecht, C. E., & Magalhaes, R. J. S. (2021). Rabies epidemiology, prevention and control in Nigeria: Scoping progress towards elimination. PLoS neglected tro tropical diseases, 15(8), e0009617., [Online]. Available: DOI: 10.1371/journal.pntd.0009617

Pattanaik, A., & Mani, R. S. (2019). WHO's new rabies recommendations: implications for high incidence countries. Current opinion in infectious diseases, 32(5), 401–406., [Online]. Available: .DOI: 10.1097/QCO.0000000000000578

Rohde, R. E., & Rupprecht, C. E. (2020). Update on lyssaviruses and rabies: will past progress play as prologue in the near term towards future elimination?. Faculty reviews, 9, 9., [Online]. Available: .DOI: 10.12703/b/9-9

Roland, S., Benjamin, E., Patrick, B. V., Juana, M., & Derrick, A. (2022). Seroprevalence and predisposing factors of rabies antibodies in unvaccinated dogs in Sierra Leone. Veterinary medicine and science, 8(6), 2345–2350. https://doi.org/, [Online]. Available: https://doi.org/.DOI: 10.1002/vms3

Rupprecht, C. E., & Salahuddin, N. (2019). Current status of human rabies prevention: remaining barriers to global biologics accessibility and disease elimination. Expert review of vaccines, 18(6), 629–640., [Online]. Available: .DOI: 10.1080/14760584.2019.1627205

Saepudin, M., Pranaka, R. N., Umboh, H. H., & Wardoyo, S. (2022). Risk factors associated with rabies incidence in rabies endemic areas in West Kalimantan. Germs, 12(4), 472–477., [Online]. Available: .DOI: 10.18683/germs.2022.1353

Salomão, C., Nacima, A., Cuamba, L., Gujral, L., Amiel, O., Baltazar, C., Cliff, J., & Gudo, E. S. (2017). Epidemiology, clinical features and risk factors for human rabies and animal bites during an outbreak of rabies in Maputo and Matola cities, Mozambique, 2014: Implications for public health interventions for rabies control. PLoS neglected tropical diseases, 11(7), e0005787., [Online]. Available: DOI: 10.1371/journal.pntd.0005787

Scholand, S. J., Quiambao, B. P., & Rupprecht, C. E. (2022). Time to Revise the WHO Categories for Severe Rabies Virus Exposures-Category IV?. Viruses, 14(5), 1111., [Online]. Available: .DOI: 10.3390/v14051111

Singh, R., Singh, K. P., Cherian, S., Saminathan, M., Kapoor, S., Manjunatha Reddy, G. B., Panda, S., & Dhama, K. (2017). Rabies - epidemiology, pathogenesis, public health concerns and advances in diagnosis and control: A comprehensive review. The Veteri nary Quarterly, 37(1), 212–251., [Online]. Available: DOI: 10.1080/01652176.2017.1343516

Smith, S. P., Wu, G., Fooks, A. R., Ma, J., & Banyard, A. C. (2019). Trying to treat the untreatable: experimental approaches to clear rabies virus infection from the CNS. The Journal of general virology, 100(8), 1171–1186. [Online]. Available: DOI: 10.1099/jgv.0.001269

Taylor, L. H., & Nel, L. H. (2015). Global epidemiology of canine rabies: past, present, and future prospects. Veterinary medicine (Auckland, N.Z.), 6, 361–371., [Online]. Available: .DOI: 10.2147/VMRR.S51147

Warrell M. J. (2018). Developments in human rabies prophylaxis. Developments in human rabies prophylaxis. Revue scientifique et technique (International Office of Epizootics), 37(2), 629–647., [Online]. Available: .DOI: 10.20506/rst.37.2.2829

Weant, K. A., & Baker, S. N. (2013). Review of human rabies prophylaxis and treatment. Critical care nursing clinics of North America, 25(2), 225–242., [Online]. Available: .DOI: 10.1016/j.ccell.2013.02.001

World Health Organization (2018). Rabies vaccines: WHO position paper, April 2018 - Recommendations. Vaccine, 36(37), 5500–5503, [Online]. Available: .DOI: 10.1016/j.vaccine.2018.06.061

Yousaf, M. Z., Qasim, M., Zia, S., Khan, M.u, Ashfaq, U. A., & Khan, S. (2012). Rabies molecular virology, diagnosis, prevention and treatment. Virology journal, 9, 50., [Online]. Available: .DOI: 10.1186/1743-422X-9-50

# Chapter 10
# Unraveling Coxsackie and Echovirus, Epidemiology, Pathogenesis, and Global Challenges: From Molecular Mechanisms to Clinical Realities and Global Health Implications

**Ali Saad Al-shammari**
https://orcid.org/0000-0002-4298-5456
*College of Medicine, University of Baghdad, Iraq*

**Hussein Mohsin Hasan**
https://orcid.org/0009-0002-5297-2664
*College of Medicine, University of Baghdad, Iraq*

**Noora Madhloom Naji Naji**
*College of Medicine, University of Nahrain, Iraq*

**Noran Muhsen Rashid Al-Gizey**
*College of Medicine, University of Baghdad, Iraq*

**Yasmeen Amer Fadhel Tawfeeq**
*Azerbaijan Medical University, Iraq*

**Raghda Amer Fadhel Tawfeeq**
*College of Medicine, University of Kirkuk, Iraq*

**Sajjad Ghanim Al-Badri**
*College of Medicine, University of Baghdad, Iraq*

**May Saad Al-Jorani**
https://orcid.org/0000-0002-2710-2600
*College of Medicine, University of Al-Mustansiriyah, Iraq*

**Nabeel Hamzah Kadhim Al-Fatlawi**
*College of Medicine, University of Baghdad, Iraq*

DOI: 10.4018/979-8-3693-1990-1.ch010

**Abdullah Muataz Taha Al-Ibraheem**
https://orcid.org/0009-0006-8575-0119
*Al-Kindy College of Medicine, University of Baghdad, Iraq*

## ABSTRACT

*This chapter delves into Coxsackie and Echovirus, pervasive enteroviruses causing a range of illnesses from mild to severe. It examines their molecular biology, epidemiology, and impact on global health, particularly in vulnerable populations like neonates. The discussion includes transmission methods, clinical challenges, and the dire need for effective treatments and preventive measures. The absence of vaccines and the difficulties in managing outbreaks, especially in underprivileged areas, are also highlighted.*

## INTRODUCTION

### Coxsackie Virus

Belongs to Enterovirus in the Picornaviridae family, with single-strand RNA, inhabiting the human digestive tract, (Muckelbauer *et al.,* 1995). Transferred through unclean hands and feces-contaminated surfaces. Usually it results in mild flu-like symptoms, occasionally leading to severe conditions. Isolated in 1948 during a study on paralytic poliomyelitis in Coxsackie, New York, (Gamble, 1962). Often asymptomatic but can cause fever, especially in young children and infants, (Stewart *et al.,* 2013). Two main serotypes, A and B, causing diseases like Herpangina and aseptic meningitis, (Wright *et al*., 1963; Swann, 1961) can lead to more severe conditions like meningitis in some cases.

### ECHO Virus

ECHO viruses are positive-sense single-stranded RNA viruses linked to various diseases, (Klein, Eggers, & Nelsen-Salz, 2000). Subset of Enterovirus B, encompassing 29 serotypes, causing skin rashes and infections. Often asymptomatic but can cause fever; severity varies based on factors like age, immune status, and viral strain, (Somekh *et al.,* 2001). This can lead to serious illnesses such as aseptic meningitis, encephalitis, paralysis, and myocarditis. Originally classified into 34 serotypes, with some reclassified as other viruses, (Rosen et al., 1970; Tyrrell, 1963). Small nonenveloped viruses with an icosahedral configuration, resistant to ether and alcohol, (Tinari *et al.,* 2005). Males appear more susceptible to clinical illness, particularly aseptic meningitis, (Codd et al., 1976). ECHO virus infection during pregnancy can lead to dangerous consequences, (Tassin *et al.,* 2014).

## General Overview

Coxsackie and echoviruses are enteroviruses, which are small RNA viruses that frequently infect the throat and gastrointestinal tract, (Pons-Salort, Parker, & Grassly, 2015). Simply said, they are common viruses that frequently result in hand-foot-and-mouth disease (a rash that causes blisters on the hands, feet, and mouth), mild flu-like illness, or no symptoms at all. A minor percentage of infections can cause major issues including viral meningitis (an infection of the brain's lining), myocarditis (inflammation of the heart), or paralysis, but the majority are moderate or asymptomatic, (Pons-Salort, Parker, & Grassly, 2015). Unwashed hands, tainted food or water, or respiratory droplets are just a few of the ways that these viruses spread among individuals, particularly in crowded or unsanitary environments. The viruses can spread widely before being discovered since many cases are difficult to identify (because of the mild symptoms). Each of the two types of coxsackieviruses, A and B, tends to cause slightly distinct diseases. Children who catch Group A Coxsackieviruses (such as strains A6, A16) are known to develop herpangina, or painful mouth blisters, and hand-foot-and-mouth disease, (Pons-Salort, Parker, & Grassly, 2015). Group B Coxsackieviruses, on the other hand, frequently attack internal organs; they have been connected to viral heart infections (myocarditis), outbreaks of chest discomfort (Bornholm syndrome), and even initiators of long-term illnesses like type 1 diabetes, (Pons-Salort, Parker, & Grassly, 2015). Echoviruses are another subset of enteroviruses that usually cause non-specific fevers, skin rashes, or colds and it is One of the most frequent causes of aseptic meningitis outbreaks (viral meningitis) worldwide.

In conclusion, public health experts closely monitor Coxsackie and Echoviruses because, although they typically only cause fever and rash in children, everyone should be aware that they can occasionally cause serious illness, particularly in newborns or those with weakened immune systems.

## EPIDEMIOLOGY AND PREVALENCE IN DEVELOPING AND DEVELOPED NATIONS

ECHO and Coxsackie viruses are prevalent throughout the year, peaking in the summer and fall in temperate regions, (Moore, 1982). Infants under one year experience higher infection rates compared to older children and adults, with males exhibiting up to a 50% higher risk than females, (Gelfand *et al.,* 1963; Wilfert *et al.,*

1975). Transmission primarily occurs through contact with virus-laden respiratory secretions and fecal matter, with enhanced risk in areas of poor sanitation, (Couch *et al.*, 1970; Midgley *et al.*, 2015). Notably, Enterovirus D70 can also be transmitted through tears, (Onorato *et al.,* 1985). Infections among household contacts, especially from infants, are notably high, (Kogon *et al.,* 1969; Chang *et al.,* 2004). The impact of individual virus serotypes varies widely, with some causing endemic diseases and others leading to large-scale outbreaks, (Gondo *et al.,* 1995; Centers for Disease Control and Prevention, 1991). Recent data from 2022 in the United States identified enterovirus D68 and human parechovirus 3 as the most prevalent serotypes, (Centers for Diease Control and Prevention, 2022). Specific serotypes like Coxsackievirus A6 and Enterovirus D68 have been linked to distinct outbreaks of atypical diseases and respiratory illnesses, respectively, (Ayscue *et al.,* 2014). Similarly, Enterovirus A71 has been associated with severe regional epidemics in the Asia-Pacific region, (Schmidt, Lennette, & Ho, 1974; Miwa *et al.,* 1980). Enteroviruses, including Echovirus and Coxsackievirus, exhibit a distinct epidemiology: they are more prevalent in warmer climates and areas with poor hygiene and overcrowding, showing a seasonal peak in warmer months as per WHO data. In cooler countries, their incidence decreases during colder periods. These viruses predominantly affect children, with the majority of infections occurring in those under 14 years old. Their clinical manifestations often involve the central nervous system, primarily presenting as aseptic meningitis, with varying symptoms depending on the virus type. Interestingly, a notable portion of group B coxsackievirus infections are associated with cardiac features. The increasing reports of these infections may indicate either the expansion of virus laboratory activities or the emergence of new diseases, with a trend towards affecting older age groups due to improved hygiene delaying virus circulation in early childhood, (Grist, Bell, & Reid, 1975), Coxsackie virus infections peaked in spring (34.6%), showing a statistically significant increase compared to other seasons. In contrast, Echo virus infections predominantly occurred in autumn and winter (62.2%), with the infection rate generally decreasing with age. However, an exception was noted for Echo viruses, which infected individuals aged 19-60 years more than younger age groups (0-6 years) (Sidiropoulou *et al.,* n.d.).

## Global Impact and Socioeconomic Burden

Global prevalence: Millions of people worldwide are infected with coxsackie and echoviruses each year, (Centers for Disease Control and Prevention, 2022).

These non-polio enteroviruses are now the most common causes of viral nerve system illnesses in the post-polio period. For instance, enteroviruses currently cause the majority of meningitis infections across all age groups in nations where bacterial meningitis and polio have been successfully prevented by immunization, (Kadambari *et al.,* 2024). Every continent reports breakouts on a regular basis, demonstrating that no area is completely immune, (Centers for Disease Control and Prevention, 2022). Importantly, a large number of illnesses affect infants and children, occasionally overburdening pediatric wards during seasonal spikes. Health burden: The public health burden is high due to the high number of infections, even if individual cases are typically mild. A common example is Hand-Foot-and-Mouth Disease (HFMD), a prevalent pediatric disease brought on by Coxsackie A16, EV-A71, and others has grown to be a significant public health concern in the Asia-Pacific region. According to a recent analysis, HFMD causes high-burden Asian countries to lose around 96,900 disability-adjusted life years (DALYs) annually, (Koh *et al.*, 2018). Practically speaking, that DALY number represents significant healthcare use and lost workdays. Large outbreaks can put a strain on healthcare systems; for example, the 2011 HFMD outbreak in Vietnam resulted in almost 200,000 recorded cases and 200 fatalities, placing a demand on hospital resources, (Nhan *et al.,* 2020). Even though enteroviral meningitis is typically self-limited, outbreaks also result in expenses for lumbar punctures, hospital stays, and infection control procedures.

> Economic burden: It is becoming more widely acknowledged that Coxsackie/Echo virus outbreaks have a negative economic impact. Hospitalized HFMD cases in just two years resulted in an estimated around $90 million US dollars in direct and indirect expenditures, according to a 2016–2017 study conducted in Vietnam, (Nhan *et al.*, 2019).

Beijing's yearly economic losses from HFMD, which include both direct medical expenses and indirect costs from missed productivity during seasonal epidemics, range from US $7.03 million to US $13.31 million, (Shen *et al.,* 2023).

The following are the average total costs per HFMD episode, according to a nationwide Chinese survey conducted in 2012–2013:

> For mild outpatients, US$201
> For mild inpatients, US $1,072
> For serious cases, US $3,051

These include caregivers' salary cuts, highlighting the strain on families when parents are forced to skip work, (Zheng *et al.,* 2017).

In addition to financial costs, outbreaks have a social cost since they disturb routines and instill anxiety (e.g., school and nursery closures during HFMD epidemics). Enterovirus infections can be fatal in neonatal units; in Europe, a recent outbreak of severe Echovirus-11 infections in newborns led to seven fatalities out of nine cases, triggering global concerns.

These catastrophes highlight the significant financial and personal costs that communities may incur from sporadic enterovirus epidemics.

## Risk Factors

Enterovirus infections in neonates, including Coxsackievirus and Echovirus, are influenced by a multitude of risk factors, encompassing a variety of neonatal and maternal health aspects, biological indicators, socioeconomic and lifestyle elements, infection-specific variables, and potential complications. The vulnerability to severe infection is notably heightened in premature infants, a risk further amplified by a maternal history of viral illness.

Biologically, certain markers such as a higher White Blood Cell (WBC) count, reduced hemoglobin levels, and elevated bilirubin levels, particularly in cases involving hepatic necrosis, are indicative of a more severe infection trajectory. Socioeconomic factors also play a significant role; lower socioeconomic status and the absence of breastfeeding are strongly correlated with increased risks of infection.

Specific serotypes of the virus, including Echovirus 11 and Coxsackievirus B, are associated with more serious infections. Neonates presenting with multi-systemic disease and hepatic necrosis are at particularly high risk. The presence of concurrent myocarditis, especially in cases of fatal hepatic necrosis, emerges as a critical risk factor, (Lin *et al*., 2003). In terms of Echovirus, specific serotypes like Echovirus 11 are closely linked to severe cases in newborns. Gender plays a role, with male infants showing a higher frequency of severe Echovirus disease. Transmission routes for Echovirus are diverse, including both vertical transmission from an infected mother and nosocomial transmission through contact with hospital staff. Furthermore, the pattern of outbreaks is influenced by geographical and climatic factors; cooler regions typically see a spike in cases during the warmer months, whereas tropical areas are prone to year-round occurrences, (Modlin, 1986). Collectively, these diverse factors contribute to a holistic understanding of the intricate dynamics and challenges inherent in managing enterovirus infections.

# ENVIRONMENTAL FACTORS IN VIRAL SPREAD

## Hygiene and Sanitation

Environmental factors are crucial in the transmission of coxsackie and echoviruses because they spread by respiratory droplets and the fecal-oral pathway. Enterovirus circulation is higher in areas with low sanitation, such as those with limited hand-washing facilities, insufficient sewage systems, or a lack of clean water. Because these viruses may live on surfaces and in water, epidemics have previously been brought on by tainted drinking water or swimming pools. Improvements in sanitation, on the other hand, are believed to postpone enterovirus exposure. Children actually tend to come into contact with these viruses later in life as nations progress and cleanliness improves, which paradoxically can result in more symptomatic illnesses (older children or adults produce larger inflammatory responses). This "hygiene delay" theory has been used to explain why teens and adults in some areas began experiencing uncommon outbreaks after missing early childhood diseases. In general, strict personal cleanliness and clean surroundings lessen (but do not completely eradicate) the spread of these resilient infections.

## Urbanization and Crowding

Rapid urbanization has produced crowded areas that are perfect for the spread of viruses. Person-to-person transmission of enteroviruses is facilitated by close contact in congested cities, childcare facilities, and educational institutions. According to a recent big study conducted in China, the incidence of enteroviral infections was more than twice as high in urban regions as in rural ones (around 2.1 times higher). Due to higher contact rates and population densities, urban children are more prone than their rural counterparts to undergo HFMD outbreaks. However, outbreaks may go unnoticed in rural areas with inadequate infrastructure. Unfortunately, the environment is ideal for enterovirus outbreaks in areas of violence or refugee camps, where overcrowding and poor sanitation coexist. Thus, infrastructure and population density are important environmental factors that influence the propagation of the Coxsackie/Echo virus.

## Climate and Seasonality

Seasonality is apparent in enteroviruses. While Coxsackie and Echo infections can spread throughout the year in tropical places (with slight surges during hotter, wet seasons), they peak in temperate climes throughout the summer and early fall. It is believed that these viruses are more stable and spread more easily in warmer, more humid environments. There is growing evidence that enterovirus epidemics may be exacerbated by climate change. According to a new study on climate modeling, in the worst-case scenarios, enterovirus outbreak sizes could rise by as much as 40% by the end of this century. The mechanism is that the geographic range and seasonal window for enterovirus transmission are expanded by hotter summers and milder winters. In summary, enterovirus epidemiology is significantly influenced by environmental factors: Uncrowded living and proper sanitation slow the spread of viruses, but urbanization and climate change are likely to make it easier for them to spread. Planning for public health must therefore take these environmental factors into account, including enhancing water and sanitation facilities and keeping an eye on how changes in the climate may affect the patterns of virus circulation.

## Pathogenesis

The Coxsackie virus, part of the Enterovirus which includes type A and B coxsackie viruses, the gastrointestinal tract is mostly affected by the Coxsackie virus, it is transferred by respiratory droplets as well as feco-oral transmission. Once within the host, the virus replicates and targets the gastrointestinal epithelium and lymphoid tissues, which could propagate to other sites. The coxsackie and adenovirus receptor (CAR), which is found on a variety of cell types, including lymphocytes, is the primary target of the virus. Following its attachment to the receptor, the virus enters the cell, releases its genetic material, Multiple organs (heart, liver, brain, kidney, lung, pancreas, spleen) become chronically infected with CVB. The majority of these tissues still have significant virus titers, (Mena *et al.,* 1999). Coxsackie viruses are encased in an icosahedral capsid, a spherical protein shell composed of twenty equilateral triangle faces. They are known as naked viruses because they lack a lipid membrane. They are positive sense single strand viruses, meaning that their RNA is Mrna. The host cell's ribosomes use this Mrna to form a single, long polyprotein chain, which is subsequently broken up by viral protease. All of this occurs in the cytoplasm of the cell host, where ribosomes are present and produce multiple viral proteins. A study found that TLR4 on mast cells and macrophages was shown to be upregulated by coxsackie virus infection right after infection. Critical pro inflammatory cytokine levels are elevated in susceptible mice, and they also have higher mast cell counts and develop chronic autoimmune heart disease, (Fairweather, Frisancho-Kiss, & Rose, 2005; Rose, 2008). Common infectious agents called coxsackie viruses have been related to the development of autoimmune conditions like type 1 diabetes and chronic autoimmune myocarditis. An improper immune reaction against self-antigens causes autoimmune disease. Tissue deterioration resulting in organ-specific or systemic disorders may arise from this. Tissue destruction is ultimately caused by the adaptive immune system, specifically autoreactive T cells or antibodies, Common human pathogens, the group B coxsackie virus (serotypes 1-6) have been associated to more serious acute illnesses like myocarditis, encephalitis, pericarditis, and meningitis in addition to mild infections, (Kaplan *et al.,* 1983). in addition to chronic illness the pathogenesis marked by immune cell infiltration that results in tissue damage, scarring, and fibrosis deposition. This ultimately causes the heart to enlarge, contractile function to be lost, and Dilated cardiomyopathy to develop, (Fairweather *et al.*, 2001). Coxsackievirus A16 Typically enters through mouth and respiratory tract replicates in mucous membranes of the throat and tonsils then spreads and causes skin lesion, with VP1–VP4 making up the icosahedron-shaped viral capsid. The RNA-dependent RNA polymerase (3D) protein causes multiple mutations during EV replication because it lacks a proofreading function. VP1, VP2, and VP3 form an extensive canyon at the surface of the capsid that serves as the receptor-binding site, (Lei *et al.*, 2015).

## Echo

Enteric cytopathic human orphan (Echo) virus belongs to a group of viruses called enteroviruses, non – polio enteroviruses lead to gastrointestinal infection, The increasing incidence of type I DM has also been linked to multiple echovirus serotypes. Recent Research has demonstrated that enterovirus infections in both groups were frequently linked to increases in islet cell antibody and/or insulin autoantibody titers, as shown by using non serotype specific EIA and RIA, (Roivainen *et al.,* 1998). the cytotoxic stage of the virus in the pancreas may directly cause β cell lysis, (Bopegamage & Petrovicová, 1994). When self-antigens and viral antigens share antigenic determinants, T cells may cross-react; this phenomenon is known as molecular mimicry, Viral infections have the potential to cause localized production of cytokines and other mediators of inflammation, which could have a direct toxic effect on β cells, (Kaufman *et al.,* 1993). Decay-accelerating factor (DAF) serves as the cellular receptor for a large number of echoviruses. Most cell surfaces contain DAF, a glycosylphosphatidylinositol-anchored complement regulatory protein. It keeps cells safe from complement attack, (He *et al.*, 2002). In molecular biology, phage display is a technique used to study interactions between proteins and DNA. Scientists can choose particular peptides that interact with binding affinities for a target interest, such as proteins or antibodies, by expressing foreign peptides on the surface of bacteriophages, Echo virus binding peptides were selected from phage display peptide libraries containing random peptides from five to nine amino acids, each peptide flanked by cysteine residues. Microtiter wells were coated with the purified viruses, (Pulli, Koivunen, & Hyypiä, 1997).

Viral replication in target organs causes cell damage and immune responses as part of the pathogenesis of echoviruses. The virus may occasionally spread to the central nervous system and cause neurological symptoms. There have been increasing outbreaks of echovirus 11 (E11), particularly in young children it has affinity for nerve tissues, exhibiting neurotropism the virus can invade and replicate in neurons, (Zhang *et al.,* 2021).

Viremia can occur when a virus enters the bloodstream. The virus spreads to different organs, including the liver, (Wang *et al.,* 2001). Hepatic venous endothelium and vascular endothelium are both affected by viruses. Important host factors involved in echovirus pathogenesis include expression of the human homologue of the neonatal Fc receptor (hFcRn), the primary receptor for echoviruses, and inhibition of type I interferon (IFN) signaling causes Severe hepatitis is a characteristic of newborn echovirus infections, (Wells *et al.*, 2021). According to studies, EV1 enters the cell quickly and travels with VLA-2 to early endosomes after binding to VLA-2 on the apical surface of polarized epithelial cells. The entry of the virus requires membrane cholesterol and dynamin GTPase but is not dependent on either caveolin or clathrin-mediated endocytosis. That demonstrates how different substances that interfere with macropinocytosis were able to prevent virus internalization and infection echo virus was found EV1 internalization into Caco-2 cells used to prevent macropinocytosis, (Krieger *et al.,* 2013).

## Genomic Variability and Its Implications

Significant genetic heterogeneity is exhibited by coxsackie and echoviruses, which has significant consequences for vaccine development, public health, and disease severity. These are fast-mutating RNA viruses that often recombine (swap genetic components) with one another. Consequently, there are more than 100 different enterovirus serotypesm (24)and fresh variations keep appearing. For instance, in the last ten years, recombination events among Coxsackie A viruses have produced novel lineages of Coxsackie A6, some of which have caused atypical outbreaks or spread more quickly, (Song *et al.,* 2020). A dominant CVA6 strain produced at least two new recombinant groups that spread over populations with various clinical symptoms, according to a Chinese study. These results demonstrate how genomic rearrangement may change a virus's pathogenicity, or capacity to cause disease. The emergent lineages in the CV-A6 case were linked to extensive HFMD outbreaks, which made the health of children more at risk,, (Song *et al.,* 2020).

Coxsackie/Echo viruses' tremendous genetic diversity has a number of practical repercussions. First, a single serotype infection typically offers little to no defense against other serotypes. Due to different viral strains, a child may contract HFMD from CV-A6 one year and then from EV-A71 or CV-A16 the next year. Because a vaccination against one enterovirus (such as EV-A71) won't protect against a variety of other co-circulating enteroviruses causing identical symptoms, this serotype diversity impedes the development of vaccines, (Zhu *et al.,* 2023).

In fact, EV71 cases decreased after China introduced an EV-A71 vaccination, but Coxsackie viruses (A6, A16, etc.) swiftly took over as the main causes of HFMD. To increase protection, researchers are currently working on multivalent vaccinations that incorporate multiple enterovirus antigens, (Zhu *et al.,* 2023). Second, the virus may adapt to evade immunization or antivirals due to genetic diversity. For example, research indicates that spontaneous mutations in the viral capsid might alter antigenicity, making it impossible for antibodies or antiviral medications to bind. This evolutionary flexibility is highlighted by the recent appearance of more neurovirulent EV-D68 clades and vaccine-escape EV-A71 strain, (Centers for Disease Control and Prevention, 2022).

Third, public health now prioritizes strong genetic surveillance. Scientists quickly sequenced the virus genomes in response to rare outbreaks; such the devastating newborn Echovirus-11 outbreak in Europe in 2022–2023. They found that the European E-11 strains in France and Italy shared nearly the same genetic makeup, indicating that a virulent lineage had expanded globally. Real-time sharing of such sequencing data facilitates the tracking of transmission and the identification of novel mutations. In conclusion, the Coxsackie and Echo viruses are always changing at the genetic level. Because of this unpredictability, we must remain watchful, updating vaccinations and diagnostic tests to reflect the evolution of the viruses and keeping an eye out for novel strains that could lead to the next outbreak, (World Health Organization, 2023).

## Symptoms and Signs

Coxsackievirus infections, which result from enteroviruses belonging to the Enterovirus genus, may present with diverse symptoms. The prevalent strains, Coxsackie A and Coxsackie B viruses, are responsible for a spectrum of illnesses such as hand, foot, and mouth disease (HFMD), herpangina, and viral myocarditis, (de Crom *et al.*, 2016). Below are typical symptoms and indicators linked with Coxsackievirus A infection.

Hand, foot, and mouth disease (HFMD) is a common viral illness that can affect infants and children as well as adults. (HFMD) is commonly associated with coxsackievirus A16 or enterovirus 71, (Woodland, 2019).The usual manifestation is discomforting vesicular rash on the oral mucosa, and subsequently, the development of papulovesicular eruptions on the palms and soles, and even the genitals and buttocks with a mild fever, generally below 383°C. This occurs after an incubation period of 3 to 5 days. Spontaneous recovery typically takes place within 7 to 10 days, (Second *et al.,* 2017).

Herpangina, the onset of herpangina is usually sudden, accompanied by elevated fever ranging from 38.9 to 40°C (102 to 104°F). Occasionally, fever can reach up to 40.6°C (105°F). The onset of fever may also be accompanied by seizures. By examination, herpangina is characterized by the presence of oral ulcers on the anterior tonsillar pillars, soft palate, buccal mucosa, or the uvula. The infection is typically self-limiting, with symptoms resolving within a week to ten days. Supportive care, including pain relief and maintaining hydration, is the primary approach to managing herpangina, (Mirand *et al.,* 2012).

It also can cause hemorrhagic conjunctivitis, a condition impacting the sclera of the eyes, typically initiates with eye discomfort, swiftly progressing to redness, watery eyes, swelling, sensitivity to light, and blurred vision, (Sklar *et al.*, 1983).

Manifestations of viral infection within the Coxsackie B category encompass symptoms such as headaches, fever, sore throat, gastrointestinal discomfort, profound fatigue, and pleurodynia or Bornholm disease which is painful spasms of the chest and upper abdomen due to irritation of the pleura and muscles, and the pain is worse with breathing associated with fever or flu-like symptoms. The pain can last from two days to two weeks, (Lal *et al.*, 2018). Both of coxsackie virus infections may cause aseptic meningitis, which is characterized by fever and irritability in infants, while in children or adults, it presents with fever, headache, stiff neck, nausea, and vomiting and encephalitis, on the other hand, is marked by confusion and seizures, with severity varying from mild to potentially fatal disease, (Rorabaugh *et al.*, 1993). The infection with this virus, especially coxsackie B virus may lead to myopericarditis, causes inflammation of the subepicardial myocardium and pericardium. Patients present with shortness of breath, chest pain, and an irregular heartbeat. The illness can last for a few hours up to a few months. Severity varies from asymptomatic to fulminant heart failure due to dilated cardiomyopathy and sometimes cardiac arrest, (Cooper, 2009). and pancreatitis, which is a rare complication presents with abdominal pain, nausea, vomiting, and elevated pancreatic enzymes amylase and lipase. Severe pancreatitis due to Coxsackie group B can lead to pancreatic beta-cell destruction and the development of type one diabetes mellitus, (Yin *et al.,* 2021).

Echovirus is another member of the enterovirus genus, part of the Picornaviridae family. So, the symptoms and signs were similar to other those seen with coxsackie virus infections, (Carrol *et al.,* 2006) echovirus infection can induce upper respiratory infections, characterized by symptoms such as a sore throat, coryza, and cough. However, the most common clinical presentation is an undifferentiated febrile illness. In infants, certain echoviruses can lead to serious lower respiratory tract disease (Ehrnst & Eriksson, 1996) echoviruses infection frequently results in generalized maculopapular eruptions. Multiple cases occur in households with young children, is mild cases present with fever, which typically persists for 24 to 36 hours.

## LABORATORY DIAGNOSIS

### COXSACKIE Virus

#### Recovery of Virus

Viruses can be isolated from throat washings during the first few days of illness and from stools during the first few weeks. In coxsackievirus A21 infections, the largest amount of virus is found in nasal secretions (Burrell, Howard, & Murphy, 2017), cases of aseptic meningitis, strains have been recovered from the cerebrospinal fluid as well as from the alimentary tract. In hemorrhagic conjunctivitis cases, A24 virus is isolated from conjunctival swabs, throat swabs, and feces, (Fredrick, 2023).

Specimens can be inoculated into tissue cultures and suckling mice. In tissue culture, a cytopathic effect appears within 5-14 days. In suckling mice, signs of illness appear usually within 1-2 weeks. Because of the difficulty of the technique, virus isolation in suckling mice is rarely attempted.

#### Nucleic Acid Detection

Methods for the direct detection of enteroviruses provide rapid and sensitive assays useful for clinical samples. Reverse transcription PCR tests can be broadly reactive (detect many serotypes) or more specific. Such assays have advantages over cell culture methods because many enteroviruses clinical isolates have poor growth characteristics. Real-time PCR assays are comparable in sensitivity to conventional PCR assays but are less labor intensive to perform, (Harvala *et al.,* 2018).

#### Serology

Neutralizing antibodies appear early during the course of infection, tend to be specific for the infecting virus, and persist for years. Serum antibodies can also be detected by other methods such as immunofluorescence. Serologic tests are difficult to evaluate (because of the multiplicity of virus types) unless the antigen used in the test has been isolated from a specific patient or during an epidemic outbreak.

### Echo Virus

It is impossible in an individual case to diagnose an echovirus infection on clinical grounds. However, in the following epidemic situations, echoviruses must be considered: summer outbreaks of aseptic meningitis and summer epidemics, especially in young children, of a febrile illness with rash, (Burrell, Howard, & Murphy, 2017; Fredrick, 2023).

The diagnosis depends on laboratory tests. Nucleic acid detection assays, such as PCR, are more rapid than virus isolation for diagnosis. Although the specific virus may not be identified by PCR, it is often not necessary to determine the specific serotype of infecting enterovirus associated with a disease, (Harvala *et al.,* 2018; World Health Organization, 2023).

Virus isolation may be accomplished from throat swabs, stools, rectal swabs, and, in aseptic meningitis, cerebrospinal fluid. Serologic tests are impractical (because of the many different viral types) except when a virus has been isolated from a patient or during an outbreak of typical clinical illness. Neutralizing and hemagglutination-inhibiting antibodies are type specific and may persist for years, (Hyypiä & Harvala, 2015).

If an agent is isolated in tissue culture, it can be tested against different pools of antisera against enteroviruses. Determination of the type of virus present is by either immunofluorescence or neutralization test. Infection with two or more enteroviruses may occur simultaneously.

## EMERGING DIAGNOSTIC AND TREATMENT STRATEGIES

Diagnostics: Molecular advances have made it possible to diagnose Coxsackie and Echovirus infections more quickly and accurately in recent years. Real-time PCR on cerebrospinal fluid (CSF) is now the gold-standard diagnostic for suspected enteroviral meningitis because it can detect enterovirus RNA with exceptional sensitivity and specificity (typically >95%), (Verstrepen *et al.*, 2001). Because these PCR findings can be obtained in a day, doctors can promptly differentiate bacterial meningitis from viral causes and avoid giving patients needless medication. Additionally, a lot of hospitals use multiplex respiratory viral panels that identify rhinoviruses and enteroviruses. It's interesting to note that this has made it possible to diagnose systemic enterovirus infections in infants early. For example, a positive "rhinovirus/enterovirus" PCR result from a nasopharyngeal swab in 2023 identified a cluster of ill neonates in California before the conclusive results of CSF and blood testing were obtained, (Musa *et al.,* 2024).

The broad PCR panel result in that case suggested enterovirus sepsis, which prompted immediate supportive care. Emergency rooms are increasingly using syndromic panels, which screen for dozens of pathogens simultaneously, to better detect Coxsackie/Echo viruses that cause neonatal encephalitis or sepsis-like illness, (Musa *et al.,* 2024). Additionally, during epidemics, specialized labs are using next-generation sequencing (NGS) techniques to identify and genotype enteroviruses.

For instance, NGS was utilized to extract the complete viral genome from patient samples during the 2023 European Echovirus-11 outbreak, allowing for the examination of whether a novel strain was present, (Fernandez-Garcia *et al.,* 2024). As part of epidemic investigations, the CDC and WHO now advise genetic characterization of enterovirus isolates (by whole-genome sequencing or VP1 sequencing) (World Health Organization, 2023). On the point-of-care front, scientists are creating quick testing for enteroviruses, such as isothermal nucleic acid amplification assays and antigen detection kits, (Lin *et al.,* 2008; Wu *et al.,* 2025). A quick bedside test for, say, Coxsackie A would be very helpful to clinicians in differentiating HFMD from comparable rashes, even though it isn't currently readily accessible. Faster, multiplexed, and more thorough testing is generally the trend in diagnostics, which translates into early enterovirus infection identification and better patient care.

## Treatment

Although supportive care is still the mainstay for Coxsackie and echovirus infections, encouraging advancements are imminent. Rest, fluids, and temperature management are the only treatments needed for the majority of mild infections (such as HFMD, herpangina, or pleurodynia), which go away on their own in a week or so. In critical care, severe symptoms (such as myocarditis, newborn sepsis, or encephalitis) are treated with organ support (circulatory support, ventilation, etc.) as required. Intravenous immunoglobulin (IVIG), which produces a pool of neutralizing antibodies, has been a conventional treatment for severe enterovirus infections in babies. IVIG is frequently administered to critically ill newborns with Coxsackie or Echo infections in an attempt to curb the virus, despite conflicting clinical findings; in the 2023 San Diego cluster, four out of five unwell neonates got IVIG, (Musa *et al.,* 2024). Notably, the mother's convalescent plasma and an experimental antiviral medication called pocapavir (a capsid-binding agent) were also administered to the sickest baby in that cluster; sadly, the infant did not survive, (Musa *et al.*, 2024).

This humanitarian application emphasizes how urgently we need potent antivirals. Scientists have investigated a number of antiviral substances that target enteroviruses within the last ten years. By binding the capsid of the virus, one such medication, pleconaril, shown activity against enteroviruses, such as Coxsackie and Echo. Nevertheless, pleconaril's development stagnated because of its limited effectiveness and a few adverse effects. Pocapavir and vapendavir, two newer-generation capsid inhibitors, have shown some promise for broad enterovirus activity after being evaluated in modest trials for poliovirus and EV-D68, respectively. In the lab, antiviral tactics that target the viral polymerase (such as ribavirin analogues) or protease (3C protease inhibitors) are also being studied. None have been approved for routine clinical use in enterovirus infections as of yet.

Most enterovirus infections are self-limited, requiring no specific therapy; care is primarily supportive. There is no immediate remedy for hand-foot-and-mouth disease, lacking antibiotics, vaccines, or magic medications. Treatment focuses on symptom alleviation, typically with ibuprofen or acetaminophen for fever, numbing sprays for mouth sores, and calamine for rashes, along with maintaining hydration and throat soothing. Preventing the spread involves frequent handwashing, avoiding close contact with symptomatic individuals, and disinfecting contaminated items and surfaces. In severe cases, particularly Echovirus infections, immune system treatments like IVIG may be considered. For life-threatening cases, IVIG and the antiviral drug pleconaril may be administered, potentially improving outcomes.

## IVIG Therapy in Neonatal Enterovirus Infection

- A prospective study with neonates showed IVIG at 750 mg/kg had modest effects on antibody titers, subtle clinical benefits, and faster cessation of viremia and viruria.
- In hepatic necrosis cases, no correlation between IVIG and clinical outcomes was found.
- Favorable outcomes were reported in a neonate with disseminated echovirus 11 infection after IVIG treatment.
- Successful IVIG treatment of myocarditis was reported in two neonates among five with CNS and cardiac complications.
- A retrospective analysis of neonatal enterovirus infection cases suggested early IVIG therapy was independently associated with survival, (Chuang & Huang, 2019).

## Pleconaril as Antiviral Drug

- Pleconaril, a capsid inhibitor, demonstrated clinical benefit in reducing headache duration and showed promise in neonatal cases.
- In a series of patients, including immunocompromised and neonates, pleconaril usage exhibited substantial clinical benefits.
- A trial with neonates indicated potential efficacy, with pleconaril-treated infants showing faster viral clearance and lower overall mortality, (Torres-Torres *et al.,* 2015).

## Pocapavir (SCH 48973, V-073)

- Pocapavir, an investigational capsid inhibitor, successfully treated severe neonatal enteroviral infections, including myocarditis.

The use of Pocapavir in a once-daily enteral regimen demonstrated no noteworthy adverse drug-related events in a premature infant with severe enteroviral sepsis. Despite the presence of multiple factors known to be linked with severe morbidity and a heightened risk of mortality, the patient was discharged with minimal residual sequelae of neonatal enteroviral infection. This case report presents valuable preliminary data for clinicians considering the utilization of pocapavir in the treatment of severe enteroviral sepsis in neonates in the future.

ECMO for Neonatal Enteroviral Myocarditis:

- ECMO was employed in neonates with cardiovascular collapse due to severe enteroviral myocarditis, showing survival in a substantial proportion, (Nikonov *et al.*, 2017).

In summary, it is crucial to highlight that despite the existence of several promising direct-action antiviral preparations, including those already approved for medical use, there is currently no globally certified and universally recognized antiviral drug for treating diseases caused by enteroviruses. Physicians often find themselves addressing the consequences of the disease rather than its root cause, leading to a loss of valuable time and an increased risk of irreversible damage in patients. The most effective measure against enteroviral infections presently is prevention. Vaccines against other dangerous representatives of the genus Enterovirus are actively under development.

Developing antiviral drugs faces significant challenges, not only scientific but also organizational and financial on a global scale. Effective prevention requires universal and continuous efforts, which remains a challenge.

Crucially, prevention does not assist those already infected, leaving them reliant on their own immune systems and symptomatic treatment. The pressing need for designing drugs directly targeting enteroviruses causing various dangerous diseases is evident. Particularly, there is a demand for drugs with a wide spectrum of specificity that can suppress enterovirus epidemics at their onset, before widespread transmission. The global development of such preparations is underway, (Young, 1973).

## Coxsackievirus and Echovirus Challenges

Coxsackievirus and Echovirus are both part of the Enterovirus genus, a group of RNA viruses. Coxsackievirus is known for causing hand, foot, and mouth disease, herpangina, and myocarditis, among other illnesses. Echovirus, on the other hand, typically causes mild febrile illnesses, but can also lead to more serious conditions like meningitis and encephalitis.

Coxsackievirus and Echovirus Challenges of infections include:

Limited Antiviral Options: Unlike bacterial infections, Coxsackievirus and Echovirus, both enteroviruses, do not have specific antiviral treatments. This lack of targeted medications means that management often focuses on symptomatic relief, which may not always be effective in preventing complications, (Brooks *et al.*, 2019).

1. **No Vaccinations Available:** There are no vaccines to prevent infections caused by Coxsackievirus and Echovirus. The absence of a preventive vaccine means that the focus is on non-pharmaceutical interventions, like hygiene practices and public health measures, which can be challenging to implement uniformly across populations, (Boily *et al.,* 2008).
2. **Impact of Wars and Conflicts**: In areas affected by war or political instability, healthcare systems often face significant strain. This can result in poor disease surveillance, limited access to healthcare services, and increased risk of spread of infectious diseases like Coxsackievirus and Echovirus, especially in crowded and unsanitary conditions, (Bruce, Zulz, & Koch, 2016).
3. **Challenges Posed by Migration:** Migration, especially in large numbers, can lead to the spread of enteroviruses. Migrants may be exposed to new strains of the virus, or they may inadvertently carry the virus to new areas. Overcrowded living conditions, often seen in refugee camps or along migration routes, are conducive to the spread of these viruses, (Gilbert *et al.,* 2006).

Effective management of Coxsackievirus and Echovirus infections requires a comprehensive approach that includes public health education, enhanced disease surveillance, and robust implementation of hygiene and sanitation practices. In the absence of specific treatments and vaccines, these preventive measures are crucial. Additionally, ensuring access to healthcare services in conflict-affected areas and among migrant populations is essential for early detection and management of these infections.

Novel research strategies to limit the spread of Echo and Coxsackie viruses involve multifaceted approaches tailored to their transmission patterns. For Echo virus, emphasizing public health education on personal hygiene, respiratory etiquette, and sanitation practices can be pivotal. Additionally, targeted vaccination campaigns and early detection measures may play a crucial role in controlling its dissemination.

In the case of Coxsackie viruses, a comprehensive strategy could include community-wide vaccination initiatives, particularly focusing on chapopulations such as children. Concurrently, promoting hygiene practices, especially handwashing and surface disinfection, can contribute significantly to reducing the transmission of

Coxsackie viruses. Public awareness campaigns regarding the modes of transmission and precautionary measures can enhance the effectiveness of these strategies.

Research endeavors should prioritize investigating the effectiveness of the mentioned strategies for Echo and Coxsackie viruses. Rigorous studies should assess the impact of public health education, vaccination initiatives, and hygiene promotion on limiting the transmission of Echo virus. Similarly, for Coxsackie viruses, research should delve into the outcomes of community-wide vaccination efforts and the influence of hygiene campaigns on reducing its prevalence. Ongoing assessment and adaptation of these strategies based on research findings are crucial for refining approaches to prevent the spread of these viruses.

## PREVENTIVE STRATEGIES AND PUBLIC HEALTH MEASURES

Since there is currently no universal vaccine and the viruses spread via everyday activities, preventing Coxsackie and Echovirus infections requires a multifaceted strategy. Important preventive measures consist of:

Hygiene and Public Education: The foundation of prevention is a focus on basic hygiene. Regular hand washing with soap can greatly reduce transmission, particularly before meals and after changing diapers or using the restroom. Virus particles can be eliminated by thoroughly cleaning shared surfaces and toys with disinfectants (enteroviruses can remain on surfaces for days). Community health education has been shown to be successful. For instance, a study conducted in rural China revealed that parents who received extensive hand hygiene training improved their hygiene habits and reduced the incidence of HFMD in young children by 50%. Children are taught cough etiquette and basic handwashing techniques by public health initiatives in childcare facilities and schools. Additionally, sick people should be encouraged to stay at home and refrain from social interaction until they have a fever and blisters resolve, especially children with HFMD, to prevent the spreading of the virus, (Guo *et al.*, 2018).

Environmental Sanitation: One long-term preventive strategy is to upgrade the infrastructure related to water, sanitation, and hygiene (WASH). Fecal-oral enterovirus transmission is decreased by providing access to clean drinking water and appropriate waste disposal. Additional levels of protection are offered in communities by keeping swimming pools clean (with proper chlorination) and routinely cleaning high-touch surfaces throughout outbreak season, (Carratalà *et al.*, 2020).

Strict infection control measures in healthcare settings, such as staff hand cleanliness and isolating newborns with enteroviral infections, can prevent the spread of hospital-related (nosocomial) infections. Clean settings are crucial for prevention since some enteroviruses, such as EV-D70, which causes eye infections, can even transmit through unchlorinated water or inadequate sanitation, (Centers for Disease Control and Prevention, 2022).

This humanitarian application emphasizes how urgently we need potent antivirals. Scientists have investigated a number of antiviral substances that target enteroviruses within the last ten years. By binding the capsid of the virus, one such medication, pleconaril, shown activity against enteroviruses, such as Coxsackie and Echo. Nevertheless, pleconaril's development stagnated because of its limited effectiveness and a few adverse effects. Pocapavir and vapendavir, two newer-generation capsid inhibitors, have shown some promise for broad enterovirus activity after being evaluated in modest trials for poliovirus and EV-D68, respectively. In the lab, antiviral tactics that target the viral polymerase (such as ribavirin analogues) or protease (3C protease inhibitors) are also being studied. None have been approved for routine clinical use in enterovirus infections as of yet, (Anasir, Zarif, & Poh, 2021; Egorova *et al.,* 2019).

Host-directed therapy is another new therapeutic approach. For instance, physicians may employ immunosuppressive medicine in addition to antiviral treatments if a patient develops fulminant Coxsackie myocarditis, which results in heart failure. Although there aren't many thorough studies, interferon treatments are also being considered for persistent enteroviral infections, such as persistent heart infections. In terms of supportive care, enhanced life support, such as heart-lung bypass (ECMO), (Li *et al.,* 2024), has been helpful in saving lives in cases of newborn enteroviral myocarditis. This is because it effectively buys the infant's immune system time to eradicate the virus. Researchers are even looking into gene silencing and small interfering RNA (siRNA) techniques that may be able to target enteroviral RNA inside human cells—a novel idea for the future, (Daliento *et al.,* 2003; Kühl *et al.,* 2012).

The focus on vaccinations and hygiene is important since it is easier to avoid infection in the first place than to treat severe instances after the fact. Nonetheless, the creation of antiviral medications continues to be a top focus in enterovirus research due to the frequent outbreaks. Fortunately, Coxsackie/Echo virus treatments are being informed by the knowledge gained from rhinovirus medication trials and polio antiviral development. In conclusion, although the majority of treatments is supportive today, the first targeted medication for these infections may be developed in the next years, which would revolutionize the way that infants with life-threatening Coxsackie/Echo virus disease are treated.

*Figure 1. Mechanism of B-cells destruction by Coxsackie virus*

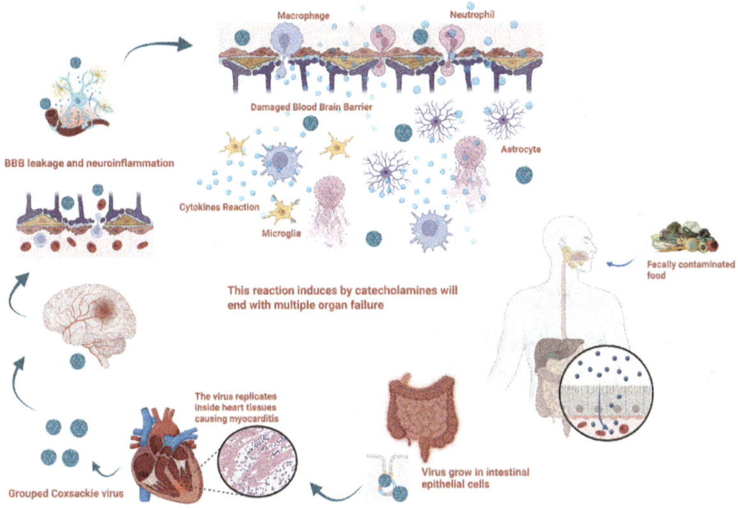


## FINAL THOUGHTS

In conclusion, Coxsackie and Echoviruses represent a significant yet often underrecognized public health concern, particularly in resource-limited settings and among vulnerable populations such as neonates. Through an exploration of their molecular characteristics, modes of transmission, and epidemiological patterns, this chapter has underscored the pressing clinical and societal challenges posed by these enteroviruses. The persistent lack of targeted vaccines and limited treatment options continue to hinder effective control and response to outbreaks. As these viruses remain prevalent and adaptable, a coordinated global effort in research, surveillance, and healthcare infrastructure is essential. Advancing our understanding and intervention strategies is not just a scientific necessity—it is a humanitarian imperative.

## REFERENCES


Anasir, M. I., Zarif, F., & Poh, C. L. (2021). Antivirals blocking entry of enteroviruses and therapeutic potential. *Journal of Biomedical Science*, *28*(1), 10. DOI: 10.1186/s12929-021-00708-8 PMID: 33451326

Ayscue, P., Van Haren, K., Sheriff, H., Waubant, E., Waldron, P., & Yagi, S. (2014). Acute flaccid paralysis with anterior myelitis - California, June 2012-June 2014. *MMWR. Morbidity and Mortality Weekly Report*, *63*(40), 903–906. PMID: 25299608

Boily, M. C., Abu-Raddad, L., Desai, K., Masse, B., Self, S., & Anderson, R. (2008). Measuring the public-health impact of candidate HIV vaccines as part of the licensing process. *The Lancet. Infectious Diseases*, *8*(3), 200–207. DOI: 10.1016/S1473-3099(07)70292-X PMID: 18291341

Bopegamage, S. A., & Petrovicová, A. (1994). In vitro infection of mouse pancreatic islet cells with coxsackie viruses. *Acta Virologica. English Ed.*, *38*(5), 251–255. PMID: 7725998

Brooks, G. F., Carroll, K. C., Butel, J. S., & Morse, S. A. (2019). *Jawetz*. Melnick & Adelberg's Medical Microbiology.

Bruce, M., Zulz, T., & Koch, A. (2016). Surveillance of infectious diseases in the Arctic. *Public Health*, *137*, 5–12. DOI: 10.1016/j.puhe.2016.06.014 PMID: 27473191

Burrell, C. J., Howard, C. R., & Murphy, F. A. (2017). *Laboratory Diagnosis of Virus Diseases. Fenner and White's Medical Virology*. Academic Press.

Carratalà, A., Bachmann, V., Julian, T. R., & Kohn, T. (2020). Adaptation of Human Enterovirus to Warm Environments Leads to Resistance against Chlorine Disinfection. *Environmental Science & Technology*, *54*(18), 11292–11300. DOI: 10.1021/acs.est.0c03199 PMID: 32875801

Carrol, E. D., Beadsworth, M. B., Jenkins, N., Ratcliffe, L., Ashton, I., Crowley, B., Nye, F. J., & Beeching, N. J. (2006). Clinical and diagnostic findings of an echovirus meningitis outbreak in the north west of England. *Postgraduate Medical Journal*, *82*(963), 60–64. DOI: 10.1136/pgmj.2005.036608 PMID: 16397083

Centers for Disease C. (2022). *Prevention. National Enterovirus Surveillance System (NESS)*. Surveillance Data.

Centers for Disease Control (CDC) (1991). Aseptic meningitis—New York State and United States, weeks 1-36, 1991. *MMWR. Morbidity and Mortality Weekly Report*, *40*(45), 773–775.

Chang, L. Y., Tsao, K. C., Hsia, S. H., Shih, S. R., Huang, C. G., & Chan, W. K. (2004). Transmission and clinical features of enterovirus 71 infections in household contacts in Taiwan. *Journal of the American Medical Association, 291*(2), 222–227. DOI: 10.1001/jama.291.2.222 PMID: 14722149

Chuang, Y.-Y., & Huang, Y.-C. (2019). Enteroviral infection in neonates. *Journal of Microbiology, Immunology, and Infection, 52*(6), 851–857. DOI: 10.1016/j.jmii.2019.08.018 PMID: 31607572

Codd, A. A., Hale, J. H., Bell, T. M., Sims, D. G., Bacon, C. J., & Gardner, P. S. (1976). Epidemic of echovirus 19 in the north-east of England. *The Journal of Hygiene, 76*(2), 307–317. DOI: 10.1017/S0022172400055200 PMID: 1063219

Cooper, L. T.Jr. (2009). Myocarditis. *The New England Journal of Medicine, 360*(15), 1526–1538. DOI: 10.1056/NEJMra0800028 PMID: 19357408

Couch, R. B., Douglas, R. G.Jr, Lindgren, K. M., Gerone, P. J., & Knight, V. (1970). Airborne transmission of respiratory infection with coxsackievirus A type 21. *American Journal of Epidemiology, 91*(1), 78–86. DOI: 10.1093/oxfordjournals.aje.a121115 PMID: 5415578

Daliento L, Calabrese F, Tona F, Caforio AL, Tarsia G, Angelini A, et al. (2003). Successful treatment of enterovirus-induced myocarditis with interferon-alpha. *The Journal of heart and lung transplantation: the official publication of the International Society for Heart Transplantation. 22*(2):214-7.

de Crom, S. C., Rossen, J. W., van Furth, A. M., & Obihara, C. C. (2016). Enterovirus and parechovirus infection in children: A brief overview. *European Journal of Pediatrics, 175*(8), 1023–1029. DOI: 10.1007/s00431-016-2725-7 PMID: 27156106

Egorova, A., Ekins, S., Schmidtke, M., & Makarov, V. (2019). Back to the future: Advances in development of broad-spectrum capsid-binding inhibitors of enteroviruses. *European Journal of Medicinal Chemistry, 178*, 606–622. DOI: 10.1016/j.ejmech.2019.06.008 PMID: 31226653

Ehrnst, A., & Eriksson, M. (1996). Echovirus Type 23 Observed as a Nosocomial Infection in Infants. *Scandinavian Journal of Infectious Diseases, 28*(2), 205–206. DOI: 10.3109/00365549609049079 PMID: 8792494

Fairweather, D., Frisancho-Kiss, S., & Rose, N. R. (2005). Viruses as adjuvants for autoimmunity: Evidence from Coxsackievirus-induced myocarditis. *Reviews in Medical Virology, 15*(1), 17–27. DOI: 10.1002/rmv.445 PMID: 15386590

Fairweather, D., Kaya, Z., Shellam, G. R., Lawson, C. M., & Rose, N. R. (2001). From Infection to Autoimmunity. *Journal of Autoimmunity*, *16*(3), 175–186. DOI: 10.1006/jaut.2000.0492 PMID: 11334481

Fernandez-Garcia MD, Garcia-Ibañez N, Camacho J, Gutierrez A, Sánchez García L, Calvo C, et al. (2024). Enhanced echovirus 11 genomic surveillance in neonatal infections in Spain following a European alert reveals new recombinant forms linked to severe cases, 2019 to 2023. *European communicable disease bulletin. 29*(44).

Fredrick, D.R. (2023). Conjunctivitis beyond the neonatal period.

Gamble, D. R. (1962). Isolation of Coxsackie viruses from normal children aged 0-5 years. *British Medical Journal*, *1*(5270), 16–18. DOI: 10.1136/bmj.1.5270.16 PMID: 13896555

Gelfand, H. M., Holguin, A. H., Marchetti, G. E., & Feorino, P. M. (1963). A continuing surveillance of enterovirus infections in healthy children in six united states cities. I. Viruses isolated during 1960 and 1961. *American Journal of Hygiene*, *78*, 358–375. PMID: 14071359

Gilbert, M., Xiao, X., Domenech, J., Lubroth, J., Martin, V., & Slingenbergh, J. (2006). Anatidae migration in the western Palearctic and spread of highly pathogenic avian influenza H5NI virus. *Emerging Infectious Diseases*, *12*(11), 1650–1656. DOI: 10.3201/eid1211.060223 PMID: 17283613

Gondo, K., Kusuhara, K., Take, H., & Ueda, K. (1995). Echovirus type 9 epidemic in Kagoshima, southern Japan: Seroepidemiology and clinical observation of aseptic meningitis. *The Pediatric Infectious Disease Journal*, *14*(9), 787–791. DOI: 10.1097/00006454-199509000-00011 PMID: 8559629

Grist, N. R., Bell, E. J., & Reid, D. (1975). The epidemiology of enteroviruses. *Scottish Medical Journal*, *20*(1), 27–31. DOI: 10.1177/003693307502000108 PMID: 1111084

Guo, N., Ma, H., Deng, J., Ma, Y., Huang, L., Guo, R., & Zhang, L. (2018). Effect of hand washing and personal hygiene on hand food mouth disease: A community intervention study. *Medicine*, *97*(51), e13144. DOI: 10.1097/MD.0000000000013144 PMID: 30572426

. Harvala H, Broberg E, Benschop K, Berginc N, Ladhani S, Susi P, et al. (2018). Recommendations for enterovirus diagnostics and characterisation within and beyond Europe. *Journal of clinical virology: the official publication of the Pan American Society for Clinical Virology.*

He, Y., Lin, F., Chipman, P. R., Bator, C. M., Baker, T. S., Shoham, M., Kuhn, R. J., Medof, M. E., & Rossmann, M. G. (2002). Structure of decay-accelerating factor bound to echovirus 7: A virus-receptor complex. *Proceedings of the National Academy of Sciences of the United States of America*, *99*(16), 10325–10329. DOI: 10.1073/pnas.152161599 PMID: 12119400

Hyypiä, T, & Harvala, H. (2015). Echoviruses. doi.org/10.1016/B978-0-12-801238-3.02562-9.

Kadambari, S., Abdullahi, F., Celma, C., & Ladhani, S. (2024). Epidemiological trends in viral meningitis in England: Prospective national surveillance, 2013-2023. *The Journal of Infection*, *89*(3), 106223. DOI: 10.1016/j.jinf.2024.106223 PMID: 38986749

Kaplan, M. H., Klein, S. W., McPhee, J., & Harper, R. G. (1983). Group B coxsackievirus infections in infants younger than three months of age: A serious childhood illness. *Reviews of Infectious Diseases*, *5*(6), 1019–1032. DOI: 10.1093/clinids/5.6.1019 PMID: 6318288

Kaufman, D. L., Clare-Salzler, M., Tian, J., Forsthuber, T., Ting, G. S., Robinson, P., Atkinson, M. A., Sercarz, E. E., Tobin, A. J., & Lehmann, P. V. (1993). Spontaneous loss of T-cell tolerance to glutamic acid decarboxylase in murine insulin-dependent diabetes. *Nature*, *366*(6450), 69–72. DOI: 10.1038/366069a0 PMID: 7694152

Klein, M., Eggers, H. J., & Nelsen-Salz, B. (2000). Echovirus-9 protein 2C binds single-stranded RNA unspecifically. *The Journal of General Virology*, *81*(Pt 10), 2481–2484. DOI: 10.1099/0022-1317-81-10-2481 PMID: 10993936

Kogon, A., Spigland, I., Frothingham, T. E., Elveback, L., Williams, C., Hall, C. E., & Fox, J. P. (1969). The virus watch program: A continuing surveillance of viral infections in metropolitan New York families. VII. Observations on viral excretion, seroimmunity, intrafamilial spread and illness association in coxsackie and echovirus infections. *American Journal of Epidemiology*, *89*(1), 51–61. DOI: 10.1093/oxfordjournals.aje.a120915 PMID: 5762818

Koh, W. M., Badaruddin, H., La, H., Chen, M. I., & Cook, A. R. (2018). Severity and burden of hand, foot and mouth disease in Asia: A modelling study. *BMJ Global Health*, *3*(1), e000442. DOI: 10.1136/bmjgh-2017-000442 PMID: 29564154

Krieger, S. E., Kim, C., Zhang, L., Marjomaki, V., & Bergelson, J. M. (2013). Echovirus 1 entry into polarized Caco-2 cells depends on dynamin, cholesterol, and cellular factors associated with macropinocytosis. *Journal of Virology*, *87*(16), 8884–8895. DOI: 10.1128/JVI.03415-12 PMID: 23740983

Kühl, U., Lassner, D., von Schlippenbach, J., Poller, W., & Schultheiss, H.-P. (2012). Interferon-Beta Improves Survival in Enterovirus-Associated Cardiomyopathy. *Journal of the American College of Cardiology*, *60*(14), 1295–1296. DOI: 10.1016/j.jacc.2012.06.026 PMID: 23017536

Lal, A., Akhtar, J., Isaac, S., Mishra, A. K., Khan, M. S., Noreldin, M., & Abraham, G. M. (2018). Unusual cause of chest pain, Bornholm disease, a forgotten entity; case report and review of literature. *Respiratory Medicine Case Reports*, *25*, 270–273. DOI: 10.1016/j.rmcr.2018.10.005 PMID: 30364740

Lei, X., Cui, S., Zhao, Z., & Wang, J. (2015). Etiology, pathogenesis, antivirals and vaccines of hand, foot, and mouth disease. *National Science Review*, *2*(3), 268–284. DOI: 10.1093/nsr/nwv038

Li, X., Sun, L., Xi, S., Hu, Y., Yu, Z., Liu, H., Sun, H., Jing, W., Yuan, L., Liu, H., & Li, T. (2024). V-A ECMO for neonatal coxsackievirus B fulminant myocarditis: A case report and literature review. *Frontiers in Cardiovascular Medicine*, *11*, 1364289. DOI: 10.3389/fcvm.2024.1364289 PMID: 38836060

Lin, T. L., Li, Y. S., Huang, C. W., Hsu, C. C., Wu, H. S., Tseng, T. C., & Yang, C.-F. (2008). Rapid and highly sensitive coxsackievirus a indirect immunofluorescence assay typing kit for enterovirus serotyping. *Journal of Clinical Microbiology*, *46*(2), 785–788. DOI: 10.1128/JCM.01114-07 PMID: 18032614

Lin, T. Y., Kao, H. T., Hsieh, S. H., Huang, Y. C., Chiu, C. H., Chou, Y. H., Yang, P.-H., Lin, R.-I., Tsao, K.-C., Hsu, K.-H., & Chang, L.-Y. (2003). Neonatal enterovirus infections: Emphasis on risk factors of severe and fatal infections. *The Pediatric Infectious Disease Journal*, *22*(10), 889–894. DOI: 10.1097/01.inf.0000091294.63706.f3 PMID: 14551490

Mena, I., Perry, C. M., Harkins, S., Rodriguez, F., Gebhard, J., & Whitton, J. L. (1999). The role of B lymphocytes in coxsackievirus B3 infection. *American Journal of Pathology*, *155*(4), 1205–1215. DOI: 10.1016/S0002-9440(10)65223-6 PMID: 10514403

Midgley, C. M., Watson, J. T., Nix, W. A., Curns, A. T., Rogers, S. L., Brown, B. A., Conover, C., Dominguez, S. R., Feikin, D. R., Gray, S., Hassan, F., Hoferka, S., Jackson, M. A., Johnson, D., Leshem, E., Miller, L., Nichols, J. B., Nyquist, A.-C., Obringer, E., & Gerber, S. I. (2015). Severe respiratory illness associated with a nationwide outbreak of enterovirus D68 in the USA (2014): A descriptive epidemiological investigation. *The Lancet. Respiratory Medicine*, *3*(11), 879–887. DOI: 10.1016/S2213-2600(15)00335-5 PMID: 26482320

. Mirand A, Henquell C, Archimbaud C, Ughetto S, Antona D, Bailly JL, et al. (2012). Outbreak of hand, foot and mouth disease/herpangina associated with coxsackievirus A6 and A10 infections in 2010, France: a large citywide, prospective observational study. *Clinical microbiology and infection: the official publication of the European Society of Clinical Microbiology and Infectious Diseases. 18*(5):E110-8.

Miwa, C., Ohtani, M., Watanabe, H., Fujimoto, J., Kinbara, K., & Tanaka, H. (1980). Epidemic of hand, foot and mouth disease in Gifu Prefecture in 1978. *Japanese Journal of Medical Science & Biology*, *33*(3), 167–180. DOI: 10.7883/yoken1952.33.167 PMID: 6259389

Modlin, J. F. (1986). Perinatal echovirus infection: Insights from a literature review of 61 cases of serious infection and 16 outbreaks in nurseries. *Reviews of Infectious Diseases*, *8*(6), 918–926. DOI: 10.1093/clinids/8.6.918 PMID: 3541126

Moore, M. (1982). Centers for Disease Control. Enteroviral disease in the United States, 1970-1979. *The Journal of Infectious Diseases*, *146*(1), 103–108. DOI: 10.1093/infdis/146.1.103 PMID: 6282988

Muckelbauer JK, Kremer M, Minor I, Diana G, Dutko FJ, Groarke J, et al. (1995). The structure of coxsackievirus B3 at 3.5 A resolution.

Musa, N., Ghoniem, A., Hsu, C. H., Patel, M. K., & Goodson, J. L. (2024). Progress Toward Measles Elimination — Eastern Mediterranean Region, 2019–2022. *MMWR. Morbidity and Mortality Weekly Report*, *73*(7), 141–145. DOI: 10.15585/mmwr.mm7307a1 PMID: 38386606

Nhan, L. N. T., Khanh, T. H., Hong, N. T. T., Van, H. M. T., Nhu, L. N. T., Ny, N. T. H., Nguyet, L. A., Thanh, T. T., Anh, N. T., Hang, V. T. T., Qui, P. T., Viet, H. L., Tung, T. H., Ha, D. Q., Tuan, H. M., Thwaites, G., Chau, N. V. V., Thwaites, L., Hung, N. T., & Tan, L. V. (2020). Clinical, etiological and epidemiological investigations of hand, foot and mouth disease in southern Vietnam during 2015 - 2018. *PLoS Neglected Tropical Diseases*, *14*(8), e0008544. DOI: 10.1371/journal.pntd.0008544 PMID: 32804980

Nhan, L. N. T., Turner, H. C., Khanh, T. H., Hung, N. T., Lien, L. B., Hong, N. T. T., Nhu, L. N. T., Ny, N. T. H., Nguyet, L. A., Thanh, T. T., Van, H. M. T., Viet, H. L., Tung, T. H., Phuong, T. T. L., Devine, A., Thwaites, G., Chau, N. V. V., Thwaites, L., van Doorn, H. R., & Tan, L. V. (2019). Economic Burden Attributed to Children Presenting to Hospitals With Hand, Foot, and Mouth Disease in Vietnam. *Open Forum Infectious Diseases*, *6*(7), ofz284. DOI: 10.1093/ofid/ofz284 PMID: 31363772

Nikonov, O. S., Chernykh, E. S., Garber, M. B., & Nikonova, E. Y. (2017). Enteroviruses: Classification, Diseases They Cause, and Approaches to Development of Antiviral Drugs. *Biochemistry (Moscow), 82*(13), 1615–1631. DOI: 10.1134/S0006297917130041 PMID: 29523062

Onorato, I. M., Morens, D. M., Schonberger, L. B., Hatch, M. H., Kaminski, R. M., & Turner, J. P. (1985). Acute hemorrhagic conjunctivitis caused by enterovirus type 70: An epidemic in American Samoa. *The American Journal of Tropical Medicine and Hygiene, 34*(5), 984–991. DOI: 10.4269/ajtmh.1985.34.984 PMID: 2994502

Pons-Salort, M., Parker, E. P., & Grassly, N. C. (2015). The epidemiology of non-polio enteroviruses: Recent advances and outstanding questions. *Current Opinion in Infectious Diseases, 28*(5), 479–487. DOI: 10.1097/QCO.0000000000000187 PMID: 26203854

Pulli, T., Koivunen, E., & Hyypiä, T. (1997). Cell-surface interactions of echovirus 22. *The Journal of Biological Chemistry, 272*(34), 21176–21180. DOI: 10.1074/jbc.272.34.21176 PMID: 9261123

Roivainen, M., Knip, M., Hyöty, H., Kulmala, P., Hiltunen, M., Vähäsalo, P., Hovi, T., & Åkerblom, H. K. (1998). Several different enterovirus serotypes can be associated with prediabetic autoimmune episodes and onset of overt IDDM. Childhood Diabetes in Finland (DiMe) Study Group. *Journal of Medical Virology, 56*(1), 74–78. DOI: 10.1002/(SICI)1096-9071(199809)56:1<74::AID-JMV12>3.0.CO;2-W PMID: 9700636

Rorabaugh, M. L., Berlin, L. E., Heldrich, F., Roberts, K., Rosenberg, L. A., Doran, T., & Modlin, J. F. (1993). Aseptic meningitis in infants younger than 2 years of age: Acute illness and neurologic complications. *Pediatrics, 92*(2), 206–211. DOI: 10.1542/peds.92.2.206 PMID: 8337018

Rose, N. R. (2008). Autoimmunity in coxsackievirus infection. *Current Topics in Microbiology and Immunology, 323*, 293–314. DOI: 10.1007/978-3-540-75546-3_14 PMID: 18357776

Rosen, L., Melnick, J. L., Schmidt, J., & Wenner, H. A. (1970). Subclassification of enteroviruses and ECHO virus type 34. Brief report. *Archiv fur die Gesamte Virusforschung, 30*(1), 89–92. DOI: 10.1007/BF01262587 PMID: 4986680

Schmidt, N. J., Lennette, E. H., & Ho, H. H. (1974). An apparently new enterovirus isolated from patients with disease of the central nervous system. *The Journal of Infectious Diseases, 129*(3), 304–309. DOI: 10.1093/infdis/129.3.304 PMID: 4361245

Second, J., Velter, C., Calès, S., Truchetet, F., Lipsker, D., & Cribier, B. (2017). Clinicopathologic analysis of atypical hand, foot, and mouth disease in adult patients. *Journal of the American Academy of Dermatology*, *76*(4), 722–729. DOI: 10.1016/j.jaad.2016.10.022 PMID: 28027826

Shen, Y., Li, S., Huo, D., Dong, S., Yang, Y., & Jia, L. (2023). Economic Burden of Hand, Foot, and Mouth Disease - Beijing Municipality, China, 2016-2019. *China CDC Weekly*, *5*(43), 953–957. PMID: 38025512

Sidiropoulou, K., Mamalis, S., Christoforidi, M., & Exindari, M. (n.d.) Epidemiological data of Coxsackie and Echo viruses in N. Greece. *Acta Microbiol Hellen*. *64*(3).

Sklar, V. E., Patriarca, P. A., Onorato, I. M., Langford, M. P., Clark, S. W., Culbertson, W. W., & Forster, R. K. (1983). Clinical findings and results of treatment in an outbreak of acute hemorrhagic conjunctivitis in southern Florida. *American Journal of Ophthalmology*, *95*(1), 45–54. DOI: 10.1016/0002-9394(83)90332-X PMID: 6849368

Somekh, E., Shohat, T., Handsher, R., & Serour, F. (2001). An outbreak of echovirus 11 in a children's home. *Epidemiology and Infection*, *126*(3), 441–444. DOI: 10.1017/S0950268801005404 PMID: 11467801

Song, Y., Zhang, Y., Han, Z., Xu, W., Xiao, J., Wang, X., Wang, J., Yang, J., Yu, Q., Yu, D., Chen, J., Huang, W., Li, J., Xie, T., Lu, H., Ji, T., Yang, Q., Yan, D., Zhu, S., & Xu, W. (2020). Genetic recombination in fast-spreading coxsackievirus A6 variants: A potential role in evolution and pathogenicity. *Virus Evolution*, *6*(2), veaa048. DOI: 10.1093/ve/veaa048 PMID: 34804589

Stewart, C. L., Chu, E. Y., Introcaso, C. E., Schaffer, A., & James, W. D. (2013). Coxsackievirus A6-induced hand-foot-mouth disease. *JAMA Dermatology*, *149*(12), 1419–1421. DOI: 10.1001/jamadermatol.2013.6777 PMID: 24172861

Swann, N. H. (1961). Epidemic pleurodynia, orchitis, and myocarditis in an adult due to Coxsackie virus, group B, type 4. *Annals of Internal Medicine*, *54*(5), 1008–1013. DOI: 10.7326/0003-4819-54-5-1008 PMID: 13774219

Tassin M, Martinovic J, Mirand A, Peigue-Lafeuille H, Picone O, Benachi A, et al. (2014). A case of congenital Echovirus 11 infection acquired early in pregnancy. *Journal of clinical virology: the official publication of the Pan American Society for Clinical Virology*. *59*(1):71-3.

Tinari, A., Pietrantoni, A., Ammendolia, M. G., Valenti, P., & Superti, F. (2005). Inhibitory activity of bovine lactoferrin against echovirus induced programmed cell death in vitro. *International Journal of Antimicrobial Agents*, *25*(5), 433–438. DOI: 10.1016/j.ijantimicag.2005.02.011 PMID: 15848300

Torres-Torres, S., Myers, A. L., Klatte, J. M., Rhoden, E. E., Oberste, M. S., Collett, M. S., & McCulloh, R. J. (2015). First use of investigational antiviral drug pocapavir (v-073) for treating neonatal enteroviral sepsis. *The Pediatric Infectious Disease Journal*, *34*(1), 52–54. DOI: 10.1097/INF.0000000000000497 PMID: 25229269

Tyrrell, D. A. (1963). Clinical clues in virus infections. *British Medical Journal*, *1*(5329), 493–496. DOI: 10.1136/bmj.1.5329.493 PMID: 13995046

Verstrepen, W. A., Kuhn, S., Kockx, M. M., Van De Vyvere, M. E., & Mertens, A. H. (2001). Rapid detection of enterovirus RNA in cerebrospinal fluid specimens with a novel single-tube real-time reverse transcription-PCR assay. *Journal of Clinical Microbiology*, *39*(11), 4093–4096. DOI: 10.1128/JCM.39.11.4093-4096.2001 PMID: 11682535

Wang, J., Atchison, R. W., Walpusk, J., & Jaffe, R. (2001). Echovirus hepatic failure in infancy: Report of four cases with speculation on the pathogenesis. *Pediatric and Developmental Pathology*, *4*(5), 454–460. DOI: 10.1007/s10024001-0043-0 PMID: 11779047

Wells, A. I., Grimes, K. A., Kim, K., Branche, E., Bakkenist, C. J., DePas, W. H., Shresta, S., & Coyne, C. B. (2021). Human FcRn expression and Type I Interferon signaling control Echovirus 11 pathogenesis in mice. *PLoS Pathogens*, *17*(1), e1009252. DOI: 10.1371/journal.ppat.1009252 PMID: 33513208

Wilfert, C. M., Lauer, B. A., Cohen, M., Costenbader, M. L., & Myers, E. (1975). An epidemic of echovirus 18 meningitis. *The Journal of Infectious Diseases*, *131*(1), 75–78. DOI: 10.1093/infdis/131.1.75 PMID: 1167369

Woodland, D. L. (2019). Hand, Foot, and Mouth Disease. *Viral Immunology*, *32*(4), 159. DOI: 10.1089/vim.2019.29037.dlw PMID: 31038400

World Health O. Disease Outbreak News: 2023-DON469. 2023.

World Health Org. (2023). Enterovirus-Echovirus 11 Infection – European Region. *Disease Outbreak News*, *7*, 2023.

Wright, H. T.Jr, Landing, B. H., Lennette, E. H., & Mc, A. R. (1963). Fatal infection in an infant associated with Coxsackie virus group A, type 16. *The New England Journal of Medicine*, *268*(19), 1041–1044. DOI: 10.1056/NEJM196305092681904 PMID: 14001956

Wu, Z., Tang, M., Li, X., Jiang, L., Ma, J., Zhou, W., & Shi, W. (2025). Simultaneous detection of Enterovirus 71 and Coxsackievirus A16 based on RT-RPA-CRISPR Cas12a/13a system. *Microchemical Journal*, *212*, 113335. DOI: 10.1016/j.microc.2025.113335

Yin, Z., Wu, Y., Zhu, R., Xu, L., Lin, Y., Yang, H., Fu, W., Huang, Q., Zhang, D., Wang, J., Wang, W., Wang, Y., Cheng, T., & Xia, N. (2021). Development of A Neonatal Mouse Model for Coxsackievirus B1 Antiviral Evaluation. *Virologica Sinica*, *36*(6), 1575–1584. DOI: 10.1007/s12250-021-00444-1 PMID: 34581960

Young, N. A. (1973). Polioviruses, coxsackieviruses, and echoviruses comparison of the genomes by RNA hybridization. *Journal of Virology*, *11*(6), 832–839. DOI: 10.1128/jvi.11.6.832-839.1973 PMID: 4351457

Zhang, G., Li, J., Sun, Q., Zhang, K., Xu, W., Zhang, Y., & Wu, G. (2021). Pathological Features of Echovirus-11-Associated Brain Damage in Mice Based on RNA-Seq Analysis. *Viruses*, *13*(12), 2477. DOI: 10.3390/v13122477 PMID: 34960747

Zheng, Y., Jit, M., Wu, J. T., Yang, J., Leung, K., Liao, Q., & Yu, H. (2017). Economic costs and health-related quality of life for hand, foot and mouth disease (HFMD) patients in China. *PLoS One*, *12*(9), e0184266. DOI: 10.1371/journal.pone.0184266 PMID: 28934232

Zhu, P., Ji, W., Li, D., Li, Z., Chen, Y., Dai, B., Han, S., Chen, S., Jin, Y., & Duan, G. (2023). Current status of hand-foot-and-mouth disease. *Journal of Biomedical Science*, *30*(1), 15. DOI: 10.1186/s12929-023-00908-4 PMID: 36829162

# Chapter 11
# Unveiling the Plague:
## Tracing History, Symptoms, Treatments, and Modern Research Perspectives

**Amarelle Chamoun**
https://orcid.org/0000-0002-3473-8922
*Faculty of Medical Sciences, Lebanese University, Beirut, Lebanon*

**Jana Mahdi**
*Faculty of Medical Sciences, Lebanese University, Beirut, Lebanon*

**Hadi Imad Farhat**
*Faculty of Medical Sciences, Lebanese University, Beirut, Lebanon*

**Tia Khadra**
*Faculty of Medical Sciences, Lebanese University, Beirut, Lebanon*

**Jana Jaber**
*Faculty of Medical Sciences, Lebanese University, Beirut, Lebanon*

## ABSTRACT

*Plague, a vector-borne illness caused by Yersinia pestis, is a serious threat to the public's health, particularly in light of its previous human outbreaks in Africa, Asia, and South America. Transmission occurs mostly by infected flea bites, causing typical painful, swollen lymph nodes known as buboes, followed by septicemic pathogen propagation. However, droplet inhalation following intimate contact with diseased mammals causes primary pneumonic plague. Clinical manifestations include bubonic and pneumonic forms, septicemia, and in rare cases, pharyngitis and meningitis. Early diagnosis and the immediate initiation of treatment can decrease mortality*

DOI: 10.4018/979-8-3693-1990-1.ch011

*rate in bubonic plague and septicemic plague to 5-50%; however, a delay in treatment can be life threatening. Majority of cases can be successfully managed with antibiotics. This chapter covers current knowledge of Y. pestis, the most important current technologies and criteria for laboratory diagnosis of plague, main challenges experienced in underdeveloped nations, and the current novel research approaches.*

## INTRODUCTION

Plague is an ancient bacteria called Yersinia pestis. It is transmitted to humans by being bitten by an infected flea or by getting in contact with an infected animal. Plague can cause a variety of symptoms, such as fever, headache, chills, muscle aches, and swelling of the lymph nodes. Plague can be lethal if left untreated.

The Justinianic Plague, which hit the Byzantine Empire and the Mediterranean region in the 6th century CE, was the most famous plague outbreak throughout history, killing approximately 25 to 50 million people; one-quarter to one-half of this population, (Eisenberg & Mordechai, 2019).

Plague outbreaks have continued throughout history, and the disease remains a public health threat to this day. Nowadays, we have seen outbreaks of plague in Africa, Asia, and the Americas, (Vallès *et al.,* 2020).

Plague can be treated with antibiotics, but early diagnosis and treatment are primordial. It is important to see a doctor right away if you think you may have been exposed, (Glatter & Finkleman, 2021).

## DISCUSSION

### Definition

Plague is a disease caused by the bacterium Yersinia pestis. It is a highly contagious and often fatal disease. It usually causes sudden and severe outbreaks, resulting in fear and devastation. Often named the "dreadful visitation," plague has haunted the human mind for decades, leaving an unforgettable mark on societies, cultures, and history, (Khan, 2004). Plague typing methods have been an effective instrument to understand and track the disease, hence facilitating the identification and differentiation of the bacterium strains. These methods have significantly contributed to our understanding of the disease, (Lindler, 2009).

Plague has left a long-lasting impact on human memory, and its recurrence throughout history serves as a reminder of the importance of learning from the past to prevent future outbreaks. All this emphasizes the critical need for research, vigilance, and public health measures to combat this ancient pest, (Metcalfe, 2013).

## Epidemiology and Prevalence in Developing and Developed Nations

Despite its historical association with medieval Europe, plague is still a global public health concern, shadowing in both developed and developing nations. The 14th-century pandemic devastated Europe with recurrent waves for centuries, highlighting the devastating potential of this disease, (Benedictow, 2019). Today, plague primarily affects wild rodents and their fleas, but human infections still occur, particularly in Africa and Asia, (Hinnebusch, 2010). However, epidemiology and prevalence vary significantly between developed and developing countries.

In developed nations, good surveillance systems and rapid antibiotic treatment have drastically reduced the weight of plague. Cases are rare, often traced to contact with infected rodents or fleas in rural areas, (Hinnebusch, 2010). Public health infrastructure plays a crucial role in early detection, isolation, and treatment, preventing outbreaks before they spiral out of control.

In contrast, developing countries often face heavier challenges. Limited access to healthcare, poverty, and preacrity of sanitation create conditions appropriate to plague transmission. Rodent populations thrive in overcrowded, unsanitary environments, while inadequate healthcare infrastructure coerce timely diagnosis and treatment, (Benedictow, 2019). This confluence of factors can lead to outbreaks that disproportionately impact vulnerable populations.

Understanding these disparities is crucial for effectively controlling the spread. While developed nations focus on maintaining surveillance and preparedness, developing nations require targeted interventions to address underlying socio-economic factors and strengthen their healthcare systems. By working on these gaps, we can work towards a future where plague is no longer a threat, regardless of a nation's development status.

## Risk Factors

Various studies have been performed to identify risk factors associated with the infection of the pathogen Yersenia pestis. The main mode of transmission is through man-to-rodent contact which constitutes the main risk factor for contracting plague in endemic areas such as Zimbabwe, (Munyenyiwa *et al.,* 2019). Activities such as hunting, the transport and disposition of dead rodents facilitates the transmission of fleas from the infected carrier rodent to humans or any other any domestic animal that may harbor them, thereby facilitating the transmission of the disease in the household such as cats at home. Case control studies have been performed and found that the factor of age older than 10 years, and resettlement are associated with a statistically significant higher risk of infection and transmission, (Manungo *et al.*, 1998). This is due to the active lifestyle of this population. In addition, living in rural areas are associated with outdoor activities in the farm such as herding cattle, farming, and hunting. These occupational exposures render this select population to venture into the bush which allows increased contact of the human population with plague reservoirs systems, (Manungo *et al.*, 1998). Additional noted activities reported in the literature include sleeping on straw mats, storing food in huts or reservoirs in the dormitory, the possession of domestic dogs and allowing them into huts where people sleep, garbage being stored inside the hut or in its vicinity, and finally cooking inside the huts, (Eisen *et al.,* 2014).

Note that there is one important element which is the diet of certain select populations that may pose a risk of contracting the plague which include preparation of rodents for food. Certain populations in Zambia are known to have rodents as part of their diet. Trapping, transporting and preparing rodents for a meal exposes this population in the household to infection by the flea vector especially with freshly trapped rodents or carcasses of rodents which increases human bites from fleas, (Nyirenda *et al.,* 2017).

## Pathogenesis

Infections caused by the organism of Yersenia Pestis can be the result of a flea bite, direct handling of infected animal tissues which would result into the formation of the bubonic plague, ingestion of infected tissues, or respiratory droplets from infected humans which would result in Pneumonic plague. Based on the route of infection, there are three categories of the plague in terms of clinical manifestation: bubonic, septicemic and pneumonic.

In bubonic plague, Yersenia pestis would colonize local and regional lymph nodes draining the infected site secondary to breach of the skin by the bite of a flea carrying the organism. The bacteria in turn would grow in numbers resulting in tender, hot, and hemorrhagic nodes so called Buboes. Sequentially, the bacteria would spread into other organs such as the liver, spleen, kidneys and other organs causing septicemia and septic shock leading to death, (Du & Wang, 2016).

As for the pneumonic plague, which carries a higher risk of mortality than its cutaneous counterpart, it is transmitted through respiratory droplets in between humans. It has a short incubation period up to 6 days, which is followed by flu like symptoms which progress rapidly into cough, difficulty breathing, and bloody sputum production. These patients progress rapidly and die from respiratory failure and severe sepsis, (Smiley, 2008).

Yersenia Pestis has multiple routes of transmission and multiple mechanisms of virulence that allow it to infect and spread enabling it to become a virulent flea-borne pathogen.

Y. pestis is characterized by a cell membrane enzyme protease that allows it to inhibit bacterial lysis which is induced by complement activation of the host's immune system called Plasminogen activator (Pla). Additionally, it grants the organism the ability to invade macrophages and lymphocytes allowing spread into loco-regional lymph nodes. Finally, it allows the induction of disseminated intravascular coagulation by acting as a cofactor leading to the generalized occlusion of blood vessels, (Mikula, Kolodziejczyk, & Goldman, 2012).

Y. pestis carries another virulent factor that allows it to spread more efficiently by its host, the flea. This factor is a hemin storage gene cluster (hms), encoding the biosynthesis of the poly-N-acetyl-glucosamine capsule which is responsible for the formation of a biofilm allowing the organism to stick to the flea's forestomach preventing it from swallowing the blood meal properly from its first prey which would push the flea to bite more hosts. During biting, a described regurgitation and swallowing of the blood meal is performed which would serve as an efficient spreading mechanism of Y. pestis by fleas, (Hinnebusch, 2005).

Another described virulence factor of Yersenia pestis is through the Yersinia outer-membrane proteins (Yops), constituting a wide variety of effectors translocated into host cells. They play pleiotropic roles during the infection as they may inhibit phagocytosis by inhibiting the Rho GTPases and thereby disrupting the actin cytoskeleton, they may down-regulate the production of pro-inflammatory cytokines and may induce cellular death, (Trosky, Liverman, & Orth, 2008). For example, the tyrosine phosphatase YopH dephosphorylates focal adhesion complex proteins of immune cells, YopE mimics GTPase-activating proteins (GAP) allowing it to down-regulate host cell Rho GTPases, cysteine protease YopT cleaves and releases membrane-bound Rho GTPases, and the acetyltransferase YopJ blocks both the mitogen-activated protein kinase (MAPK) and the nuclear factor-κB (NF-κB) signaling pathways, allowing it to inhibit pro-inflammatory cytokine production, (Persson *et al.,* 1997).

Finally, Y. pestis is characterized by anti-inflammatory mechanisms which allow it to grow without being attacked by the host immune system and triggering an inflammatory reaction at the early stage of infection. It induces the production of the anti-inflammatory cytokine IL-10 via an interaction with TLR2 of the host immune system. The Yop effectors can also inhibit phagocytosis, disrupt the cytoskeleton, and down-regulate the host inflammatory responses, (Demeure *et al.,* 2019).

## Clinical Manifestations

Yersinia pestis infection or 'black death' is fatal with an estimated mortality of 60% to 100% in untreated patients, (Campbell, 1995). Plague may present as any of three possible syndromes, (Prentice & Rahalison, 2007).

### Bubonic Plague

It is the most common form of plague accounting for 80% to 95% of cases (Prentice & Rahalison, 2007) (Daya & Nakamura, 2005). It characteristically manifests with tender, often erythematous swellings known as 'buboes' in lymph node-bearing regions, typically, though not exclusively, in the inguinal region. This presentation is preceded by prodromal symptoms, including an abrupt onset of fever, chills, fatigue, and headache, occasionally accompanied by lymphadenopathy. Axillary, cervical, or epitrochlear buboes may occur in patients with bubonic plague associated with cat exposure, (Gage *et al.,* 2000).

While the flea bite is typically subtle, if it occurs on an extremity, it may be linked to swelling of lymph nodes in the corresponding draining region. Moreover, various cutaneous manifestations may also occur; for instance, some patients may develop pustules, eschars, or necrotic lesions resembling ecthyma gangrenosum, (Welty *et al.,* 1985).

If left untreated, around 50% of cases develop a sequela of sepsis and, potentially, shock (Prentice & Rahalison, 2007) due to disseminated infection. This is often complicated by pneumonia, referred to as secondary pneumonic plague, and meningitis, (Warren *et al.,* 2011).

### Pneumonic Plague

It is the most aggressive and life-threatening form of plague (26); it is rapidly fatal if management is not initiated early in the course of the disease, (Ratsitorahina *et al.,* 2000). It can be either primary or secondary.

**Primary Pneumonic Plague**. Unlike Bubonic plague, which is transmitted through the bite of an infected flea or exposure to infected material through a break in the skin, primary pneumonic plague —a rare form (Ratsitorahina *et al.,* 2000)— is acquired by inhalation of respiratory secretions or aerosolized droplets from infected host, or by laboratory exposure. It typically presents with sudden onset of dyspnea, high fever, pleuritic chest pain, and cough that may be accompanied by characteristic bloody sputum. Gastrointestinal symptoms such as vomiting, diarrhea, and abdominal pain, are common, (Hull, Montes, & Mann, 1986).

**Secondary Pneumonic Plague**. It is the result of pulmonary bacterial seeding from a bubo or other source via hematogenous route. Presentation is similar to that of primary pneumonic plague. Patients typically develop secondary pneumonic plague when treatment for bubonic infection is delayed.

### Septicemic Plague

It typically presents as a sequela of bubonic plague. Nonetheless, 10% to 20% of cases manifest without a preceding bubo (Prentice & Rahalison, 2007), presenting a diagnostic challenge due to the nonspecific nature of other symptoms like hyperpyrexia, profound fatigue, and gastrointestinal symptoms. Septic complications ranging from hypotension to multi-organ failure develop later in the course of the disease; a small percentage of patients develop petechiae and purpura as a result of disseminated intravascular coagulation, (Butler, 1994).

Pharyngitis, tonsillitis, and anterior cervical lymphadenitis are less common manifestations of the black death, (Butler, 1994) (Crook & Tempest, 1993).

## DIAGNOSIS

The foundation for an accurate diagnosis of plague rests on maintaining a high index of clinical suspicion. Physicians residing in endemic regions must remain vigilant, especially if a patient mentions contact with rodents or any other animal vector within the preceding 10 days, for presentation of regional lymphadenitis accompanied with fever and hypotension, (Ratsitorahina *et al.,* 2000). Moreover, when encountering a case involving pneumonia, hemoptysis, and sputum containing gram-negative rods, it is prudent to consider the possibility of plague.

While complete blood counts may exhibit similarities across various infectious diseases, a white blood cell count exceeding 20,000/microL and the presence of thrombocytopenia serve as valuable diagnostic indicators for identifying plague in endemic areas, (Butler *et al.*, 1974).

Chest x-ray findings in pneumonic plague can be nonspecific, yet some patients may exhibit hilar or mediastinal adenopathy, potentially offering a clue to the presence of plague, (Alsofrom, Mettler, & Mann, 1981).

The definitive identification of Y. pestis is established by isolation of the organism in culture or by serologic testing, (Prentice & Rahalison, 2007) (Human Plague, n.d.). Multiple additional tests are accessible to support the diagnosis.

## DIAGNOSTIC MODALITIES

### Culture and Staining

Clinical samples used can be either bubo aspirates, respiratory tract specimens, blood, pharyngeal swabs, or urine, (Barbieri *et al.*, 2020). Y. pestis has the capacity to thrive on nutrient-rich, non-selective brain heart infusion agar (BHIA); nevertheless, the use of MacConkey agar and CIN medium is recommended (Rasoamanana *et al.,* 1996) to restrict the proliferation of potentially contaminating bacteria within the sample. Employing Wright-Giemsa stain on sampled blood reveals rod-shaped organisms in as much as 40 percent of cases.

### Serology

This test relies on the detection of a capsule-like antigen expressed exclusively by Y. pestis bacteria. Serologic testing requires the acquisition of an acute and a convalescent serum sample spaced 1-2 weeks apart; a minimum fourfold rise in antibody titers to the F-1 pestis antigen is suggestive of the diagnosis, (Human Plague, n.d.). Alternatively, a single titer exceeding 1:16 using the passive hemagglutination test strongly suggests the diagnosis, (Butler, 1994).

### Rapid Tests

A rapid diagnostic test capable of detecting Y. pestis F1 antigen in the sputum or serum within 15 minutes (27,36).

### Molecular Testing

Polymerase chain reaction (PCR) can be utilized for the provisional identification of Y. pestis.

## TREATMENT

The most effective treatment for plague infection consists of two major approaches: specific antibiotics and nonspecific supportive treatments such as anti-shock treatment. In fact, prior to the use of antibiotics, the overall mortality rate of plague infection was estimated to be higher than fifty percent, with nearly 100 lethality established for untreated cases of primary plague meningitis, septicemia, and pneumonia; nonetheless, after the use of antibiotics in plague management, the mortality rate attributed to bubonic plague and septicemic plague declined to 5-50%, (Nikiforov *et al.*, 2016). Early detection with timely administration of efficient antibiotics is critical, as multiple studies have indicated that delaying antibiotic initiation or anti-shock therapy implementation by more than 24 hours can be life-threatening for patients, since it is correlated with higher levels of bacterial biomass and a further severe subsequent inflammatory response resulting from endotoxin release triggered by both lytic and non-lytic antimicrobials, (Yang, 2017) (Nau & Eiffert, 2002). Streptomycin and gentamicin are the most effective antibiotics against Y. pestis, and as such, streptomycin is the first-line antibiotic for most cases of plague treatment; both can be used and are recommended among all adults, which includes pregnant women, immunocompromised patients, and children (though lower dosages may be required in some cases), (Rosario-Acevedo *et al.,* 2021). Chloramphenicol is another effective treatment for bubonic or septicemic plague that can be utilized with aminoglycosides, (Dennis, 2005) (Rosario-Acevedo *et al.,* 2021). Doxycycline and tetracycline are appropriate alternative antibacterial treatments for individuals with simple plague and can also be administered in combination with other antibiotics or in people who are intolerant to aminoglycosides, (Rosario-Acevedo *et al.,* 2021). Antibiotic medication should be endured for 10 days in all cases, (Nikiforov *et al.,* 2016). All of these medications are provided parenterally when treating a small number of plague patients, whereas oral antibiotic treatment has been utilized during a plague epidemic involving a large number of patients and individuals who may have come into contact with the plague. In such instances, doxycycline at a dose of 100 mg twice day or ciprofloxacin at a dose of 500 mg twice daily are recommended, (Jullien & Garner, 2019). Furthermore, most Y. pestis isolates from all over the world are streptomycin-sensitive; nonetheless, a multidrug-resistant (MDR) strain was discovered from Madagascar, (Galimand *et al.*, 1997). Fortunately, this MDR strain has never reappeared naturally in this region or elsewhere in the world. If infection by such a strain occurs, the above-mentioned antibiotics should be avoided in the selection of effective treatments, (Yang, 2017).

Shock and extensive diffuse intravascular coagulation (DIC) characterize severe cases of plague, necessitating supportive anti-shock therapy, which includes infusion therapy, administration of vasopressors and corticosteroids, inotropy, and respiratory support, (Anisimov & Amoako, 2006). In severe cases, shock therapy is started by early fluid resuscitation and the prompt commencement of mechanical breathing, (Nikiforov *et al.,* 2016) (Anisimov & Amoako, 2006). Infusion treatment is performed using a balanced combination of crystalloids and colloids, with the possibility of adding vasopressors, which include norepinephrine and dopamine, or Steroids, that can also be used to restore hemodynamics to their normal state, (Nikiforov *et al.,* 2016). Ionotropic Dobutamine is widely used for plague patients suffering from cardiac depression, which is characteristic in severe plague infections.

Lastly, DIC-related bleeding should most likely be treated with replacement therapy, such as platelets for thrombocytopenia, cryoprecipitate for hypofibrinogenemia, and fresh frozen plasma for low coagulation factors, (Anisimov & Amoako, 2006).

In terms of prevention, pneumonic plague is very easy to prevent given that wearing a face mask or by simply covering one's mouth with a jacket can successfully prevent transmission, (Wang *et al.*, 2011). A patient with suspected pneumonic or bubonic plague and subsequent pneumonic or septicemic plague, on the other hand, should be isolated, (Yang, 2017). Apart from physical protection, the WHO Expert Committee on Plague, suggested antimicrobial prophylaxis with tetracycline, streptomycin, and chloramphenicol. There is still no effective vaccination for plague prevention, however some countries, such as China and Russia, utilize a live attenuated vaccine, (Wang *et al.*, 2013) (WHO, 1970).

## NOVEL RESEARCH STRATEGIES

The World Health Organization Expert Committee on Plague has designated antibiotics such as tetracycline and streptomycin as the 'gold standard' treatment for plague. However, concerns about the emergence of antibiotic-resistant Y. pestis strains have prompted the search for alternatives to antibiotics. Researchers have looked into alternatives such as immunotherapy, non-pathogen-specific immunomodulatory therapy, phage therapy, bacteriocin therapy, and treatment with virulence factor inhibitors, (Anisimov & Amoako, 2006).

Recent research has looked into the efficacy of phage therapy against Yersinia pestis. In mouse models of pneumonic plague, phage treatment, particularly with the well-characterized A1122 and PST phages, showed some success in delaying mortality and providing protection. These phages were chosen for their known specificity to Y. pestis as well as their ability to target multiple receptors, reducing the possibility of phage-resistant mutants emerging. However, difficulties were encountered during in vivo experiments, most notably in maintaining phage activity within the bloodstream and organs, possibly due to interference by blood components that hampered phage-bacterial interactions. Furthermore, the presence of phages in the spleen and liver in the absence of effective bacterial clearance indicated potential difficulties in phage accessibility to bacteria within these organs. Despite this, the phage cocktail demonstrated a remarkable synergistic effect when combined with the antibiotic ceftriaxone. This combined approach also triggered the development of adaptive immunity in surviving animals, increasing the efficacy of the treatment. These findings highlight the potential for emergency use, even in acute infections such as pneumonic plague, implying a synergistic effect between phages and antibiotics that could be investigated and optimized to combat highly resistant pathogens. Further research into phage efficacy in the presence of blood components, as well as their ability to supplement antibiotic therapy, holds promise for alternative treatments against multidrug-resistant pathogens, (Vagima *et al.,* 2022).

Moreover, there is evidence that Pseudomonas aeruginosa, an opportunistic pathogen that causes severe pneumonia in immunocompromised patients, and Yersinia pestis use a virulence mechanism that is highly homologous, the type III secretion system. Both Yersinia and Pseudomonas have type III secretion systems that contain a protein called V-antigen, which can be used as a target for immunotherapy, (Sawa & Wiener-Kronish, 2004).

When it comes to vaccines, the search for new antigens from Y. pestis is an ongoing effort in the development of plague vaccines, (Sun, 2016). While promising in animal models, the F1/LcrV-based subunit vaccine primarily induces a humoral immune response. Its effectiveness in humans has yet to be determined, but it has the potential to benefit populations living in plague-prone areas. Because of its reliance on humoral immunity, periodic boosters may be required. Future plague vaccines should aim to elicit strong cell-mediated immunity as well as humoral responses, as both are critical to vaccine effectiveness, (Verma & Tuteja, 2016). Another novel strategy is nanotechnology, which has transformed plague vaccine development by tackling major obstacles such as immunogenicity and stability. Several novel approaches based on nanocarrier-based systems have been investigated, demonstrating their ability to efficiently deliver Y. pestis antigens while also stimulating robust immune responses. Nanostructural vaccine particles loaded with Y. pestis antigens demonstrated stability, pH-responsive loading, and efficient immune presentation. Biodegradable polyanhydride nanoparticles encapsulating F1-V antigens induced persistent antibody responses, whereas Y. pestis F1-antigen decorated gold nanoparticles elicited strong IgG antibody responses. Furthermore, bacteriophage T4 DNA nanoparticles delivering the F1-V plague vaccine demonstrated promising results in eliciting both antibody and cellular immune responses, suggesting new avenues for plague vaccine design and genetic therapies.

Several studies have looked into new adjuvants to improve the efficacy of plague vaccines. Protollin, a Proteosome-based adjuvant, outperformed Alhydrogel in inducing potent immune responses, resulting in significant protection against Y. pestis aerosol challenges. Intranasal vaccination with IL-12-adjuvanted inactivated Y. pestis CO92 provided complete protection in mice against lethal Y. pestis challenges, with reduced pulmonary pathology and pro-inflammatory cytokines. The use of Y. pestis LcrV protein fused to anti-DEC antibody, along with poly IC adjuvant, to target dendritic cells via the DEC-205 receptor induced robust mucosal cellular immunity, high frequencies of IFN--secreting CD4+ T cells, and improved survival after a Y. pestis pulmonary challenge. Furthermore, when combined with alum, SA-4-1BBL, a Th1 adjuvant, improved cellular responses and generated a balanced

Th1/Th2 immune response, providing better protection against Y. pestis bubonic challenges than individual adjuvants. These findings highlight the potential of these adjuvants to improve the efficacy of plague vaccines, opening up new avenues for further development and application against other pathogens.

Plant-based technology has emerged as a low-cost method of producing vaccine antigens, showing promise in the development of vaccines against a variety of diseases. Researchers used Nicotiana benthamiana to create plague antigens F1, V, and the fusion protein F1-V, which elicited systemic immune responses and provided protection against virulent Y. pestis challenges in guinea pigs via subcutaneous immunization. They successfully induced mucosal immune responses in mice using tomatoes as an oral vaccine delivery system, revealing increased antibody concentrations after an oral boost with transgenic tomato fruits containing F1-V antigen. Zera technology also improved protein accumulation, with Zera-F1-V accumulation outperforming F1-V without Zera fusion across multiple host plant systems. Furthermore, studies in N. benthamiana showed that F1, LcrV, and F1-LcrV antigens synthesized with a thermostable carrier molecule inducing high titers of protective antibodies against Y. pestis in Cynomolgus Macaques, providing complete protection against aerosolized Y. pestis challenges. Chloroplast engineering in lettuce and carrot plants also resulted in the successful expression of the F1-V fusion antigen, which elicited systemic humoral responses in mice following subcutaneous immunization. These plant-based strategies demonstrate the potential for low-cost and easily accessible plague vaccine development, (Sun, 2016).

## CONCLUSION

Plague, a historically significant and long-lasting infectious disease caused by Yersinia pestis, continues to be a public-health threat in many parts of the world. This article has given a comprehensive overview of plague, including epidemiology, transmission, clinical manifestations, diagnosis, treatment, challenges, and emerging research strategies. The disease, which is typically spread by fleas or direct contact with infected animals, manifests in three forms: bubonic, septicemic, and pneumonic, with each having distinct clinical features ranging from swollen lymph nodes to severe respiratory symptoms. Diagnosis of the plague is based on clinical suspicion, which is supported by laboratory tests such as culture, PCR, and serology, and treatment is based on antibiotics and supportive care. Outbreaks in endemic areas, antibiotic resistance, and limited access to healthcare resources, particularly in vulnerable communities, continue to pose difficulties in plague management. New research strategies, such as vaccine development, novel antimicrobial therapies, and advanced diagnostic tools, provide hope for more effective control and prevention.

Finally, plague continues to be a source of concern due to its rapid spread and severe consequences. Improved surveillance, healthcare infrastructure, and global collaboration are required to develop innovative interventions and mitigate the impact of this ancient yet persistent infectious threat.

## REFERENCES


Alsofrom, D. J., Mettler, F. A.Jr, & Mann, J. M. (1981). Radiographic manifestations of plaque in New Mexico, 1975-1980. A review of 42 proved cases. *Radiology*, *139*(3), 561–565. DOI: 10.1148/radiology.139.3.7232721 PMID: 7232721

Anisimov, A. P., & Amoako, K. K. (2006). Treatment of plague: Promising alternatives to antibiotics. *Journal of Medical Microbiology*, *55*(Pt 11), 1461–1475. DOI: 10.1099/jmm.0.46697-0 PMID: 17030904

Barbieri, R., Signoli, M., Chevé, D., Costedoat, C., Tzortzis, S., Aboudharam, G., Raoult, D., & Drancourt, M. (2020). Yersinia pestis: The Natural History of Plague. *Clinical Microbiology Reviews*, *34*(1), e00044–e19. DOI: 10.1128/CMR.00044-19 PMID: 33298527

Benedictow, O. J. (2019). Epidemiology of Plague: Problems with the Use of Mathematical Epidemiological Models in Plague Research and the Question of Transmission by Human Fleas and Lice. The Canadian Journal of Infectious Diseases & Medical Microbiology =. *The Canadian Journal of Infectious Diseases & Medical Microbiology*, *1542024*, 1–20. Advance online publication. DOI: 10.1155/2019/1542024 PMID: 31531149

Butler, T. (1994). Yersinia infections: Centennial of the discovery of the plague bacillus. *Clinical Infectious Diseases*, *19*(4), 655–661. DOI: 10.1093/clinids/19.4.655 PMID: 7803628

Butler, T., Bell, W. R., Linh, N. N., Tiep, N. D., & Arnold, K.Clinical and Hematologic Aspects. (1974). Yersinia pestis infection in Vietnam. I. Clinical and hematologic aspects. *The Journal of Infectious Diseases*, *129*(Suppl), S78–S84. DOI: 10.1093/infdis/129.Supplement_1.S78 PMID: 4825250

Campbell, G. L., & Hughes, J. M. (1995). Plague in India: A New Warning from an Old Nemesis. *Annals of Internal Medicine*, *122*(2), 151–153. DOI: 10.7326/0003-4819-122-2-199501150-00014 PMID: 7992992

Chanteau, S., Rahalison, L., Ralafiarisoa, L., Foulon, J., Ratsitorahina, M., Ratsifasoamanana, L., Carniel, É., & Nato, F. (2003). Development and testing of a rapid diagnostic test for bubonic and pneumonic plague. The Lancet. https://www.semanticscholar.org/paper/Development-and-testing-of-a-rapid-diagnostic-test-Chanteau-Rahalison/0ad30482641f56f661161362b49e68f47bea8ee6

Crook, L. D., & Tempest, B. (1992). Plague. A clinical review of 27 cases. *Archives of Internal Medicine*, *152*(6), 1253–1256. DOI: 10.1001/archinte.1992.00400180107017 PMID: 1599354

. Daya, M., & Nakamura, Y. (2005). Pulmonary disease from biological agents: Anthrax, plague, Q fever, and tularemia. Critical Care Clinics, 21(4), 747–763, vii. DOI: 10.1016/j.ccc.2005.06.009

Demeure, C. E., Dussurget, O., Mas Fiol, G., Le Guern, A.-S., Savin, C., & Pizarro-Cerdá, J. (2019). Yersinia pestis and plague: An updated view on evolution, virulence determinants, immune subversion, vaccination, and diagnostics. *Genes and Immunity*, *20*(5), 357–370. DOI: 10.1038/s41435-019-0065-0 PMID: 30940874

Dennis, D. T. (2005). Plague as a Biological Weapon. In Fong, I. W., & Alibek, K. (Eds.), *Bioterrorism and Infectious Agents: A New Dilemma for the 21st Century* (pp. 37–70). Springer US., DOI: 10.1007/0-387-23685-6_2

Du, Z., & Wang, X. (2016). Pathology and Pathogenesis of Yersinia pestis. *Advances in Experimental Medicine and Biology*, *918*, 193–222. DOI: 10.1007/978-94-024-0890-4_7 PMID: 27722864

Eisen, R. J., MacMillan, K., Atiku, L. A., Mpanga, J. T., Zielinski-Gutierrez, E., Graham, C. B., Boegler, K. A., Enscore, R. E., & Gage, K. L. (2014). Identification of Risk Factors for Plague in the West Nile Region of Uganda. *The American Journal of Tropical Medicine and Hygiene*, *90*(6), 1047–1058. DOI: 10.4269/ajtmh.14-0035 PMID: 24686743

Eisenberg, M., & Mordechai, L. (2019). The Justinianic Plague: An interdisciplinary review. *Byzantine and Modern Greek Studies*, *43*(2), 156–180. DOI: 10.1017/byz.2019.10

Expert, W. H. O. (1970). Committee on plague. Fourth report. *World Health Organization Technical Report Series*, *447*, 1–25. PMID: 4986823

Gage, K. L., Dennis, D. T., Orloski, K. A., Ettestad, P., Brown, T. L., Reynolds, P. J., Pape, W. J., Fritz, C. L., Carter, L. G., & Stein, J. D. (2000). Cases of Cat-Associated Human Plague in the Western US, 1977-1998. *Clinical Infectious Diseases*, *30*(6), 893–900. DOI: 10.1086/313804 PMID: 10852811

Galimand, M., Guiyoule, A., Gerbaud, G., Rasoamanana, B., Chanteau, S., Carniel, E., & Courvalin, P. (1997). Multidrug Resistance in Yersinia pestis Mediated by a Transferable Plasmid. *The New England Journal of Medicine*, *337*(10), 677–681. DOI: 10.1056/NEJM199709043371004 PMID: 9278464

Glatter, K. A., & Finkelman, P. (2021). History of the Plague: An Ancient Pandemic for the Age of COVID-19. *The American Journal of Medicine*, *134*(2), 176–181. DOI: 10.1016/j.amjmed.2020.08.019 PMID: 32979306

Hinnebusch, B. J. (2005). The evolution of flea-borne transmission in Yersinia pestis. *Current Issues in Molecular Biology*, *7*(2), 197–212. PMID: 16053250

Hinnebusch, B. J. (2010). Plague in the 21st Century: Global Public Health Challenges and Goals. In V. St. Georgiev (Ed.), *National Institute of Allergy and Infectious Diseases, NIH: Volume 3: Intramural Research* (pp. 87–94). Humana Press. DOI: 10.1007/978-1-60761-512-5_9

Hull, H. F., Montes, J. M., & Mann, J. M. (1986). Plague masquerading as gastrointestinal illness. *The Western Journal of Medicine*, *145*(4), 485–487. PMID: 3788132

Human Plague—United States. 1993-1994. (n.d.). Retrieved December 15, 2023, from https://www.cdc.gov/mmwr/preview/mmwrhtml/00026077.htm

Jullien, S., & Garner, P. (2019). Web Annex A. Antibiotics for treating plague [executive summary]. *Systematic Reviews.*

Khan, I. A. (2004). Plague: The dreadful visitation occupying the human mind for centuries. *Transactions of the Royal Society of Tropical Medicine and Hygiene*, *98*(5), 270–277. DOI: 10.1016/S0035-9203(03)00059-2 PMID: 15109549

Lindler, L. E. (2009). Typing methods for the plague pathogen, Yersinia pestis. *Journal of AOAC International*, *92*(4), 1174–1183. DOI: 10.1093/jaoac/92.4.1174 PMID: 19714987

Manungo, P., Peterson, D. E., Todd, C. H., Mthamo, N., & Pazvakavambwa, B. (1998). Risk factors for contracting plague in Nkayi district, Zimbabwe. *The Central African Journal of Medicine*, *44*(7), 173–176. PMID: 10028191

Metcalfe, S. (2013). History lessons. *Australian Family Physician*, *42*(8), 519. PMID: 24133699

Mikula, K. M., Kolodziejczyk, R., & Goldman, A. (2012). Yersinia infection tools-characterization of structure and function of adhesins. *Frontiers in Cellular and Infection Microbiology*, *2*, 169. DOI: 10.3389/fcimb.2012.00169 PMID: 23316485

Munyenyiwa, A., Zimba, M., Nhiwatiwa, T., & Barson, M. (2019). Plague in Zimbabwe from 1974 to 2018: A review article. *PLoS Neglected Tropical Diseases*, *13*(11), e0007761. DOI: 10.1371/journal.pntd.0007761 PMID: 31751348

Nau, R., & Eiffert, H. (2002). Modulation of Release of Proinflammatory Bacterial Compounds by Antibacterials: Potential Impact on Course of Inflammation and Outcome in Sepsis and Meningitis. *Clinical Microbiology Reviews*, *15*(1), 95–110. DOI: 10.1128/CMR.15.1.95-110.2002 PMID: 11781269

Nikiforov, V. V., Gao, H., Zhou, L., & Anisimov, A. (2016). Plague: Clinics, Diagnosis and Treatment. In Yang, R., & Anisimov, A. (Eds.), *Yersinia pestis: Retrospective and Perspective* (pp. 293–312). Springer Netherlands., DOI: 10.1007/978-94-024-0890-4_11

Nyirenda, S. S., Hang'ombe, B. M., Machang'u, R., Mwanza, J., & Kilonzo, B. S. (2017). Identification of Risk Factors Associated with Transmission of Plague Disease in Eastern Zambia. *The American Journal of Tropical Medicine and Hygiene*, *97*(3), 826–830. DOI: 10.4269/ajtmh.16-0990 PMID: 28722614

Pechous, R. D., Sivaraman, V., Stasulli, N. M., & Goldman, W. E. (2016). Pneumonic Plague: The Darker Side of Yersinia pestis. *Trends in Microbiology*, *24*(3), 190–197. DOI: 10.1016/j.tim.2015.11.008 PMID: 26698952

Persson, C., Carballeira, N., Wolf-Watz, H., & Fällman, M. (1997). The PTPase YopH inhibits uptake of Yersinia, tyrosine phosphorylation of p130Cas and FAK, and the associated accumulation of these proteins in peripheral focal adhesions. *The EMBO Journal*, *16*(9), 2307–2318. DOI: 10.1093/emboj/16.9.2307 PMID: 9171345

Prentice, M. B., & Rahalison, L. (2007). Plague. *Lancet*, *369*(9568), 1196–1207. DOI: 10.1016/S0140-6736(07)60566-2 PMID: 17416264

Rasoamanana, B., Rahalison, L., Raharimanana, C., & Chanteau, S. (1996). Comparison of Yersinia CIN agar and mouse inoculation assay for the diagnosis of plague. *Transactions of the Royal Society of Tropical Medicine and Hygiene*, *90*(6), 651. DOI: 10.1016/S0035-9203(96)90420-4 PMID: 9015505

Ratsitorahina, M., Chanteau, S., Rahalison, L., Ratsifasoamanana, L., & Boisier, P. (2000). Epidemiological and diagnostic aspects of the outbreak of pneumonic plague in Madagascar. *Lancet*, *355*(9198), 111–113. DOI: 10.1016/S0140-6736(99)05163-6 PMID: 10675169

Rosario-Acevedo, R., Biryukov, S. S., Bozue, J. A., & Cote, C. K. (2021). Plague Prevention and Therapy: Perspectives on Current and Future Strategies. *Biomedicines*, *9*(10), 10. Advance online publication. DOI: 10.3390/biomedicines9101421 PMID: 34680537

. Sawa, T., & Wiener-Kronish, J. P. (2004). A therapeutic strategy against the shared virulence mechanism utilized by both Yersinia pestis and Pseudomonas aeruginosa. Anesthesiology Clinics of North America, 22(3), 591–606, viii–ix. DOI: 10.1016/j.atc.2004.05.002

Smiley, S. T. (2008). Immune defense against pneumonic plague. *Immunological Reviews*, *225*(1), 256–271. DOI: 10.1111/j.1600-065X.2008.00674.x PMID: 18837787

Sun, W. (2016). Chapter 12 Plague vaccines: Status and future. *Advances in Experimental Medicine and Biology*, *918*, 313–360. DOI: 10.1007/978-94-024-0890-4_12 PMID: 27722869

Trosky, J. E., Liverman, A. D. B., & Orth, K. (2008). Yersinia outer proteins: Yops. *Cellular Microbiology*, *10*(3), 557–565. DOI: 10.1111/j.1462-5822.2007.01109.x PMID: 18081726

Vagima, Y., Gur, D., Aftalion, M., Moses, S., Levy, Y., Makovitzki, A., Holtzman, T., Oren, Z., Segula, Y., Fatelevich, E., Tidhar, A., Zauberman, A., Rotem, S., Mamroud, E., & Steinberger-Levy, I. (2022). Phage Therapy Potentiates Second-Line Antibiotic Treatment against Pneumonic Plague. *Viruses*, *14*(4), 688. DOI: 10.3390/v14040688 PMID: 35458417

Vallès, X., Stenseth, N. C., Demeure, C., Horby, P., Mead, P. S., Cabanillas, O., Ratsitorahina, M., Rajerison, M., Andrianaivoarimanana, V., Ramasindrazana, B., Pizarro-Cerda, J., Scholz, H. C., Girod, R., Hinnebusch, B. J., Vigan-Womas, I., Fontanet, A., Wagner, D. M., Telfer, S., Yazdanpanah, Y., & Baril, L. (2020). Human plague: An old scourge that needs new answers. *PLoS Neglected Tropical Diseases*, *14*(8), e0008251. DOI: 10.1371/journal.pntd.0008251 PMID: 32853251

Verma, S. K., & Tuteja, U. (2016). Plague Vaccine Development: Current Research and Future Trends. *Frontiers in Immunology*, *7*, 602. DOI: 10.3389/fimmu.2016.00602 PMID: 28018363

Wang, H., Cui, Y., Wang, Z., Wang, X., Guo, Z., Yan, Y., Li, C., Cui, B., Xiao, X., Yang, Y., Qi, Z., Wang, G., Wei, B., Yu, S., He, D., Chen, H., Chen, G., Song, Y., & Yang, R. (2011). A Dog-Associated Primary Pneumonic Plague in Qinghai Province, China. *Clinical Infectious Diseases*, *52*(2), 185–190. DOI: 10.1093/cid/ciq107 PMID: 21288842

Wang, X., Zhang, X., Zhou, D., & Yang, R. (2013). Live-attenuated Yersinia pestis vaccines. *Expert Review of Vaccines*, *12*(6), 677–686. DOI: 10.1586/erv.13.42 PMID: 23750796

Warren, R., Lockman, H., Barnewall, R., Krile, R., Blanco, O. B., Vasconcelos, D., Price, J., House, R. V., Bolanowksi, M. A., & Fellows, P. (2011). Cynomolgus macaque model for pneumonic plague. *Microbial Pathogenesis*, *50*(1), 12–22. DOI: 10.1016/j.micpath.2010.10.002 PMID: 21040776

Welty, T., Grabman, J., Kompare, E., Wood, G., Welty, E., Duzen, J. V., Rudd, P., & Poland, J. (1985). Nineteen cases of plague in Arizona. A spectrum including ecthyma gangrenosum due to plague and plague in pregnancy. The Western Journal of Medicine. https://www.semanticscholar.org/paper/Nineteen-cases-of-plague-in-Arizona.-A-spectrum-due-Welty-Grabman/e8e04e8f9b02b4e4f735e5637e027c5d36563340

Yang, R. (2017). Plague: Recognition, Treatment, and Prevention. Journal of Clinical Microbiology, 56(1). DOI: 10.1128/JCM.01519-17

# Chapter 12
# Decoding Cholera:
## From Symptoms to Breakthroughs in Treatment and Research

**Amarelle Chamoun**
https://orcid.org/0000-0002-3473-8922
*Faculty of Medical Sciences, Lebanese University, Beirut, Lebanon*

**Jana Mahdi**
*Faculty of Medical Sciences, Lebanese University, Beirut, Lebanon*

**Jana Jaber**
*Faculty of Medical Sciences, Lebanese University, Beirut, Lebanon*

**Hadi Imad Farhat**
*Faculty of Medical Sciences, Lebanese University, Beirut, Lebanon*

**Tia Khadra**
*Faculty of Medical Sciences, Lebanese University, Beirut, Lebanon*

## ABSTRACT

*Cholera, resulting from Gram-negative bacteria Vibrio cholerae, is an ongoing concern to public health, generating widespread infections, particularly in developing countries, leading to significant morbidity and mortality annually. Some strains can produce an enterotoxin, significantly contributing to the disease. Contamination occurs by ingestion, direct contact with a patient, or contaminated water and food. As a consequence of the toxin-induced fluid intestinal leakage, patients present with acute watery diarrhea and vomiting. Diagnosis is established by recognition of the bacteria in a stool specimen. Severity of dehydration defines the prognosis, which can be lethal in only a few hours if intensive rehydration is not administered*

DOI: 10.4018/979-8-3693-1990-1.ch012

*immediately. During outbreaks or in endemic areas, oral cholera vaccines are important components of an integrated control package. This chapter presents the epidemiology, pathophysiology, diagnosis, clinical signs and symptoms, treatment options for V. cholerae patients, challenges, and the current most novel research approaches.*

## INTRODUCTION

Cholera, caused by the bacterium *Vibrio cholerae*, is an ancient disease that has haunted humanity for centuries (Mercer, 2021). It is transmitted mainly through the consumption of contaminated food and water (Sack et al., 2004), and characterized by profuse watery diarrhea, vomiting, and abdominal cramps. In severe cases, it can lead to muscle cramps, hypotension and shock (Segura, 2022).

The first recorded cholera outbreak surged in India during the 16th century. From there, the disease spread rapidly across Asia and Europe. During the 19th century, cholera emerged as a global pandemic, killing millions of people worldwide (Mercer, 2021). Since then, there have been seven large pandemics worldwide over the last two centuries, such as in Zimbabwe (2008-2009), Haiti (2010-2012), and Yemen (2016-2020).

Despite advances in healthcare, cholera remains a pressing global health concern. Today, it is responsible for an estimated 1 to 4 million cases and 21,000 to 143,000 deaths annually. According to the World Health Organization (WHO), both the number of infections and the geographic spread of cholera have increased since 2021, with the majority of cases occurring in Africa and the Eastern Mediterranean. This persistent crisis is largely driven by poor socioeconomic conditions, including inadequate access to clean water, sanitation, and housing. In 2015, the economic burden of cholera was estimated to be $130 million (Asantewaa et al., 2024).

The modern understanding of cholera transmission can be traced back to 1854, during a severe outbreak in London, when Dr. John Snow, an obstetrician and anesthesiologist, identified contaminated water as the mode of transmission. His work laid the foundation for modern epidemiology and public health infrastructure, emphasizing the role of clean water and sanitation in disease prevention (Azman et al., 2013).

Despite its long and devastating history, cholera is both preventable and treatable. By understanding the epidemiology, pathogenesis, clinical features, diagnosis, treatment, and prevention of cholera, we can develop and implement effective strategies to overcome this disease and reduce its global burden.

## DISCUSSION

### Definition

Cholera is a highly contagious and life-threatening gastrointestinal tract infection caused by the bacterium *Vibrio cholerae*. It is primarily transmitted through the ingestion of contaminated water and food (Sack et al., 2021). This pathogen produces toxins that lead to rapid and severe fluid loss through profuse watery diarrhea (Parsi, 2001), which can quickly result in dehydration, electrolyte imbalances, and in severe cases, shock and death if not promptly treated (Mercer, 2021).

Cholera has long been a major public health concern, responsible for numerous outbreaks and epidemics worldwide (Mercer, 2021), causing widespread illness and death in affected communities. Effective prevention and control measures such as access to clean drinking water, improved sanitation practices, and vaccination, have played a crucial role in reducing the incidence and impact of cholera in many parts of the world (Sack et al., 2004). However, cholera remains a persistent threat in many regions with inadequate sanitation infrastructure and limited access to healthcare systems (Mercer, 2021).

### Epidemiology and Prevalence in Developing and Developed Nations

The epidemiology and prevalence of cholera shows huge disparities between developing and developed nations due to the profound impact of socio-economic factors and healthcare infrastructure.

To this day, cholera remains a persistent public health challenge in developing countries, with prevalence rates accounting for up to 90% of all reported cases globally. Between 1990 and 2019, cholera outbreaks have been alarmingly frequent in these regions, leading to a significantly higher number of cases and increased mortality rates (Igere & Ekundayo, 2019).

Cholera continues to pose a serious public health threat in Africa, with Malawi experiencing its worst outbreak in two decades and countries such as Nigeria, Ethiopia, and Kenya also struggling to control the disease. Between December 2023 and January 2024, multiple African nations reported 667,000 cholera cases and 4,000 related deaths, and over the past 20 years, sub-Saharan Africa has recorded more than 2.6 million cases and 60,000 deaths (Akingbola, Abiodun, & Ojo, 2025).

On the other hand, developed countries have largely succeeded in stabilizing the prevalence of cholera. Here, cholera is a rare occurrence, composing only a minor fraction of all diarrheal diseases. This huge reduction in cholera prevalence in developed regions can be attributed to two factors: improved sanitation and access to clean drinking water. These constitutional advancements in infrastructure reduced the number of cholera cases by as much as 90% in comparison to previous decades (Crowcroft, 1994). Moreover, vaccination has played an essential role in reducing the spread of cholera in developed nations. Research has shown that the efficacy of cholera vaccines has reached approximately 75%, pointing out their significant contribution to cholera containment and prevention (Durham et al., 1998).

These numbers underline the critical importance of many factors such as socio-economic conditions, healthcare infrastructure, and vaccination programs in determining the epidemiology and prevalence of cholera, pointing to the burden of this disease held by developing and developed nations.

## Risk Factors

### General Risk Factors

Risk factors associated with cholera infection may be limited to the individual, which include the consumption of water from street vendors (Sinclair et al., 1982), dipping hands into water stored within the household, showering in rivers (Acosta, Galindo, & Kimario, 2001), consuming food remnants (Swerdlow, Malegna, & Begkoyian, 1997), ingesting meals cooked up by a food handler who has recently experienced illness (Holmberg, Harris, & Kay, 1984), neglecting hand washing with soap prior to eating (Hutin, Luby, & Paquet, 2003), and having a close familial connection with an affected individual (Hattis, LaRocque, & Paquet, 2003). Notably, among household contacts of cholera patients, the risk of cholera infection was primarily linked to the quality of household water and the approaches taken in water treatment (Burrowes, Perin, & Monira, 2017).

On a larger scale, factors contributing to the risk of infection encompass rainfall, seasonal variations, inadequate sanitation, voyages, disagreements, dispersal of citizens, inadequate infection control measures by the healthcare system, and residing near polluted water sources. Furthermore, the risk of cholera transmission extends to practices like consuming unwashed fruits or vegetables (Dureab, Jahn, & Krisam, 2019) Moreover, keeping water in storage vessels was linked with a three-fold elevation in the likelihood of acquiring cholera (Qase4rah et al., 2021).

### Specific Drivers of Cholera Outbreaks in Low- and Middle-Income Countries

Since the seventh cholera pandemic began in 1961, the disease has become widespread in many low- and middle-income nations in Africa, Asia, and South America. According to Asantewaa et al., the majority of reported outbreaks occurred in Africa (74%), followed by Asia (26%), with Yemen experiencing the largest outbreak with over 2.3 million suspected cases between 2016 and 2022, driven primarily by conflict-related disruptions to healthcare and sanitation infrastructure. Similarly, ongoing conflicts in Nigeria, the Democratic Republic of the Congo, Syria, and other areas have exacerbated cholera outbreaks by limiting access to clean water and sanitation. Moreover, natural disasters such as cyclones and floods often damage water infrastructure and displace populations, creating ideal conditions for cholera outbreaks, as seen in Mozambique and Malawi. In rural areas, the use of contaminated water sources, like rivers and hand-dug wells, combined with poor sanitation, open defecation, and rainfall runoff increases the risk of transmission. Unimproved latrines and lack of hygiene awareness in countries like India, Ghana, and Uganda further compound the issue. Additionally, foodborne transmission in these countries, especially through improperly cooked seafood, vegetables, cold rice, and street-vended food, remains a major concern. Person-to-person spread, particularly in overcrowded households, also sustains cholera transmission in endemic areas (Asantewaa et al., 2024).

## Pathogenesis

Cholera manifests as a severe secretory diarrhea that can lead to mortality within hours of symptoms (Centers for Disease Control and Prevention, 2010). The rate of fluid loss may surpass 1% of the total body weight within an hour. Infection typically necessitates the ingestion of substantial inoculum, with a consistent disease manifestation requiring between 10 and 10 (Acosta, Galindo, & Kimario, 2023) viable organisms. This is due to the destruction of the majority of *V. cholera* by gastric acidity. After enduring the acidic gastric environment, *V. cholera* enters the gut lumen of the small intestine. In this environment, signals from both bile and mucus induce *V.cholera* to initiate the expression of virulence factor, leading to symptomatic infection (Weil, Becker, & Harris, 2019). Upon reaching the intestine, it employs a single sheathed flagellum for propulsion, penetrating the mucus barrier to adhere to the small intestinal mucosal surface (Freter, O'Brien, & Macsai, 1981). The bacterium preferably colonizes the mid-to-distal small intestine, forming clonal microcolonies in villous crypts (Millet et al., 2014). In addition, it encounters a dense layer of glycosylated proteins, known as mucins. This mucus, housing commensal bacteria, triggers *V. cholerae*'s detection mechanisms. The presence of mucin activates *V. cholerae*'s type VI secretion system (T6SS), acting as a molecular syringe to deliver toxic proteins to nearby bacteria (Bachmann et al., 2015) [25]. Also, this will trigger the ToxR regulon, a pivotal control center in the signaling pathway governing virulence through modulation of CT and toxin-coregulated pilus (TCP) expression (Peterson & Gellings, 2018). All cholera-causing strains carry the ToxR regulon and the necessary equipment to release TCP and CT. TCP, a vital factor for colonization, takes the form of a flexible type IV pilus (Holmgren et al., 1975). It consists of TcpA, a repetitive arrangement of its main structure. In addition, TCP functions as the receptor for the lysogenic bacteriophage CTXϕ, which encodes CT, which is an AB5-subunit toxin (Waldor & Mekalanos, 1996) [28]. Both the enzymatic catalytic A subunit (CtxA) and a pentamer of B subunits (CtxB) are components of the CT structure. The pentamer of B subunits binds to monosialoganglioside GM1 on the apical surface of epithelium (Waldor & <ekalanos, 1996; Cassel & Pfeuffer, 1978), initiating endocytosis. CtxA then breaks free from the endosome to ribosylate the G-protein-regulated adenylyl cyclase on the cell's basolateral membrane (Cassel & Pfeuffer, 1978). This cascade leads to depletion of chloride (Cl-) and substantial fluid secretion into the small intestine, suppressing the absorptive capability of the large intestine's capacity and leading to intense watery diarrhea (Kaper, Morris, & Levine, 1995). Starting with a surge in numbers within the small intestine, *V. cholerae* populations densely flourish, prompting the organisms to disengage from the intestinal surface and depart the host (Qadri, Bhuiyan, & Dutta, 2004). In case of severe cholera, the host expels 10 (Durham et al., 1998)[9] organisms per ml of stool and vomit, sustaining this ongoing release for multiple days when antibiotic treatment is ineffective (Yen, 1964). Beyond the host's excretion, these organisms endure as highly infectious for up to 24 hours. Notably, organisms shed by humans demonstrate greater infectivity compared to their aquatic counterparts (Ellis, La-Rocque, & Uddin, 2015). This pathogenic progression emphasizes pivotal stages in the lifecycle of *V. cholerae* and the intricacies of infection within the human host.

## Clinical Manifestations

Contracting *V. cholerae* may lead to a range of conditions, ranging from asymptomatic colonization of the intestines to the development of severe diarrhea (Weil, Khan, & Chowdhury, 2009). Cholera is an acute gastrointestinal illness characterized by watery diarrhea, induced by toxin-producing strains of the Gram-negative Bacterium *Vibrio cholerae* O1 and O139. The manifestations of cholera caused by the two mentioned serotypes are clinically indistinguishable. The median incubation period of toxigenic cholera is estimated to be 36 hours. However, several factors including host susceptibility, gastric pH, and size of ingested inoculum may affect said period which can range from a few hours to as long as five days. It must be noted that the incubation period did not differ by a clinically significant margin between strains (except O1 El Tor Ogawa) (Azman et al., 2013).

The most common clinical manifestations of cholera are:

**Diarrhea**: The spectrum of *V. cholerae* infections manifests in varying degrees of diarrhea, ranging from mild and self-limiting cases to severe forms necessitating hospitalization. While the milder presentations closely resemble other diarrheal illnesses clinically, the severe variant, referred to as "cholera gravis," stands out distinctly. Cholera gravis is characterized by the passage of abundant "rice-water" stool, often emitting a fishy odor, resulting in a rapid loss of fluids and electrolytes leading to possible hypovolemic shock within 24 hours of symptom onset (Rodriguez & Kahwaji, 2023), a characteristic not observed in other diarrheal illnesses. Notably, in adults, the volume of stool can escalate to 1 liter per hour, and in children, may reach up to 20 cc/kg/hour (Harris, Ivers, & Ferraro, 2011) [37]. Moreover, in comparison to alternative causes of childhood diarrheal illness, cholera patients' stools exhibit a heightened concentration of sodium (Molla et al., 1981), and during the initial phases of the disease, it may contain fecal matter and bile (Harris et al., 2012).

**Other Gastrointestinal Symptoms**: In the early stages of the disease, abdominal discomfort, borborygmi, and vomiting are common. Emesis is often watery and can commence either prior to or following the initiation of diarrhea.

**Manifestations of Hypovolemia and Electrolyte Loss:** Due to the rapid loss of fluids and electrolytes in severe cholera cases, the high mortality rate, ranging from 50 to 70 percent in untreated patients, is attributed to dehydration and abnormalities in electrolyte levels (Lindenbaum, greenough, & Islam, 1967; Siddique, Akram, & Zaman, 1995). Patients that succumb to the illness before seeking treatment usually undergo a median duration of 12 hours between the commencement of symptoms and death (Centers for Disease Control and Prevention, 2010). Dehydrated patients may present with dry mucous membranes, sunken eyes, cold clammy skin with decreased turgor, lethargy, and oliguria. Renal failure with acute tubular necrosis may occur as urine output decreases. Diminished peripheral pulses can also be present in the late course of the disease due to hypotension. Patients may also become acidotic and the etiology is twofold: the loss of bicarbonate in stools and the release of lactic acid as a result of poor perfusion. Such patients may present with rapid shallow breaths (Kassmaul respirations), tachycardia and confusion. Hypokalemia and hypocalcemia due to electrolyte wasting can lead to muscle cramping and weakness (Harris et al., 2012).

**Other Complications**: "Cholera sicca" is a severe and unusual form of the disease in which fluid accumulates in the intestinal lumen leading to possible circulatory collapse and even death even in the absence of diarrhea (Harris et al., 2012). Children may present with symptoms of severe hypoglycemia or coma due to the depletion of glycogen stores and inadequate gluconeogenesis. In the setting of vomiting, aspiration pneumonia has been described as a frequent comorbidity among children and has been associated with mortality (Ryan, Dhar, & Khan, 2000). It must be noted that although cholera is not usually associated with long-term complications, younger children are susceptible to the development of chronic enteropathy and malnutrition (Chowdhury et al., 2022). Fever and bacteremia are rare.

## Diagnosis

Given the acute progression of symptoms, accurate diagnosis relies heavily on correlating clinical presentation with laboratory confirmation. Cholera must be suspected in cases of profuse watery diarrhea, particularly in patients experiencing rapid and severe volume depletion. Even though such manifestation might also be caused by other infectious agents such as rotavirus and norovirus (Aj, Ba, & Dc, 2013; Carlson et al., 1978), mostly reported in children, *Vibrio cholera* is specific to patients aged five or older (Organization WH, 2023). Physicians should also consider its diagnosis if there's a history of travel to cholera-endemic areas.

Despite the availability of several diagnostic tools for accurate diagnosis, the urgency and severity associated with cholera underscore the importance of initiating treatment as soon as possible based on clinical suspicion to avoid complications. This marks clinical suspicion as the cornerstone of diagnosis of cholera. The definitive identification of *V. cholerae* involves isolating the bacterium from stool cultures. However, in regions where stool cultures may not be readily accessible, various rapid tests are available to support the diagnosis.

**Stool Culture**: Stool culture is the gold standard for definitive laboratory diagnosis of cholera, as it has been reported to effectively detect *V. cholerae* in stool samples in 45% of cases, even prior to the onset of the diarrhea (Cash et al., 1974). *V. cholerae* can be isolated and detected in the stool sample by utilizing certain selective media like taurocholate tellurite gelatin agar or thiosulfate-citrate-bile salts-sucrose (TCBS) agar. Enrichment in alkaline peptone water enhances viability and facilitates isolation of the specimen. Additionally, the serogroup and serotype of the microorganism can be determined through the application of specific antibodies (Organization WH, 2003).

**Rapid Tests**: Tests such as Cholkit and Crystal VC utilize immunochromatographic lateral flow devices, also known as dipsticks, to detect the presence of *V. cholerae* antigens in stool specimens. Although less accurate than stool cultures, a recent study showed the sensitivity of the antigen-testing modalities was 98% for both, with 97% and 98% specificity, respectively (Sayeed, Islam, & Hossain, 2018). These tests are particularly valuable when the culture's sensitivity is reduced because viable bacteria are no longer being excreted

in the stool. Specifically a negative stool culture may be observed in the setting of antibiotic administration and/or coinfection with lytic bacteriophage (Alexandrova, Haque, & Rodriguez, 2019; Nelson, Grembi, & Chao, 2020).
**Molecular Tests**: Polymerase chain reactions (PCR) can be used on dried fecal spots to test for presence of cholera enterotoxins.
**Dark-Field Microscopy**: Magnification of cholera watery stools under a dark-field microscope would reveal mobile comma-shaped bacteria. Although specific, the lack of sensitivity of this technique makes it unreliable.

## Treatment

### Fluid Replacement

Rehydration is critical for cholera treatment since it replaces lost fluids and electrolytes, successfully addressing the extreme dehydration caused by this serious illness (Mandal, Mandal, & Pal, 2011). This approach depends on the concept that cholera is a self-limiting illness, hence, if the patient is able to endure the significant fluid loss caused by cholera toxin, the infection eventually will resolve in a duration of a few days. In fact, it is reported that oral rehydration treatment (ORT) lowered cholera mortality by more than 97%, and that over 99 percent of patients on ORT survived V. cholerae infections (Hsueh & Waters, 2019).

According to WHO guidelines, the fluid therapy for a patient with suspected or confirmed cholera is directed by the degree of hypovolemia on physical examination ((ear, nose, and throat), skin pinch, pulse, and mental status) and classified as: none (<5 percent of body weight), some (5 to 10%), or severe (>10%)).

Given an average loss of 20 mL/kg per hour in cholera patients, rehydration must begin immediately (Rodriguez & Kahwaji, 2023). Most mild to severe cholera patients can be treated with oral rehydration solution (ORS). The WHO and UNICEF currently recommend low-osmolarity ORS, which is prepared in 1,000 mL of sterile water and contains salt, chloride, potassium, citrate, and anhydrous glucose. This improved ORS formula is safe and lowers hypertonicity and stool output (Chowdhury et al., 2022). Another ORS solution that has been utilized as a glucose replacement is rice-based saline (i.e., rice powder), with the goal of not only enhancing fluid absorption but also lowering diarrheal volume and length. For instance, a study demonstrated that the rice-based ORT decreased stool volumes by 36% when compared to the glucose ORT (Butler, 2017; Molla, Ahmed, & Greenough, 1985). Rice-based ORS are regarded as an affordable and more acceptable option by patients. It is important to note that homemade ORS may also be made by combining 1/2 teaspoon of salt and 6 tablespoons of sugar in 1,000 mL of sterile water (Chowdhury et al., 2022). Nonetheless, any solution including salt, water, and glucose has been shown to promote sodium reabsorption via the SGLT symporter in the intestinal wall and might be a life-saving measure (Wright, Loo, & Hirayama, 2011).

However, patients with recurrent vomiting (more than three times in one hour) or diarrhea may rapidly advance to severe dehydration if only treated with ORS. In some cases, a combination of intravenous treatment and ORS may be required. Intravenous fluids are often recommended for critically dehydrated individuals or for patients incapable of tolerating oral fluids (Health (UK), 2023) [58]. Intravenous fluids should be delivered as soon as possible to restore circulation. An initial fluid intake of 100 mL/kg should be administered during the next three hours (or five hours in children), with 30 mL/kg administered during the first half-hour (or first hour for children). The WHO recommends Ringer's lactate solution over regular saline in cholera patients since it provides greater concentrations of potassium and bicarbonate (Rodriguez & Kahwaji, 2023). Another commonly utilized solution is the "Dhaka solution" or "cholera saline," which includes a higher amount of glucose, potassium, and bicarbonate than Ringer's lactate solution and can prevent adverse effects including electrolyte imbalances (Chowdhury et al., 2022). As previously noted, the ORS should be implemented in conjunction with intravenous therapy since it provides more electrolytes and glucose than regular intravenous therapy (Davies, Bowman, & Luby, 2017). In severely dehydrated individuals, an immediate IV fluid infusion at a bolus dosage may also be recommended. Patients with severe cholera need to be monitored using a cholera cot if feasible possible. This enables for surveillance of ongoing fluid loss so proper fluid replacement can be taken (Rodriguez & Kahwaji, 2023; Chowdhury et al., 2022).

## Antibiotics

In addition to appropriate hydration, antibiotic therapy is also suggested for severe cholera patients, patients who necessitate hospitalization, or in cases of epidemic conditions. The primary goal of antibiotics is to shorten the length and severity of infectious illness and to limit transmission to other people (researchgate.net, n.d.) [60].

Multiple studies have shown that antibiotics minimize the duration of hospitalization by shortening the duration of infectious diarrhea (from 5 days to 1 or 2 days), reducing stool volume (up to 50%), and decreasing the need for rehydration fluids (Chowdhury et al., 2022) [43].

Antibiotic selection should take into account local antibiotic susceptibility patterns. Adults should use doxycycline or tetracycline as first-line therapy, while children and pregnant people should use azithromycin. The current guidelines recommend a single oral dosage of 300 mg doxycycline or 12.5 mg/kg tetracycline six hours each day for three days (Sharifi-Mood & Metanat, 2014). Several investigations comparing tetracycline to doxycycline found no significant differences in clinical outcome (Khan, Bennish, & seas, 1996). However, it has also been indicated that a single 300-mg dosage of doxycycline is similar to multiple tetracycline doses (Hsueh & Waters, 2019; Khan, Bennish, 7 Seas, 1996). A single dosage of 20 mg azithromycin can relieve diarrheal symptoms in less than 48 hours, 24 hours faster than ciprofloxacin, and reduce vomiting frequency while permitting passage of an average of 36 stools with volumes of roughly 5 L (Hsueh & Waters, 2019).

## Challenges in Low Income and Resource-Limited Settings

### Rising Antibiotic Resistance and Limited Drug Availability

Bacterial resistance to antimicrobial drugs poses a serious global public health threat, especially in the context of managing cholera, where antibiotic therapy is a key component. The emergence and spread of multidrug-resistant *V. cholerae* strains present challenges to effective treatment.

In Africa, there was an increased resistance of *V. cholerae* O1 serotype strains to co-trimoxazole, chloramphenicol, ampicillin, and tetracycline (Chowdhury et al., 2022). Moreover, reduced susceptibility to multiple antibiotics such as ciprofloxacin, tetracycline, streptomycin, and azithromycin was seen in India. A 2025 Indian study reported 40% resistance to ciprofloxacin and 20% to azithromycin among V. cholerae isolates from an outbreak. Similar resistance trends have been reported in the Democratic Republic of Congo, Ghana, and South Asian countries such as Bangladesh, Indonesia, and Vietnam (Chowdhury et al., 2022).

*V. cholerae* AFR13 7PET strain resistant to ten antibiotics, including azithromycin and ciprofloxacin, two key treatments, was identified for the first time during the 2018–2019 cholera outbreak in Yemen. Genomic tracking has since revealed its spread to Lebanon (2022), Kenya (2023), and Tanzania and the Comoros Islands, including Mayotte, in 2024. Notably, Mayotte experienced an outbreak of 221 cases caused by this highly drug-resistant strain between March and July 2024. Ongoing real-time surveillance of the emerging highly drug-resistant AFR13 7PET strain is crucial, as it may acquire an additional gene conferring resistance to tetracycline, which could undermine the effectiveness of current oral antibiotic treatment guidelines (Rouard, Collet, & Njamkepo, 2024).

This growing resistance, especially to first-line treatments like ciprofloxacin, doxycycline, and azithromycin, complicates cholera management, prolongs outbreaks, and increases mortality, especially in resource-limited areas (Samal et al., 2025).

It's important to mention that the current effective treatments for MDR *V. cholerae* with Cp resistance are third generation cephalosporins such as ceftriaxone (Cf) and cefotaxime (Ct), which are highly costly and of limited availability in developing countries (Mandal, Mandal, & Pal, 2011). In contrast, countries with stronger healthcare systems can better manage resistant strains through improved diagnostics and surveillance. This further emphasizes the urgent need for coordinated global AMR strategies (Samal et al., 2025).

## Economic Impact of Cholera Outbreaks

Cost-of-illness studies are essential for assessing the economic impact of diseases and estimating the potential savings or benefits if a disease were eradicated. These studies play a crucial role in shaping public health policy, particularly in resource-limited settings where the economic burden of endemic diseases, which frequently lead to large outbreaks due to poor social conditions, is often not well understood. A study conducted in Somalia in 2023 highlighted the economic impact of cholera treatment on both healthcare facilities and households, with an average cost for households affected by cholera was $33.94, and health facility costs averaging $82.65, for a total of US $116.59. These estimates are consistent with similar studies in other places like Matlab, Kolkata, Beira, Zanzibar, Malawi, and Bangladesh, as well as a model-based estimate for Somalia in 2021. Despite cholera treatment being provided at minimal cost in Somalia, additional expenses, such as transportation, special diets, and caregiving, can increase the financial burden. Over half of the households had to borrow money or use savings to cover these costs, a trend consistent with other studies. The stigma surrounding cholera also worsens the psychological toll, with some families facing social discrimination and trauma, including the loss of a household member. The effects extend beyond households to local economies, where cholera disrupts productivity across sectors, leading to broader economic losses. In 2015, the total economic burden of cholera in Somalia was estimated at US$3.29 million, with an expected increase to US$4.35 million in 2024. Moreover, it's important to mention how the economic burden on families extends beyond medical costs, such as lost wages and disrupted education, where a single cholera case can result in about four days of lost income, which is problematic for families relying on daily wages in informal employment. The economic strain is worse for households where the patient or caregiver is the primary breadwinner. Cholera also disrupts education, as affected children may miss school, leading to potential long-term societal costs. In a low-income country like Somalia, where primary school enrollment is below 30%, such absences can negatively affect educational achievement and worsen economic disparities. Moreover, the study highlighted that 45% of the cholera patients in their sample were children under 5 years, focusing on how early exposure can have lasting effects on children's growth and development, particularly their adult height (Figuereo, Yoon, & Kaddu, 2024).

In Zambia, most cholera treatment costs are covered by the health system, while household costs were primarily related to transport, food, and communication. Cost-effectiveness analysis showed that vaccinating a single homogeneous population at risk is cost-effective, with the cost per case averted ranging from US$352 to US$532, depending on age and vaccine effectiveness. The study also found that costs decrease when vaccine effectiveness increases, and that cost-effectiveness is influenced by cholera incidence. The study highlights the varied costs associated with cholera vaccination campaigns (OCVs), with delivery costs differing by country and setting. For example, in Lusaka, Zambia in 2017, a single dose of Shancol vaccine cost US$1.72 per person, with 80% of that cost attributed to the vaccine purchase. In Hue City, Vietnam, the cost per vaccinated person was lower at US$1.07, with 90% spent on the vaccine itself. However, the total cost of campaigns can be high, as seen in Hue, where the total cost of the campaign reached US$1,152,291. Integrating OCVs into routine health services could help reduce costs over time (Tembo, Simuyandi, & Chiyenu, 2019)

## Prevention

In regions where cholera is endemic, the WHO recommends cholera vaccination as an integral component of the national cholera control program in addition to WaSH (Organization WH, 2010). Several studies have demonstrated that introducing vaccinations early in an outbreak provides 79% protection from cholera, and as much as one dose of the cholera vaccine decreases the risk greatly (Chowdhury et al., 2022). In recent years, oral cholera vaccine (OCV) has emerged as a critical and cost-effective strategy for cholera prevention and control in both emergency and non-emergency settings. The WHO has currently pre-qualified three dead, whole-cell (WC) OCVs for purchase by United Nations organizations and are accessible for worldwide use: Shanchol, Euvichol, and Dukoral (Buliva et al., 2022) [68]. In accordance with the manufacturers, Shanchol™ and Euvichol® must be given orally in two liquid doses separated by 14 days in individuals aged ≥1 year. Based on findings from earlier research, these vaccinations increase the formation of both antibacterial and anti-toxin antibodies, including IgA antibodies generated locally in the intestines, and have been reported to provide both direct and herd protection (Buliva et al., 2022; Wierzba, 2019).

Community Health Workers (CHWs) play a vital role in cholera treatment and prevention, especially in resource-limited settings with poor healthcare access. As many individuals with cholera symptoms do not seek healthcare, often because they believe their condition is not severe enough, CHWs can bridge this gap by promoting awareness, safe practices, improving health-seeking behaviors, and referring suspected cases to treatment centers. CHWs have also been instrumental in past cholera vaccination campaigns, such as in Somalia, although vaccination rates among the study sample were low, with only 6% of patients having received the cholera vaccine[65]. Moreover, between 2017 and 2020, seven rounds of OCV campaigns were conducted in Cox's Bazar, Bangladesh, targeting both refugees and host communities. Over 1.5 million people were vaccinated, with the campaigns achieving high acceptance and successful disease prevention, with no cholera outbreaks detected in the camps after the vaccination efforts (Khan, Islam, & Khan, 2023).

While OCVs play a critical role in outbreak prevention, long-term control also requires sustained improvements in sanitation and hygiene. In Haiti, a large-scale hygiene initiative led by UNICEF and supported by the Government of Japan has shown the critical role of community mobilization in cholera prevention and response. Implemented in Artibonite and Centre regions, the Community Approach for Total Sanitation (CATS) enabled over 9,000 households to build latrines and handwashing stations, significantly reducing the risk of cholera transmission. Hygiene education campaigns and awareness reached more than 60,000 people, promoting behavior change such as ending open defecation. During the 2023 cholera resurgence, UNICEF rapidly distributed chlorine, hygiene kits, water tanks, and medical supplies, highlighting how community-driven efforts can strengthen preparedness and mitigate outbreak (Unicef,org, n.d.).

Integrating cholera treatment centers with proactive measures like monitoring, risk communication, community engagement via CHWs, WASH activities, and OCV campaigns can help public health authorities and humanitarian organizations tailor vaccination strategies to meet the specific needs of the population during outbreaks (Figuereo, Yoon, & Kaddu, 2024).

Nigeria has made significant progress in enhancing its public health response to infectious diseases, including improved cholera outbreak management. After implementing the National Action Plan for Health Security and a One Health approach, the country's overall epidemic preparedness score increased from 39% in 2017 to 54% in 2023 Improved monitoring systems, maintained by the Nigeria Centre for Disease Control (NCDC), allow for early detection and response to epidemics. Moreover, the creation of a new National Reference Laboratory has improved diagnostic capabilities, allowing for faster detection of cholera patients. Border surveillance and entry point inspections have been strengthened to help prevent cross-border transmission of cholera, which is crucial in crisis or displacement circumstances. Additionally, community engagement through trusted leaders has also improved public adoption of hygiene practices, reducing transmission risk. Additionally, Nigeria’s investment in training public health personnel ensures a rapid, skilled response to outbreaks.

Together, these improvements enhance Nigeria's capacity to detect, contain, and reduce the impact of cholera and similar infectious diseases.

Despite notable advancements, public health systems in countries like Nigeria face several weaknesses that hinder effective outbreak response, such as limited and inconsistent domestic funding for epidemic preparedness that affect the availability of essential supplies, equipment, and personnel, especially in rural areas. Other factors include the lack of adequate infrastructure in local governments, sufficient trained staff, emergency response mechanisms, coordination between public health and security authorities with no formal agreements and collaboration protocols, inadequate biosafety and biosecurity frameworks, outdated surveillance equipment, and logistical barriers to reaching remote areas (Jonah et al., 2024).

School-based hygiene education and community-led health initiatives in Bangladesh have also shown significant effects. Active hygiene committees, strong leadership, and student engagement contribute to the success of these programs. Children act as hygiene ambassadors, spreading essential practices to their families. Oral rehydration efforts, such as door-to-door training, have reduced child mortality from diarrheal diseases. These examples demonstrate how community-driven and school-based interventions can strengthen household resilience, build public trust, and play a crucial role in cholera prevention and outbreak response strategies (Sultana et al., 2023).

## Novel Research Strategies

*V. cholerae* can acquire antibiotic resistance genes from resistant bacteria and share them with other bacteria via mobile genetic elements. It may share this gene with other enteric pathogens in the human gut, complicating treatment for a variety of illnesses. As such, we are in need of a novel treatment strategy for the management of this disease (Sarwar et al., 2017) [74]. One novel and intriguing strategy for cholera therapy is inhibiting cholera toxin binding to receptors of the intestine. This therapy, combined with anti-secretory agents such as inhibitors of enkephalinase and of the cystic fibrosis transmembrane conductance regulator, could provide a new treatment option to manage severe diarrhea associated to cholera (Thiagarajah & Verkman, 2005). Nanoparticles (NPs) have recently gained favor as an alternative to antibiotics, since unlike antiobiotics that act on a specific target only, NPs kill pathogens by direct contact with the bacteria cell wall, making bacteria less likely to acquire resistance to them. Cholera toxin works by attaching to a receptor called GM1, causing a chain reaction that results in diarrhea. Because antibiotics do not neutralize the already-produced poison, current treatments focus on recovery rather than cure. Studies are investigating the ability of several chemicals to limit cholera toxin activity, with oral zinc ZnO NPs appearing as a promising contender.

The World Health Organization recommends ZnO paired with ORS as an effective therapy for reducing cholera morbidity and mortality. Research has shown that ZnO NPs bind to cholera toxin, thus preventing it from attaching to the GM1 receptor, thus blocking the very first critical step in CT-induced diarrhea. According to biophysical studies, ZnO NPs cause structural changes in the toxin, which affect its ability to interact with the GM1 receptor. Moreover, it exerts anti-Vibrio activity by producing reactive oxygen species and disrupting the bacterial membrane, resulting in membrane depolarization, enhanced permeabilization, protein leakage, and DNA damage. Furthermore, the study shows that ZnO NPs effectively reduce the effects of cholera toxin (CT) on cells, preventing the formation of vacuoles associated with toxin exposure. Importantly, the concentration of ZnO NPs used has no effect on bacterial growth or cell viability, implying their potential as a cholera prevention strategy. However, more research is needed before ZnO NPs can be considered a definitive treatment for cholera in humans (Sarwar et al., 2017).

Another therapeutic strategy is linoleic acid, which has been shown to be a potent negative effector of V. cholerae virulence, inhibiting virulence gene expression by acting on the major virulence transcription regulator protein, ToxT. ToxT promotes the expression of the two major virulence factors required for disease, CT and toxin-coregulated pilus (TCP). A conjugated form of linoleic acid (CLA) is currently available as a dietary supplement and is generally regarded as safe by the United States Food and Drug Administration (FDA), and as such, may be safe for human consumption without the need for extensive clinical trials. According to research, using the essential fatty acid CLA to inhibit CT production in cholera has several advantages. Unlike antibiotics, CLA does not inhibit bacterial growth, reducing the likelihood of bacteria developing resistance. Furthermore, CLA treatment appears to alleviate cholera symptoms without disrupting the natural balance of bacteria in the gut, which is a common issue with antibiotic therapy and can lead to vulnerability to other pathogens such as Clostridium difficile. Cost is an important consideration, particularly in areas where cholera is prevalent. CLA softgels is inexpensive in the United States, and if produced in low-income countries, the costs are expected to be even lower. CLA has been shown in vitro and in vivo to effectively reduce CT production and subsequent secretory diarrhea. This evidence suggests that CLA supplementation could be used to supplement current cholera rehydration therapy. Further research will be conducted to determine the feasibility and efficacy of incorporating CLA into cholera treatment protocols (Withey et al., 2015).

In conclusion, the emergence of new therapies, such as CLA and nanoparticles, demonstrates promising avenues for replacing antibiotics, mitigating antibiotic resistance, and paving the way for novel approaches to overcoming the challenges posed by cholera.

## Emerging Technologies

In recent years, emerging technologies, such as artificial intelligence, have begun to play a transformative role in the early detection, surveillance, and management of cholera outbreaks.

### Surveillance Tools and Smartphone Applications

Smartphone applications are increasingly being used to improve cholera risk assessment and management in endemic regions. For instance, Nusrat et al. (2024) developed a high-resolution geospatial model using satellite remote sensing to assess cholera transmission risk in Matlab, Bangladesh. The model tracks seasonal environmental changes and their impact on water access, generating monthly cholera risk maps. A smartphone app was created to disseminate these maps to rural populations, helping health workers identify at-risk areas and allocate resources effectively. It also educates users on cholera prevention through safe water practices and WASH protocols, offering a novel approach for early disease warning and management (Nusrat, Akanda, & Islam, 2024).

### Artificial Intelligence (AI)

AI is transforming cholera diagnostics by improving speed, accuracy, and accessibility, especially in low-resource settings. Key advancements include AI-driven biosensors for real-time toxin detection, genomic tools for outbreak tracking, and CRISPR-based diagnostics for precise testing. Predictive analytics and metagenomic sequencing help identify cholera hotspots and improve field testing. These technologies enhance detection, surveillance, and outbreak response, particularly in regions like India, Bangladesh, and Africa. However, challenges remain in countries like Nigeria, where data quality, inconsistent collection methods, and limited infrastructure hinder AI integration. As such, successful AI deployment requires investment in technology, workforce training, and overcoming ethical and sustainability issues, including data protection and public trust concerns (Akingbola, Abiodun, & Ojo, 2025).

## CONCLUSION

Cholera remains a global health threat, particularly in areas with limited resources and inadequate sanitation. This article has discussed the causes and clinical symptoms of cholera, as well as diagnostic methods, treatment, and ongoing challenges. The disease, which is primarily spread by contaminated water and poor sanitation, causes severe dehydration and can be fatal if not treated quickly. *V. cholerae* infection can be detected through clinical examination and specific laboratory tests. Although rehydration therapy and antibiotics are the primary treatments for severe cases, issues such as antimicrobial resistance and limited healthcare access in vulnerable areas persist. Ongoing research into improved diagnostics, vaccines, and targeted therapies is encouraging. However, collaborative efforts are required to effectively combat cholera, with a focus on clean water access, sanitation, and strengthened healthcare systems in high-risk areas. To summarize, while progress has been made, more coordinated global action is needed to reduce the impact of cholera, implement preventive measures, and develop long-term strategies to alleviate its burden on affected communities around the world.

## REFERENCES


Acosta, C., Galindo, C., Kimario, J., Senkoro, K., Urassa, H., Casals, C., Corachán, M., Eseko, N., Tanner, M., Mshinda, H., Lwilla, F., Vila, J., & Alonso, P. L. (2001). Cholera outbreak in southern Tanzania: Risk factors and patterns of transmission. *Emerging Infectious Diseases, 7*(3, Suppl), 583–587. https://ora.ox.ac.uk/objects/uuid:dd75b112-5f7a-41f6-81c6-4ac32a37b1f3. DOI: 10.3201/eid0707.010741 PMID: 11485679

Akingbola, A., Abiodun, A., Ojo, O., Jessica, O. U., Alao, U. H., Owolabi, A. O., & Chuku, J. (2025). Cholera outbreak in Nigeria: History, review of socioeconomic and meteorological drivers, diagnostic challenges, and artificial intelligence integration. *Global Health, Epidemiology and Genomics, 2025*(1), 8898076. Advance online publication. DOI: 10.1155/ghe3/8898076 PMID: 40469257

Alexandrova, L., Haque, F., Rodriguez, P., Marrazzo, A. C., Grembi, J. A., Ramachandran, V., Hryckowian, A. J., Adams, C. M., Siddique, M. S. A., Khan, A. I., Qadri, F., Andrews, J. R., Rahman, M., Spormann, A. M., Schoolnik, G. K., Chien, A., & Nelson, E. J. (2019). Identification of widespread antibiotic exposure in patients with cholera correlates with clinically relevant microbiota changes. *The Journal of Infectious Diseases, 220*(10), 1655–1666. DOI: 10.1093/infdis/jiz299 PMID: 31192364

Asantewaa, A. A., Odoom, A., Owusu-Okyere, G., & Donkor, E. S. (2024). Cholera outbreaks in low- and middle-income countries in the last decade: A systematic review and meta-analysis. *Microorganisms, 12*(12), 2504. Advance online publication. DOI: 10.3390/microorganisms12122504 PMID: 39770707

Azman, A. S., Rudolph, K. E., Cummings, D. A. T., & Lessler, J. (2013). The incubation period of cholera: A systematic review. *The Journal of Infection, 66*(5), 432–438. DOI: 10.1016/j.jinf.2012.11.013 PMID: 23201968

Bachmann, V., Kostiuk, B., Unterweger, D., Diaz-Satizabal, L., Ogg, S., & Pukatzki, S. (2015). Bile salts modulate the mucin-activated type VI secretion system of pandemic *Vibrio cholerae. PLoS Neglected Tropical Diseases, 9*(8), e0004031. Advance online publication. DOI: 10.1371/journal.pntd.0004031 PMID: 26317760

Buliva, E., Elnossery, S., Okwarah, P., Tayyab, M., Brennan, R., & Abubakar, A. (2022). Cholera prevention, control strategies, challenges and World Health Organization initiatives in the Eastern Mediterranean Region: A narrative review. SSRN *Electronic Journal*. DOI: 10.2139/ssrn.4268747

Burrowes, V., Perin, J., Monira, S., Sack, D. A., Rashid, M., Mahamud, T., Rahman, Z., Mustafiz, M., Bhuyian, S. I., Begum, F., Zohura, F., Biswas, S., Parvin, T., Hasan, T., Zhang, X., Sack, B. R., Saif-Ur-Rahman, K. M., Alam, M., & George, C. M. (2017). Risk factors for household transmission of *Vibrio cholerae* in Dhaka, Bangladesh (CHoBI7 Trial). *The American Journal of Tropical Medicine and Hygiene, 96*(6), 1382–1387. DOI: 10.4269/ajtmh.16-0871 PMID: 28719281

Carlson, J. A., Middleton, P. J., Szymanski, M. T., Huber, J., & Petric, M. (1978). Fatal rotavirus gastroenteritis: An analysis of 21 cases. *American Journal of Diseases of Children, 132*(5), 477–479. DOI: 10.1001/archpedi.1978.02120300037006 PMID: 206132

Cash, R. A., Music, S. I., Libonati, J. P., Snyder, M. J., Wenzel, R. P., & Hornick, R. B. (1974). Response of man to infection with *Vibrio cholerae*. I. Clinical, serologic, and bacteriologic responses to a known inoculum. *The Journal of Infectious Diseases, 129*(1), 45–52. DOI: 10.1093/infdis/129.1.45 PMID: 4809112

Cassel, D., & Pfeuffer, T. (1978). Mechanism of cholera toxin action: Covalent modification of the guanyl nucleotide-binding protein of the adenylate cyclase system. *Proceedings of the National Academy of Sciences of the United States of America, 75*(6), 2669–2673. DOI: 10.1073/pnas.75.6.2669 PMID: 208069

Centers for Disease Control and Prevention. (2010). Update: Outbreak of cholera—Haiti, 2010. *MMWR. Morbidity and Mortality Weekly Report, 59*(48), 1586–1590. PMID: 21150867

Chowdhury, F., Ross, A. G., Islam, M. T., McMillan, N. A. J., & Qadri, F. (2022). Diagnosis, management, and future control of cholera. *Clinical Microbiology Reviews, 35*(3), e0021121. Advance online publication. DOI: 10.1128/cmr.00211-21 PMID: 35726607

Crowcroft, N. S. (1994). Cholera: Current epidemiology. *Communicable Disease Report. CDR Review, 4*(13), R157–R164. PMID: 7531564

Davies, H. G., Bowman, C., & Luby, S. P. (2017). Cholera—Management and success. *The Journal of Infection, 74*(Suppl 1), S66–S73. DOI: 10.1016/S0163-4453(17)30194-9 PMID: 28646965

Dureab, F., Jahn, A., Krisam, J., Dureab, A., Zain, O., Al-Awlaqi, S., & Müller, O. (2019). Risk factors associated with the recent cholera outbreak in Yemen: A case-control study. *Epidemiology and Health, 41*, e2019015. Advance online publication. DOI: 10.4178/epih.e2019015 PMID: 31010279

Durham, L. K., Longini, I. M., Halloran, M. E., Clemens, J. D., Nizam, A., & Rao, M. (1998). Estimation of vaccine efficacy in the presence of waning: Application to cholera vaccines. *American Journal of Epidemiology*, *147*(10), 948–959. DOI: 10.1093/oxfordjournals.aje.a009385 PMID: 9596473

Ellis, C. N., LaRocque, R. C., Uddin, T., Krastins, B., Mayo-Smith, L. M., Sarracino, D., Karlsson, E. K., Rahman, A., Shirin, T., Bhuiyan, T. R., Chowdhury, F., Khan, A. I., Ryan, E. T., Calderwood, S. B., Qadri, F., & Harris, J. B. (2015). Comparative proteomic analysis reveals activation of mucosal innate immune signaling pathways during cholera. *Infection and Immunity*, *83*(3), 1089–1103. DOI: 10.1128/IAI.02765-14 PMID: 25561705

Figuereo, S., Yoon, I., Kaddu, S. S., Lubogo, M., Baruch, J., Hossain, A. A., Mohamed, S. I., Abubakar, A. H. A., Mohamud, K. M., & Malik, S. M. M. R. (2024). Cost of cholera for households and health facilities, Somalia. *Journal of Epidemiology and Global Health*, *14*(3), 1219–1230. DOI: 10.1007/s44197-024-00278-6 PMID: 39023718

Freter, R., O'Brien, P. C., & Macsai, M. S. (1981). Role of chemotaxis in the association of motile bacteria with intestinal mucosa: In vivo studies. *Infection and Immunity*, *34*(1), 234–240. DOI: 10.1128/iai.34.1.234-240.1981 PMID: 7298185

Harris, J. B., Ivers, L. C., & Ferraro, M. J. (2011). Case 19-2011: A 4-year-old Haitian boy with vomiting and diarrhea. *The New England Journal of Medicine*, *364*(25), 2452–2461. DOI: 10.1056/NEJMcpc1100927 PMID: 21696312

Harris, J. B., LaRocque, R. C., Chowdhury, F., Khan, A. I., Logvinenko, T., Faruque, A. S. G., Ryan, E. T., Qadri, F., & Calderwood, S. B. (2008). Susceptibility to *Vibrio cholerae* infection in a cohort of household contacts of patients with cholera in Bangladesh. *PLoS Neglected Tropical Diseases*, *2*(4), e221. Advance online publication. DOI: 10.1371/journal.pntd.0000221 PMID: 18398491

Harris, J. B., LaRocque, R. C., Qadri, F., Ryan, E. T., & Calderwood, S. B. (2012). Cholera. *Lancet*, *379*(9835), 2466–2476. DOI: 10.1016/S0140-6736(12)60436-X PMID: 22748592

Holmberg, S. D., Harris, J. R., & Kay, D. E.. (1984). Foodborne transmission of cholera in Micronesian households. *Lancet*, *1*(8372), 325–328. DOI: 10.1016/S0140-6736(84)90370-2 PMID: 6141390

Holmgren, J., Lönnroth, I., Månsson, J., & Svennerholm, L. (1975). Interaction of cholera toxin and membrane GM1 ganglioside of small intestine. *Proceedings of the National Academy of Sciences of the United States of America*, *72*(7), 2520–2524. DOI: 10.1073/pnas.72.7.2520 PMID: 1058471

Hsueh, B. Y., & Waters, C. M. (2019). Combating cholera. *F1000Research, 8*, Article 589. DOI: 10.12688/f1000research.18093.1

Hutin, Y., Luby, S., & Paquet, C. (2003). A large cholera outbreak in Kano City, Nigeria: The importance of hand washing with soap and the danger of street-vended water. *Journal of Water and Health*, *1*(1), 45–52. DOI: 10.2166/wh.2003.0006 PMID: 15384272

Igere, B. E., & Ekundayo, T. C. (2020). Global mapping of cholera *Vibrio* and outbreaks in the Pre-Millennium Development Goals (MDG)/Sustainable Development Goals (SDG) and MDGs/SDGs era of 1990–2019. *Microbial Pathogenesis*, *149*, 104319. Advance online publication. DOI: 10.1016/j.micpath.2020.104319 PMID: 32579993

Jonah, J. H., Samuel, G., Abdullahi, M. I., Emmanuel, E. A., Danladi, S. S., & Ekwuluo, C. E. (2024). Nigeria's public health response to disease outbreaks: A review of strengths and weaknesses. *Journal of Public Health in Africa*, *15*(1), 773. Advance online publication. DOI: 10.4102/jphia.v15i1.773 PMID: 40503462

Kaper, J. B., Morris, J. G.Jr, & Levine, M. M. (1995). Cholera. *Clinical Microbiology Reviews*, *8*(1), 48–86. DOI: 10.1128/CMR.8.1.48 PMID: 7704895

Khan, A. I., Islam, M. T., Khan, Z. H., Tanvir, N. A., Amin, M. A., Khan, I. I., Bhuiyan, A. T. M. R. H., Hasan, A. S. M. M., Islam, M. S., Bari, T. I. A., Rahman, A., Islam, M. N., & Qadri, F. (2023). Implementation and delivery of oral cholera vaccination campaigns in humanitarian crisis settings among Rohingya Myanmar nationals in Cox's Bazar, Bangladesh. *Vaccines*, *11*(4), 843. Advance online publication. DOI: 10.3390/vaccines11040843 PMID: 37112756

Khan, W. A., Bennish, M. L., Seas, C., Khan, E. H., Ronan, A., Dhar, U., Busch, W., & Salam, M. A. (1996). Randomised controlled comparison of single-dose ciprofloxacin and doxycycline for cholera caused by *Vibrio cholerae* 01 or 0139. *Lancet*, *348*(9023), 296–300. DOI: 10.1016/S0140-6736(96)01180-4 PMID: 8709688

Liamis, G., Filippatos, T. D., & Elisaf, M. S. (2015). Correction of hypovolemia with crystalloid fluids: Individualizing infusion therapy. *Postgraduate Medicine*, *127*(4), 405–412. DOI: 10.1080/00325481.2015.1029421 PMID: 25812486

Lindenbaum, J., Greenough, W. B., & Islam, M. R. (1967). Antibiotic therapy of cholera. *Bulletin of the World Health Organization*, *36*(6), 871–883. PMID: 4865453

Mandal, S., Mandal, M. D., & Pal, N. K. (2011). Cholera: A great global concern. *Asian Pacific Journal of Tropical Medicine*, *4*(7), 573–580. DOI: 10.1016/S1995-7645(11)60149-1 PMID: 21803312

Mercer, A. (2021). Protection against severe infectious disease in the past. *Pathogens and Global Health, 115*(3), 151–167. DOI: 10.1080/20477724.2021.1878443 PMID: 33573529

Millet, Y. A., Alvarez, D., Ringgaard, S., von Andrian, U. H., Davis, B. M., & Waldor, M. K. (2014). Insights into *Vibrio cholerae* intestinal colonization from monitoring fluorescently labeled bacteria. *PLoS Pathogens, 10*(10), e1004405. Advance online publication. DOI: 10.1371/journal.ppat.1004405 PMID: 25275396

Molla, A. M., Ahmed, S. M., & Greenough, W. B. (1985). Rice-based oral rehydration solution decreases the stool volume in acute diarrhoea. *Bulletin of the World Health Organization, 63*(4), 751–756. PMID: 3910298

Molla, A. M., Rahman, M., Sarker, S. A., Sack, D. A., & Molla, A. (1981). Stool electrolyte content and purging rates in diarrhea caused by rotavirus, enterotoxigenic *E. coli*, and *V. cholerae* in children. *The Journal of Pediatrics, 98*(5), 835–838. DOI: 10.1016/S0022-3476(81)80863-3 PMID: 6262471

National Collaborating Centre for Women's and Children's Health (UK). (2009). Fluid management. In *Diarrhoea and vomiting caused by gastroenteritis: Diagnosis, assessment and management in children younger than 5 years*. RCOG Press. https://www.ncbi.nlm.nih.gov/books/NBK63837/

Nelson, E. J., Grembi, J. A., Chao, D. L., Andrews, J. R., Alexandrova, L., Rodriguez, P. H., Ramachandran, V. V., Sayeed, M. A., Wamala, J. F., Debes, A. K., Sack, D. A., Hryckowian, A. J., Haque, F., Khatun, S., Rahman, M., Chien, A., Spormann, A. M., & Schoolnik, G. K. (2020). Gold standard cholera diagnostics are tarnished by lytic bacteriophage and antibiotics. *Journal of Clinical Microbiology, 58*(9), e00412–e00420. DOI: 10.1128/JCM.00412-20 PMID: 32611794

Nusrat, F., Akanda, A. S., Islam, A., & et al. (2024). Satellite-derived, smartphone-delivered geospatial cholera risk information for vulnerable populations. *GeoHealth, 8*(11), Article e2024GH001039. DOI: 10.1029/2024GH001039

Ojeda Rodriguez, J. A., & Kahwaji, C. I. (2023). *Vibrio cholerae* infection. In *StatPearls*. StatPearls Publishing., https://www.ncbi.nlm.nih.gov/books/NBK526099/

Parsi, V. K. (2001). Cholera. *Primary Care Update for Ob/Gyns, 8*(3), 106–109. DOI: 10.1016/S1068-607X(00)00086-X PMID: 11378428

Peterson, K. M., & Gellings, P. S. (2018). Multiple intraintestinal signals coordinate the regulation of *Vibrio cholerae* virulence determinants. *Pathogens and Disease, 76*(1), ftx126. Advance online publication. DOI: 10.1093/femspd/ftx126 PMID: 29315383

Qadri, F., Bhuiyan, T. R., & Dutta, K. K.. (2004). Acute dehydrating disease caused by *Vibrio cholerae* serogroups O1 and O139 induce increases in innate cells and inflammatory mediators at the mucosal surface of the gut. *Gut, 53*(1), 62–69. DOI: 10.1136/gut.53.1.62 PMID: 14684578

Qaserah, A. M., Al Amad, M. A., Al Serouri, A. A., & Khader, Y. S. (2021). Risk factors of cholera transmission in Al Hudaydah, Yemen: Case-control study. *JMIR Public Health and Surveillance, 7*(7), e27627. Advance online publication. DOI: 10.2196/27627 PMID: 36260393

Rouard, C., Collet, L., Njamkepo, E., Jenkins, C., Sacheli, R., Benoit-Cattin, T., Figoni, J., & Weill, F.-X. (2024). Long-distance spread of a highly drug-resistant epidemic cholera strain. *The New England Journal of Medicine, 391*(23), 2271–2273. DOI: 10.1056/NEJMc2408761 PMID: 39665659

Ryan, E. T., Dhar, U., Khan, W. A., Salam, M. A., Faruque, A. S., Fuchs, G. J., Calderwood, S. B., & Bennish, M. L. (2000). Mortality, morbidity, and microbiology of endemic cholera among hospitalized patients in Dhaka, Bangladesh. *The American Journal of Tropical Medicine and Hygiene, 63*(1–2), 12–20. DOI: 10.4269/ajtmh.2000.63.12 PMID: 11357989

Sack, D. A., Sack, R. B., Nair, G. B., & Siddique, A. K. (2004). Cholera. *The Lancet, 363*(9404), 223–233. https.//DOI: 10.1016/S0140-6736(03)15328-7

Samal, D., Turuk, J., Nayak, S. R., Pany, S., Pal, B. B., & Pati, S. (2025). Genomic insights into the dynamic antibiotic resistance landscape of *Vibrio cholerae* during the cholera outbreak 2022 in Odisha, India. *Scientific Reports, 15*(1), 1503. Advance online publication. DOI: 10.1038/s41598-024-81596-4 PMID: 39789042

Sarwar, S., Ali, A., Pal, M., & Chakrabarti, P. (2017). Zinc oxide nanoparticles provide anti-cholera activity by disrupting the interaction of cholera toxin with the human GM1 receptor. *The Journal of Biological Chemistry, 292*(44), 18303–18311. DOI: 10.1074/jbc.M117.793240 PMID: 28882894

Sayeed, M. A., Islam, K., Hossain, M., Akter, N. J., Alam, M. N., Sultana, N., Khanam, F., Kelly, M., Charles, R. C., Kováč, P., Xu, P., Andrews, J. R., Calderwood, S. B., Amin, J., Ryan, E. T., & Qadri, F. (2018). Development of a new dipstick (Cholkit) for rapid detection of *Vibrio cholerae* O1 in acute watery diarrheal stools. *PLoS Neglected Tropical Diseases, 12*(3), e0006286. Advance online publication. DOI: 10.1371/journal.pntd.0006286 PMID: 29538377

Segura, A. (2023). Epidemics and epidemiology: Back to the future. *Gaceta Sanitaria, 37*, 102277. Advance online publication. DOI: 10.1016/j.gaceta.2022.102277 PMID: 36508988

Sharifi-Mood, B., & Metanat, M. (2014). Diagnosis, clinical management, prevention, and control of cholera: A review study. *International Journal of Infection, 1*(1), Article 18303. Devicehttps://DOI: 10.17795/iji-18303

Shirai, H., Nishibuchi, M., Ramamurthy, T., Bhattacharya, S. K., Pal, S. C., & Takeda, Y. (1991). Polymerase chain reaction for detection of the cholera enterotoxin operon of *Vibrio cholerae*. *Journal of Clinical Microbiology*, *29*(11), 2517–2521. DOI: 10.1128/jcm.29.11.2517-2521.1991 PMID: 1774258

Siddique, A. K., Akram, K., Zaman, K., Laston, S., Salam, A., Majumdar, R. N., Islam, M. S., & Fronczak, N. (1995). Why treatment centres failed to prevent cholera deaths among Rwandan refugees in Goma, Zaire. *Lancet*, *345*(8946), 359–361. DOI: 10.1016/S0140-6736(95)90344-5 PMID: 7646639

Sinclair, G., Mphahlele, M. J., Duvenhage, H., Nichol, R., Whitehorn, A., & Küstner, H. (1982). Determination of the mode of transmission of cholera in Lebowa: An epidemiological investigation. *South African Medical Journal*, *62*(21), 753–755. https://www.semanticscholar.org/paper/Determination-of-the-mode-of-transmission-of-in-An-Sinclair-Mphahlele/1a6da890dee4498ec8cfebff884cdb585aaa55e8 PMID: 7135139

Sultana, F., Khan, S. M., Rahman, M., Winch, P. J., Luby, S. P., & Unicomb, L. (2023). Sustaining an elementary school-based hygiene intervention in Bangladesh by forming 'hygiene committees': A pilot study. *Journal of Water, Sanitation, and Hygiene for Development : a Journal of the International Water Association*, *13*(10), 749–763. DOI: 10.2166/washdev.2023.191

Swerdlow, D. L., Malenga, G., Begkoyian, G., Nyangulu, D., Toole, M., Waldman, R. J., Puhr, D. N. D., & Tauxe, R. V. (1997). Epidemic cholera among refugees in Malawi, Africa: Treatment and transmission. *Epidemiology and Infection*, *118*(3), 207–214. DOI: 10.1017/S0950268896007352 PMID: 9207730

Tembo, T., Simuyandi, M., Chiyenu, K., Sharma, A., Chilyabanyama, O. N., Mbwili-Muleya, C., Mazaba, M. L., & Chilengi, R. (2019). Evaluating the costs of cholera illness and cost-effectiveness of a single dose oral vaccination campaign in Lusaka, Zambia. *PLoS One*, *14*(5), e0215972. Advance online publication. DOI: 10.1371/journal.pone.0215972 PMID: 31150406

Thiagarajah, J. R., & Verkman, A. S. (2005). New drug targets for cholera therapy. *Trends in Pharmacological Sciences*, *26*(4), 172–175. DOI: 10.1016/j.tips.2005.02.003 PMID: 15808339

Tulchinsky, T. H. (2018). John Snow, cholera, the Broad Street Pump; Waterborne diseases then and now. In *Case studies in public health* (pp. 77–99). Academic Press., DOI: 10.1016/B978-0-12-804571-8.00017-2

UNICEF. (2025, June 16). The hygiene revolution in Haiti: Towards a healthier future through community mobilization. https://www.unicef.org/haiti/en/stories/hygiene-revolution-haiti-towards-healthier-future-through-community-mobilization

Waldor, M. K., & Mekalanos, J. J. (1996). Lysogenic conversion by a filamentous phage encoding cholera toxin. *Science*, *272*(5270), 1910–1914. DOI: 10.1126/science.272.5270.1910 PMID: 8658163

Weil, A. A., Becker, R. L., & Harris, J. B. (2019). *Vibrio cholerae* at the intersection of immunity and the microbiome. *MSphere*, *4*(6), e00597–e19. DOI: 10.1128/mSphere.00597-19 PMID: 31776240

Weil, A. A., Khan, A. I., Chowdhury, F., LaRocque, R. C., Faruque, A. S. G., Ryan, E. T., Calderwood, S. B., Qadri, F., & Harris, J. B. (2009). Clinical outcomes in household contacts of patients with cholera in Bangladesh. *Clinical Infectious Diseases*, *49*(10), 1473–1479. DOI: 10.1086/644779 PMID: 19842974

Wierzba, T. F. (2019). Oral cholera vaccines and their impact on the global burden of disease. *Human Vaccines & Immunotherapeutics*, *15*(6), 1294–1301. DOI: 10.1080/21645515.2018.1504155 PMID: 30183486

Withey, J. H., Nag, D., Plecha, S. C., Sinha, R., & Koley, H. (2015). Conjugated linoleic acid reduces cholera toxin production *in vitro* and *in vivo* by inhibiting *Vibrio cholerae* ToxT activity. *Antimicrobial Agents and Chemotherapy*, *59*(12), 7471–7476. DOI: 10.1128/AAC.01029-15 PMID: 26392502

World Health Organization. (2003). *Manual for the laboratory identification and antimicrobial susceptibility testing of bacterial pathogens of public health importance in the developing world: Haemophilus influenzae, Neisseria meningitidis, Streptococcus pneumoniae, Neisseria gonorrhoea, Salmonella serotype Typhi, Shigella, and Vibrio cholerae*. https://iris.who.int/handle/10665/68554

World Health Organization. (2005). *The treatment of diarrhoea: A manual for physicians and other senior health workers*. https://iris.who.int/handle/10665/43209

World Health Organization. (2010). Cholera vaccines: WHO position paper. *Weekly Epidemiological Record*, *85*(13), 117–128. PMID: 20349546

Wright, E. M., Loo, D. D. F., & Hirayama, B. A. (2011). Biology of human sodium glucose transporters. *Physiological Reviews*, *91*(2), 733–794. DOI: 10.1152/physrev.00055.2009 PMID: 21527736

Yen, C. H. (1964). A recent study of cholera with reference to an outbreak in Taiwan in 1962. *Bulletin of the World Health Organization*, *30*(6), 811–825. PMID: 14215187

# Chapter 13
# M. Lyme

**Sohaila Mourad Bassyouni**
*Alexandria University, Egypt*

**Farida Mohamed Ragab**
*Cairo University, Egypt*

**Youssef Atef Mohamed Atttia**
*Ain Shams University, Egypt*

**Zeina Hisham Gamaleldin**
*Cairo University, Egypt*

## ABSTRACT

*Lyme disease is a tick-borne illness caused by the spirochete Borrelia burgdorferi. In 1975, it was discovered in the United States during an outbreak of arthritis in Lyme, Connecticut. The presence of the spirochete, ticks as carriers, and animals like mice and deer as hosts are all necessary for the disease to manifest. The life cycle of a deer tick lasts two years. Borrelia types and strains all contribute to the vast diversity of clinical symptoms seen across the world. Timely identification and treatment are critical since delayed or ineffective treatment can result in persistent Lyme disease with severe symptoms. Diagnostic issues, as well as the lack of conclusive clearance tests, add to the difficulties in illness treatment. Raising awareness, improving diagnosis, and advocating for breakthroughs in research and treatment are all vital steps in tackling the terrible impact of Lyme disease on individuals and communities.*

DOI: 10.4018/979-8-3693-1990-1.ch013

# INTRODUCTION

## Overview

Lyme disease is a systemic illness caused by the tick-borne spirochete Borrelia burgdorferi. Lyme disease was discovered in the United States in 1975, following a mysterious epidemic of arthritis in Lyme, Connecticut, which alerted the State Health Department and the Yale Rheumatology Clinic to a high prevalence of juvenile rheumatoid arthritis (JRA) among family members and neighbours. The symptoms and indicators displayed by these people (such as severe headaches, skin lesions, and neurologic impairments) were not typical of JRA. This led to a retrospective review and the discovery of Lyme arthritis, eventually dubbed Lyme disease. Lyme disease requires the presence of at least three interconnected elements: the spirochete (Borrelia burgdorferi), ticks capable of spreading it, and animals (such as mice and deer) that provide food for the ticks at different stages of development. Lyme disease is spread in the United States by the tick species known as the "deer tick": Ixodes scapularis in the East and Mid-West and Ixodes pacificus in the West.

The tick goes through four phases of development: egg, larva, nymph, and adult. The completion of these phases is projected to take two years. Mature ticks feed on large animals, usually deer, in the autumn and early spring. Female ticks will leave their host to deposit their eggs on the ground. In the summer, these eggs hatch into larvae, which feed on mice, other small animals, and birds until early October. The larvae hibernate until the next spring, when they moult into nymphs. The nymphs feed on small animals and birds in late spring and summer before moulting into adults in the autumn, completing the two-year life cycle, (Steere, 1989).

Furthermore, while both Lyme disease and syphilis (bacterial infection) are chronic illnesses with pathology mostly caused by inflammatory reactions, their symptoms are distinct. In addition to these differences, the clinical signs of Lyme disease differed geographically. This is assumed to be due, in part, to geographical differences in the predominant Lyme disease agents. Borrelia garinii, which is common in Eurasia, has been related to neurologic disease, whereas Borrelia burgdorferi, the most common species discovered in the United States, has been linked to arthritis. Changes in symptoms and inflammation severity associated with certain B. burgdorferi strains have been observed.

The particular variations between species and strains that cause the various clinical manifestations are just now being recognised. Despite a high degree of genetic similarity across pathogenic treponemes, there are significant clinical differences in the illnesses they produce (syphilis, bejel, yaws, and pinta). At the molecular level, the discrepancies revealed in these spirochetal infections represent significant disparities in infection patterns, tissue tropisms, and host-pathogen interactions, (Klempner *et al.*, 2001).

## Importance of Studying

Lyme disease is regarded to be curable if treated early with a single antibiotic administered for a few weeks, which in this case should be roughly six to eight weeks. Most people, however, are bitten by nymphs and go unnoticed, and a correct diagnosis can take years. Co-infections are frequently overlooked, and there is no diagnostic test that verifies Lyme organism clearance even when effectively treated. Add to that a lot of faulty research or a lack of expertise, which has resulted in horrible recommendations, such as requiring a tick to be adhered to for no less than 48 hours for the virus may be transmitted. There are additional ways to get Lyme disease. Aside from being bitten by an infected tick, other risk factors include blood transfusion, intercourse, and trans-placental transmission. Lyme disease that is not treated promptly or just partially, or that is persistent, may make humans and animals exceedingly unwell, sometimes leaving them crippled, mentally ill, or dead. Furthermore, persons who have Lyme disease frequently have a co-infection that may not respond to the brief course of a single antibiotic given for a few weeks, (Lantos, 2015).

Headache is the most prevalent symptom of Lyme meningitis. Patients may have photo- and phonosensitivity, although fever and meningismus are unlikely. The CSF analysis revealed lymphocytic pleocytosis, mildly elevated protein levels, and normal glucose levels. In infants with Lyme meningitis, papilledema caused by intracranial hypertension has been observed, and it can develop in adults in rare cases. Each year, the Centers for Disease Control and Prevention reports around 30,000 cases that fulfil the stringent epidemiologic case definition in the United States. The real number of events is definitely higher, but it's difficult to say by how much.

In early June, a 39-year-old father and his 18-year-old daughter arrived for a neurology assessment after returning from a vacation in Cape Cod, Massachusetts. They were aware that they were in a Lyme disease-endemic area and wore insect repellent, hiked in long-sleeved shirts and pants, and checked for ticks often. A family member and his golden retriever stopped them on the way. Soon after arriving home, the father developed a headache with photosensitivity, and his daughter followed him to the appointment since she awakened with slight right facial weakness. The father had minor meningismus but was afebrile when evaluated. Due to Bell's phenomenon, his daughter was unable to grin on the right side and had difficulty closing her eyes.

He couldn't recall any nonpruritic targetoid skin lesions. Because the father had symptoms and signs of meningitis, a lumbar puncture and CSF analysis were conducted, which revealed a lymphocytic pleocytosis of 100 cells/mm3, protein of

70 mg/dL, glucose of 45 mg/dL, and oligoclonal bands. His daughter did not get a lumbar puncture. They were administered 100 mg of doxycycline orally twice a day for 28 days. Both the father's and daughter's serum enzyme-linked immunosorbent assay (ELISA) for Borrelia burgdorferi antibody returned positive findings 48 hours later; confirmation testing with Western blot IgM on the first test was positive, and IgG was positive on the second test four weeks later. During the family's stay at the Cape Cod residence, Ixodes ticks were discovered on the dog, (Roos, 2021).

### Purpose and Scope of the Chapter

Many clinicians, whether in denial or nihilism, believe Lyme disease is restricted to a few specific regions, and that most areas are devoid of Lyme-transmitting organisms. Many people in healthcare, from Australia to Canada, ignore or avoid the reality of this sickness entirely. The scale of the Borrelia infestation in the Australian tick population has been known for almost two decades (Wills & Barry 1991), yet practically the entire medical community in Australia is still in denial. These data show that certain tick species are frequently responsible for human and animal tick attacks in this country, where Borrelia species spirochetes are widespread. In Australia, these bacteria are suspected to be the causative agents of Lyme disease, based on structural and antigenic evidence. Wills and Barry discovered Borrelia in 42% of the ticks they examined. For unexplained reasons, it's reasonable to presume public health officials didn't want to learn that there are congenital and gestational transfer instances, or that there is verified proof Lyme may be an STD (transferred between sexually active couples). The Infectious Diseases Society of America (IDSA) produced guidelines for Lyme disease diagnosis and treatment. The aforementioned recommendations were not amended to account for the incidence of chronic Lyme disease, which has been described in over 300 peer-reviewed articles.

## THE BASICS OF LYME DISEASE

A tick bite can transmit the bacterial infection known as Lyme disease, sometimes known as borreliosis. The human body can be exposed to the Lyme disease-causing bacteria Borrelia burgdorferi through the skin or mucous membranes. Numerous organs and systems, including the skin, joints, heart, neurological system, and blood vessels, can be impacted by Lyme disease. Often appearing a few weeks after a tick bite, erythema migraines is the most common indication of Lyme disease. Some individuals, however, can simply have minor symptoms or none at all. Lyme disease can result in major side effects like arthritis, nerve damage, facial paralysis, and cardiac issues if treatment is not received, (Steere, 1989).

Lyme disease is diagnosed by laboratory testing and clinical presentation. Blood samples are tested in the lab for antibodies against Borrelia burgdorferi, and on occasion, PCR or culture are used to confirm the presence of the bacteria in the blood or tissues, (Klempner *et al.,* 2001).

. Antibiotics are typically used for a few weeks or months as part of the treatment for Lyme disease. Nevertheless, a small percentage of individuals may acquire chronic Lyme disease (CLD), a condition in which treatment with antibiotics may not resolve or worsen symptoms. Diagnosing and treating CLD can be challenging, necessitating extra testing and therapies, (Lantos, 2015). The bacterium Borrelia burgdorferi in North America and Borrelia afzelii or Borrelia garinii in Europe and Asia are the main causes of Lyme borreliosis, which is primarily transmitted by tick bites and primarily affects temperate parts of the northern hemisphere. The initial symptom of infection is usually erythema migrans, a developing skin lesion often referred to as stage 1. If neglected, stage 1 can be followed by stage 2 or stage 3 infection, which is mostly arthritis in North America or acrodermatitis chronica atrophicans in Europe, and early disseminated infection, particularly in situations with neurological abnormalities.

However, any of these signs and symptoms could be the first signs of the illness. In order to evade immune clearance, the bacteria can move across the tissues of the host and adhere to specific cells. But in the end, these organisms are destroyed by both innate and adaptive immune responses, and most of the inflammatory symptoms associated with the infection disappear. Except for those who have erythema migrans, the diagnosis of Lyme borreliosis is based on a unique clinical constellation of signs and symptoms with serological evidence of infection. Most of the time, all infection symptoms can be resolved with the right antibiotic regimen; nevertheless, in certain cases, the illness may result in post-infectious sequelae. The main method of preventing tick bites and contracting Lyme borreliosis is by taking personal preventive measures, (Roos, 2021).

Humans are typically exposed to Borrelia burgdorferi by Ixodes ticks. The life cycle of these ticks lasts two years and includes the following distinct developmental stages: egg, larva, nymph, and adult. In late summer, the eggs hatch into larvae, which subsequently feed on small animals, often acquiring B. burgdorferi infection.

They go through a second feeding after moulting into nymphs, usually in the spring or early summer, when they can spread the virus to a new host. Eventually, nymphs moult into adult ticks; this usually happens in mid-October or early-November, when adult female ticks begin feeding, mainly on large mammals.

Although white-footed mice and other small mammals can serve as asymptomatic reservoirs for Borrelia burgdorferi, deer are essential as the primary hosts of adult ticks. However, B. burgdorferi cannot survive in deer reservoirs. The geographic distribution, density, and prevalence of infected vector ticks influence the risk of contracting Lyme disease in the United States. The northeastern and north central states record the greatest number of cases of Lyme disease. Similar endemic regions exist in Europe and Asia. Notably, infected nymph ticks, owing to their minute size (resembling a poppy seed), are responsible for the majority of infections. These infections mostly happen in May through August, which is also the time when human outdoor exposure increases and nymph tick activity peaks. Although adult ticks are also capable of spreading the disease, it is easier to identify them due to their greater size (about the same as a sesame seed).

Research conducted in laboratories has indicated that a minimum attachment duration of 36 to 48 hours is required for the effective transmission of B. burgdorferi by ticks, (Hinckley *et al.,* 2014). For Lyme disease, there are two different kinds of diagnostic methods: direct and indirect. Direct methods involve culturing the bacterium Borrelia burgdorferi from skin lesions or blood samples, but these tests are not routinely available. Although it is not standardized, PCR testing for B. burgdorferi DNA in synovial fluid and cerebral fluid (CSF) appears promising. Based on measuring the antibody response against B. burgdorferi, indirect approaches are developed. The currently approved diagnostic method is antibody testing utilizing Western blot (WB) and enzyme-linked immunosorbent assay (ELISA). A two-step algorithm is used, with WB confirming a positive ELISA result. New serologic assays based on recombinant peptides are being developed. FDA-approved tests targeting specific proteins have shown effectiveness in diagnosing early-stage Lyme disease. However, seronegative results can occur in early-stage disease, and clinical suspicion should guide treatment decisions.

Most patients with late-stage and early-disseminated illness seroconvert after four weeks. Persistently positive test results do not necessarily indicate active infection and may reflect protective immunity. It is important to use diagnostic testing judiciously, a over-testing and misinterpretation can lead to unnecessary treatment. While false positive results are more prevalent when testing people who have a low chance of having Lyme disease, false negative results can also happen early in the disease, (Barclay *et al*., 2012). The frequency of Lyme disease is still rising even though primary and secondary prevention strategies are becoming more widely recognized. The goal of primary prevention is to lessen the likelihood of coming into contact with ticks in order to reduce the number of new cases of Lyme disease. The goal of secondary prevention is to stop the infection from spreading or lessen the severity of the disease in people who have been bitten by infected ticks. Despite the availability of various preventive strategies with varying costs, acceptability, and effectiveness, their adoption has generally been low. Research conducted in regions where Lyme disease is prevalent reveals that many individuals do not take precautions to minimize their infection risk, despite being well-informed about the disease's symptoms and transmission. Increasing people's confidence in their capacity to engage in preventative behaviors ought to be the goal of new prevention initiatives, (Richardson *et al.*, 2019).

## CLINICAL MANIFESTATION OF LYME

### Unique Symptoms and Presentation

Clinical indications of Lyme disease can be categorized into three stages to aid in diagnosis. The first stage, called the early localised stage, manifests in the first few weeks following inoculation and is characterized by erythema migrans at the site of the tick bite. Fever, headaches, excessive fatigue, aches and pains in the muscles, and swollen lymph nodes are some other signs and symptoms of stage 1. Weeks to months after exposure, the early disseminated stage manifests as many erythema migrans lesions, borrelial lymphocytoma, lyme neuroborreliosis, carditis, and, in rare instances, lyme arthritis. Atrophic acrodermatitis chronica, Lyme arthritis, and neurological symptoms are characteristics of the late disseminated stage (Lyme Disease: A Rigorous Review of Diagnostic Criteria and Treatment, n.d.). These indications and symptoms vary based on geographic region and species (Alberto *et al.*, 2019).

#### Neurological Implications

When the central or peripheral nerve systems are infected by the Lyme disease bacterium, neurological signs of the disease appear.

#### Cranial Nerve Involvement

Brain injury can result in facial palsy, or droop, on one or both sides of the face. Patients may experience radiculoneuropathy, which results in numbness, tingling, “shooting” pain, or weakness in the arms or legs, when the peripheral nerves are affected. Central nervous system involvement: The symptoms of Lyme meningitis that can occur when the central nervous system is affected include fever, headache, light sensitivity, and stiff neck. Numbness, pain, weakness, facial palsy/droop (paralysis of the facial muscles), visual disturbances, and meningitis symptoms such as fever, stiff neck, and severe headache are common in early disseminated Lyme disease (What Are Some Unusual Symptoms of Lyme Disease?, n.d.). Cranial neuritis (most commonly a unilateral or bilateral facial nerve palsy), meningitis, and radiculoneuritis are the most frequent neurologic consequences of Lyme disease. These might happen separately or simultaneously.

## Cranial Neuritis

The development of unilateral or bilateral cranial nerve VII palsy is one of the most prevalent neurological signs of Lyme disease. As a consequence, patients have less motor neuron facial weakness. Lyme disease was revealed to be the cause of facial nerve palsy in 4.7% of 559 people in a Lyme disease-endemic area. The majority of individuals with Lyme disease-induced facial nerve palsy had headaches and presented between July and September. Cranial nerves III, IV, VI, and VIII are impacted less frequently. Based on the observation of CSF lymphocytic pleocytosis in persons with cranial neuritis, the pathophysiology of cranial neuritis in Lyme disease is thought to be attributable to mild meningitis.

## Meningitis

Headache is the most common symptom of Lyme meningitis. Patients may also experience sensitivity to light and sound, but fever and meningismus (stiff neck) may be minor or absent. Lyme meningitis can be diagnosed through examination of cerebrospinal fluid (CSF), which may show an increase in lymphocytes, slightly elevated protein levels and normal glucose concentration. In some cases of Lyme meningitis, especially in children, papilledema (swelling of the optic disk) caused by increased pressure within the skull has been reported. However, this is rare in adults.

## Radiculoneuritis

Lyme disease in the nervous system can cause pain and weakness in one or more limbs. Initially, it was believed to be a radiculitis or plexitis, but further testing on experimentally infected rhesus macaque monkeys showed that it is a mononeuropathy multiplex (Roos, 2021).

## Cardiovascular and Musculoskeletal Involvement: Cardiac Implications

Lyme carditis is an uncommon Lyme disease manifestation that affects 1.5% to 10% of patients in North America and 0.5% to 4% of cases in Europe (Wang et al., 1999). Although both genders are affected equally by Lyme disease, Lyme carditis is more common in men, with a pathogen sex ratio of roughly 3:1. Furthermore, those between the ages of 20 and 40 are more likely to get Lyme carditis (Radesich et al., 2022).Lyme disease's cardiac consequences can be divided into two categories: conduction abnormalities and other heart diseases (Lelovas et al., 2008).

## Conduction Disturbances

Atrioventricular (AV) block is the type of conduction issue that occurs most frequently. According to Van der Linde, in 105 cases, third-degree AV blockages were detected in 49 percent of Lyme carditis patients, while second- and first-degree AV blocks were found in 16 percent and 12 percent of cases, respectively. Another study found that during the course of their disease, 98% of those with AV conduction anomalies experienced first-degree AV block, with 40% exhibiting Weckebach periodicity and 50% experiencing total AV block. The transition from first to third degree AV block can occur in minutes. Patients with first-degree AV block and a PR interval larger than 0.3 seconds have a higher risk of developing complete AV block. Conduction blockages are common at or above the AV node, particularly in the AV conduction system. However, anomalies in sinoatrial and intraatrial conduction have been found. After 6 weeks, AV obstructions normally resolve, most likely owing to the healing of underlying inflammation. People with AV blockages, sinoatrial and intraatrial conduction anomalies are expected to have a good prognosis.

## Other Cardiac Complications

Lyme disease can cause cardiac involvement in some situations, such as endocarditis, myocarditis, pericarditis, or pancarditis. Pericarditis, for example, has been associated to Lyme disease and can result in pericardial effusion, which is defined by exudate containing few neutrophils and lymphocytes. After pericardiocentesis and the use of anti-Borrelia burgdorferi medications, the effusion may resolve. B. burgdorferi was isolated from the myocardium of a patient with unexplained dilated cardiomyopathy in one case. Following that, individuals with dilated cardiomyopathy who tested positive for Borrelia burgdorferi were given ceftriaxone and saw a significant improvement in left ventricular ejection fraction. An untreated Lyme disease patient with late-onset carditis experienced varied diffuse T wave inversions at first. The left ventricular ejection fraction was low, and X-rays of the chest demonstrated cardiomegaly. All of the symptoms decreased once antibiotics against

Borrelia were taken, indicating that this might be a case of dilating cardiomyopathy in its early stages.

The precise process by which Lyme illness affects the conduction system is unknown. It has been proposed, however, that the spirochete directly enters cardiac tissues or that the infection causes an inflammatory response, or both. According to studies, there is a discrepancy between the amount of Borreliae organisms discovered at histology and the intensity of the inflammatory response, suggesting that an immunologic component of the host response is involved. An autoimmune-mediated mechanism was established in a mouse model with Lyme carditis and arthritis. Cross- reactive IgM antibodies, which were triggered by B. burgdorferi antigens, are thought to respond to self-components via a mechanism known as mimicry (Lelovas *et al.,* 2008).

## LYME ARTHRITIS

Arthritis is a major feature of Lyme disease, which is of particular concern to orthopaedic surgeons. Arthritis is the most visible symptom of late-stage Lyme disease, appearing in around 60% of untreated individuals months after the infection begins. B. burgdorferi spirochetes disseminate and infect synovial joints after the first tick bite, generating an inflammatory reaction in the synovial tissue. Synovial hypertrophy, vascular proliferation, and mononuclear cell infiltration are all part of this reaction. The synovial fluid also contains cytokines, complement, immune complexes, and neutrophils. Furthermore, B. burgdorferi has been demonstrated to boost chondrocytes' manufacture of matrix metalloproteinases (MMPs). MMPs are responsible for the degradation of collagen, proteoglycans, and extracellular matrix proteins. Chronic Lyme arthritis patients may have increased MMP levels in their synovial fluid, which leads to cartilage degradation. However, the exact mechanism via which B. burgdorferi causes joint damage is not known (Smith *et al.,* 2011).

Lyme arthritis usually affects only one main joint for a short time. The most usually afflicted joint is the knee, which accounts for up to 90% of all cases. Other joints that may be affected include the elbow, ankle, hip, and wrist. Joint effusions might be severe and out of proportion to the patient's symptoms. Fever has been recorded in 22% to 51% of Lyme arthritis youngsters. Even with effective antibiotic therapy, 50% of patients develop recurrent arthritis over a period of months to years, affecting the same or other joints. Erythema migrans does not occur or is underreported in the majority of arthritis patients (Smith *et al.,* 2011).

## Psychological and Cognitive Effect

Lyme disease is the underlying cause of a variety of mental health illnesses, including developmental issues, depression, anxiety, schizoaffective disorder, bipolar illness, eating and sleeping difficulties, dementia, seizures, suicide, and panic disorder. Lyme disease can interfere with a child's natural growth, resulting in disorders like ADHD or learning issues. More than 60 sources have recorded cases of newborn Lyme disease transmission since 1985. Lyme disease underdiagnosis and inadequate treatment can result in despair and anxiety, with research finding a 98% post-infection depression incidence compared to 0% pre-infection. There is a substantial geographical association between the frequency of Lyme disease and schizophrenia in the United States, and schizoaffective disorder is commonly reported in Lyme disease patients. In Lyme disease patients, bipolar disorder is often shown as rapid cycling, with mood instability described. Some Lyme disease patients may develop eating and sleeping issues, such as anorexia nervosa, bulimia, and excessive weight gain. Sleep problems, particularly insomnia, have also been connected to Lyme disease. Lyme disease can result in neurological problems such as memory loss, disorientation, and personality or mood changes. According to some research, Lyme disease can induce a quickly advancing form of dementia that mostly affects the frontal lobe of the brain.

Seizures can arise as a result of neurological abnormalities caused by Lyme disease, and the prevalence of seizure disorders is increased when there is a considerable delay in both recognizing and properly treating Lyme illness. Lyme disease's persistent discomfort and mental toll can lead to suicidal thoughts or actions, and indirect estimates suggest that the condition is responsible for roughly 1,200 suicides in the United States each year. For the first time, patients with Lyme disease may have panic attacks that linger for hours at a time (The Impact of Lyme Disease on Mental Health: Understanding the Connection and Seeking Support, n.d.).

# DIAGNOSIS AND LABORATORY TESTING OF LIME

## Methods for Detecting Borrelia Burgdorferi Directly

Due to low spirochete counts in clinical samples, laboratory methods for B. burgdorferi detection are restricted. Culture and PCR are the primary direct diagnostic modalities, with histopathology employed to rule out other illnesses (Müllegger & Glatz, 2008). Due to the lack of organisms, detection is challenging and time-consuming. Warthin- starry, silver stains, focus-floating microscopy, and immunofluorescence tests are used, however, they need special expertise. Antigen testing is not indicated for the diagnosis of Lyme disease (Klempner *et al.,* 2001).

## Culture

Culture is not a commonly used diagnostic approach for Lyme disease due to its low sensitivity, lengthy incubation period, and need on a particular medium and expertise. In contrast, culture remains the gold standard for confirming the diagnosis of B. burgdorferi, a disease-causing Borrelia bacterium. Because B. burgdorferi has a limited metabolic capacity, it requires complicated growth mediums such as BSK and MKP (Rui-Sablji *et al.,* 2006). The possibility of growing B. Borrelia burgdorferi diagnosis is reliant on the specimen, sickness stage, laboratory skill, and genotype. Skin biopsies acquired by EM demonstrated a sensitivity of 40 to 60%, and positive cultures were associated with shorter disease duration and smaller lesions (Ogrinc *et al.*, 2013). The sensitivity of 9-ml plasma samples grown from untreated patients with early and disseminated disease is around 40%, but it may be increased to 75% by analysing culture aliquots with a sensitive PCR. More validation is needed for a new serum culture test (Maraspin *et al.*, 2011).

## PCR

Although there is more variation due to methodology, gene targets, and primer sets, the sensitivity of PCR techniques for B. burgdorferi DNA detection in skin or blood samples is equivalent to culture methods (Liveris et al., 2012). Sensitivity may be reduced by optimal culture techniques, particularly for plasma samples (Li *et al.,* 2011). PCR is commonly used to identify Lyme arthritis, although its sensitivity in cerebral fluid samples is low (Mygland et al., 2010).

## Indirect Methods

The bulk of Lyme disease laboratory tests rely on antibody responses in serum, and antibody-based assays are the only accepted diagnostic method. However, correct test use is a major challenge, with the United States doing 3.4 million serologic tests each year, much above the anticipated 300,000 cases (Hinckley *et al.,* 2014). The CDC recommended a two-tier strategy to boost specificity in 1995, using enzyme immunoassays or indirect immunofluorescence methods. This treatment only applies to Lyme disease contracted in the United States.

Specialty laboratories that offer non-validated Lyme diagnostic tests are discouraged because to the reduction in sensitivity and specificity. It is not recommended to screen for antibodies in synovial fluid or cerebral fluid (Barclay *et al.,* 2012).

Although the current two-tier technique is successful, it has limitations such as poor sensitivity during early infections, subjective interpretation, and confusion..

Most Lyme disease tests use whole cell sonicate (WCS) from grown Borrelia burgdorferi, which can result in false-positive results because to cross-reactive antigens and differences in protein expression (Gomes-Solecki *et al.,* 2000). The C6 peptide has improved sensitivity and specificity, particularly in persons with different illnesses. Other recombinant and synthetic antigens, such as conserved portions of OspC, have been studied for use in serodiagnosis. These peptides can be used in single or multi-peptide investigations (Burbelo *et al.*, 2010).

The sensitivity of antibody-based tests increases with infection duration, with a latency between initial infection and detection of sufficient antibodies (Arnaboldi *et al.*, 2013). Patients with EM who present early are more likely to have bad outcomes, although fewer than half of all EM patients have positive outcomes. Serological testing is very beneficial in those with advanced Lyme disease. Seropositivity is more common in convalescent patients than in those with solitary EM lesions (Philipp *et al.,* 2005).

## Intrathecal Antibody Production

Anti-B. burgdorferi antibodies in the central nervous system must be detected via serum and cerebrospinal fluid analysis. In Europe, integrate antibody production is regarded as the gold standard for Lyme neuroborreliosis diagnosis (Ogrinc *et al.,* 2013). However, due to the lack of a gold standard, case definitions, tests, and retrospective review, interpretation is difficult. In acute Lyme neuroborreliosis, intrathecal antibody sensitivity is roughly 50% (Steere *et al.,* 1990).

## CXCL13

CXCL13 is a B cell chemoattractant chemokine found in the cerebral fluid of people with acute Lyme neuroborreliosis and may be beneficial in some treatment settings46,98,99. This test is no longer widely used by doctors (Bremell *et al.,* 2013).

## Other Tests

Cell proliferation, ELISPOT, cytokine measurements, complement split products, and lymphocyte transformation assays are ineffective for detecting Lyme disease in humans. Xenodiagnosis, which employs a natural tick vector, is an experimental test with prospective therapeutic applications (Marques *et al.,* 2009).

## LYME DISEASE TREATMENT

### Early Disease

Erythema migrans resolves spontaneously without antibiotic intervention; nevertheless, treatment approaches serve to shorten the length of the illness and prevent development to late-stage disease (Steere, 1989). The majority of people in the early stages of the illness get well with oral antibiotics (Steere *et al.,* 2016). Adult regimens for erythema migrans, excluding pregnant women, include either doxycycline at 100 mg orally twice daily for 10-21 days or amoxicillin at 250-500 mg orally thrice daily for 10-21 days. Doxycycline has not shown a significant advantage in avoiding neurological symptoms (Strle *et al.,* 2018). Cefuroxime axetil is an alternative to doxycycline or amoxicillin when they are not available. Doxycycline at 1- 2 mg/kg twice daily or amoxicillin at 25-50 mg/kg thrice daily are suggested doses for children with permanent dentition, with amoxicillin being effective for those under 8 years old (Steere *et al.,* 2016; "Treatment of Lyme Disease," 2016).

A comprehensive study undertaken by Waddell LA, Greig J, Lindsay LR, et al. shows that treated women with gestational Lyme disease had better foetal outcomes than untreated peers (Waddell et al., 2018). Furthermore, two further data show that persons receiving antitumor necrosis factor alpha or rituximab treatment and then getting early Lyme disease may develop antibiotic resistance. Nonetheless, this group eventually has a favourable prognosis (Maraspin, Bogovi, Rojko, Ogrinc, *et al.,* 2019; Maraspin, Bogovi, Rojko, Rui-Sablji, *et al.*, 2019).

Both doxycycline and amoxicillin exhibit notable in-vitro efficacy against all Lyme borrelial genospecies prevalent in North America and Europe (Wormser et al., 2006). There is currently no substantiated evidence indicating the emergence of drug resistance (Steere *et al.*, 2016). While doxycycline may possess superior central nervous system (CNS) penetration compared to amoxicillin, it does not demonstrate superiority in the treatment of early neurologic Lyme disease (Strle *et al.*, 2018). Doxycycline also proves effective against Anaplasma phagocytophilum, the causative agent of human granulocytic anaplasmosis, which is a potential co-infection (Sanchez *et al.,* 2016). Noteworthy variability exists in susceptibility to macrolide antibiotics, including erythromycin (Terekhova *et al.,* 2002). Azithromycin, while active in vitro, demonstrates lower efficacy than amoxicillin (Luft et al., 1996). Conversely, first- generation cephalosporins, quinolone antibiotics, and sulfa drugs are deemed ineffective (Steere, 1989). B. Neurological disease:

The existing body of data does not adequately define the best antibiotic regimen for treating Lyme neuroborreliosis (Cadavid et al., 2016; Dersch et al., 2015). In a prospective, double-blind European study, oral doxycycline at a daily dosage of 200 mg was shown to be as effective as intravenous ceftriaxone at a daily dosage of 2 g in the early stages of neurological Lyme disease, with no instances of failure (Ljstad et al., 2008). Clinicians typically administer oral doxycycline, amoxicillin, or cefuroxime axetil for mild neurological signs such as isolated facial nerve palsy, in accordance with treatment options used for other early Lyme disease presentations (Steere *et al.*, 2016). Individuals with Lyme meningitis, on the other hand, frequently require hospitalization and get intravenous ceftriaxone at 2 g for 14 days, followed by a transition to oral doxycycline upon hospital discharge to finish a total antibiotic course of 14 days (Steere *et al.,* 2016). In the setting of Lyme encephalomyelitis, a rare subgroup of patients normally receives a full course of intravenous ceftriaxone, delivered for 14 to 28 days (Sanchez et al., 2016). C. Lyme arthritis:

Most Lyme arthritis patients are normally treated with either doxycycline at a daily dose of 100 mg orally, twice daily, for 28 days, or amoxicillin at a daily dosage of 500 mg orally, three times daily, for the same period (Lantos *et al.,* 2021). Despite effective therapy, some patients may have residual inflammatory joint results that last longer than the 28-day treatment window. In such circumstances, arthritis often resolves over many months, and supplementary therapies such as nonsteroidal anti-inflammatory medication and physical therapy may be helpful. When patients do not respond favourably, a comprehensive evaluation is required to uncover any confounding variables that are contributing to therapy failure.

Although Lyme arthritis usually cures without causing permanent joint damage, some individuals may endure chronic joint pain due to premorbid osteoarthritis rather than Lyme illness. Others may experience discomfort or functional restrictions as a result of joint deconditioning, leaving them resistant to additional antibiotic medication. A second 28-day course of oral antibiotic treatment may be considered for patients with persistent synovial inflammation (Arvikar & Steere, 2015). Importantly, no data exists to support the efficacy of switching from one oral medication to another (e.g., doxycycline to amoxicillin) during a subsequent round of antibiotic therapy to enhance results.

The best usefulness and time of intra-articular corticosteroid injection for Lyme arthritis patients who are resistant to antibiotic therapy need to be clarified. Experts typically urge caution, discouraging the use of intra-articular corticosteroid injections during the early phase of antibiotic treatment due to cases of delayed arthritis remission (Bentas *et al.,* 2000; Dattwyler *et al.,* 1988). Furthermore, for patients with Lyme disease facial palsy, oral corticosteroid treatment has been linked to a possible delay in resolution (Jowett et al., 2017; Wormser *et al.*, 2018).

Despite these cautionary remarks, recent observational studies in the paediatric population suggest that intra-articular corticosteroid injection may contribute to the resolution of persistent joint inflammation, eliminating the need for additional interventions (Horton et al., 2019; Nimmrich *et al.,* 2014).

In cases where chronic synovial inflammation remains after two cycles of 28-day oral antibiotic treatment, intravenous ceftriaxone at a dose of 2 g for 14-28 days is considered (Dattwyler et al., 1988; Sanchez et al., 2016). Antibiotic refractoriness warrants investigation of disease-modifying antirheumatic medications, including methotrexate (Arvikar & Steere, 2015; Grillon *et al.,* 2019). In situations where this fails, arthroscopic synovectomy emerges as an effective method for treating antibiotic- refractory Lyme arthritis of the knee (Schoen, 2020). D. Lyme Carditis:

Lyme carditis causes varied degrees of atrioventricular block, which is often well- tolerated despite known deaths. Due to the repeated development to total heart block, hospitalisation for intensive cardiac monitoring is mandatory for Lyme carditis patients (Robinson *et al.,* 2015; Steere *et al.*, 2016; Three Sudden Cardiac Deaths Associated with Lyme Carditis — United States, November 2012-July 2013, n.d.). Despite the ongoing ambiguity about the impact of antibiotic medication on the intrinsic course of conduction system disorders, its prudent use is advised. Patients with first-degree heart block and a PR interval of less than 0.3 seconds are treated with an oral regimen, which is consistent with the typical therapy for persons in the early stages of Lyme disease. For patients with more severe atrioventricular block with a PR interval greater than 0.3 seconds, the best treatment is intravenous ceftriaxone along with careful cardiac monitoring. Because conduction system anomalies in Lyme carditis are temporary, even in cases of full cardiac block, the placement of a permanent pacemaker is discouraged (Sanchez *et al.,* 2016; Steere *et al.,* 2016).

## CHRONIC LYME DISEASE CONTROVERSY

The majority of patients benefit from antibiotic therapy; nevertheless, a fraction reports chronic or recurring nonspecific symptoms after treatment (Lantos et al., 2021). Depending on their degree and influence on everyday functioning, these symptoms are referred to as post-treatment Lyme disease symptoms (PTLDS) or syndrome (PTLDS) (Turk *et al.,* 2019). This group of people suffering with PTLDS is a subset of the larger category known as "chronic Lyme disease" (CLD). It is worth noting that the phrase "chronic Lyme disease" is avoided in academic literature and mainstream medical discourse due to a lack of precise criteria and consensus on its definition, since it might refer to a wide range of individuals.

These people, like fibromyalgia sufferers, continue to have similar subjective symptoms including fatigue, generalized pain, and worry. Another subset is diagnosed with 'chronic Lyme illness,' despite the absence of supporting clinical signs of Lyme disease or laboratory evidence of exposure (Lantos, 2015). Despite repeated findings demonstrating their lack of effectiveness and possibility for adverse outcomes, these patients are sometimes subjected to long-term antibiotic or unconventional therapy

(Berende *et al.*, 2016, 2019; De Wilde *et al.,* 2017; Lantos et al., 2015; Marzec *et al.,* 2017). It is critical to recognize the issue of Lyme disease misdiagnosis and incorrect treatment. When possible, understanding the underlying causes of these symptoms might protect patients from unnecessary procedures and improve overall results.

## PREVENTION

Education, using repellent such as DEET and lemon oil eucalyptus, wearing protective cloths (long pants, long-sleeved shirts and closed shoes), vaccination, deer reduction, wearing light-colored cloths, removal of attached ticks, full body examination, showering using wash cloth, domestic strategies such as having a fence or a stone wall, and administrating a single dose of 200 mg of doxycycline (4.4 mg per kg in children) within 72 h following a high- risk tick bite may have an impact on decreasing the prevalence of Lyme disease (Lantos et al., 2021; Richardson *et al.*, 2019).

## CONCLUSION

The Lyme disease chapter shed light on the intricacies of this systemic illness caused by the spirochete Borrelia burgdorferi. We have gained a better understanding of this complex condition by researching its origins, transmission, clinical manifestations, diagnostic issues, and therapy options. Lyme disease, which was first identified in the United States in the 1970s, has since become a serious public health concern. The discovery of an arthritis epidemic in Lyme, Connecticut, led to the discovery of Lyme disease, which manifested with unusual symptoms not typical of juvenile rheumatoid arthritis. This discovery cleared the path for more study into the disease's aetiology and transmission.

The presence of the Borrelia burgdorferi spirochete, ticks capable of spreading it, and animals such as mice and deer that act as hosts for these ticks are all important points mentioned in this chapter. Understanding the life cycle of the primary Lyme disease vector is crucial to understanding the illness's epidemiology and regional changes in prevalence. Furthermore, the chapter emphasizes the significance of early Lyme disease identification and treatment. Prompt antibiotic therapy during the early stages of infection can result in a favorable outcome.

The issue, however, is appropriate diagnosis, since many instances go unnoticed, resulting in delayed or ineffective treatment. This can lead to chronic Lyme disease, which can have serious and long-term consequences for individuals. The consequences of Lyme disease go beyond physical health. Chronic Lyme disease can have serious physical, mental, and social consequences. Patients may face functional limitations, mental health difficulties, and a worse quality of life. Furthermore, the absence of specific diagnostic testing to establish the clearance of the Lyme organism complicates illness treatment.

Raising awareness of Lyme disease and pushing for its treatment are critical in overcoming its issues. We can enhance early detection and proper therapy by educating healthcare professionals and the general public about the various clinical presentations, transmission mechanisms, and prevention actions. Furthermore, encouraging collaboration among healthcare practitioners, academics, politicians, and patient advocacy organizations is critical for progressing research, diagnostic tools, and treatment alternatives.

Finally, the chapter emphasizes the intricacies of Lyme disease and the importance of continuing efforts to address its impact on individuals and communities. We can improve Lyme disease management and outcomes by working to improve diagnostic methods, treatment alternatives, and supportive care. We can strive towards a future where Lyme disease is successfully avoided, identified, and managed via improved awareness, research, and activism, eventually improving the lives of individuals impacted by this difficult condition.

## REFERENCES


. Alberto, J., Garza, C., Cruz-valadez, E. De, Ocampo-candiani, J., & Welsh, O. (2019). Clinical spectrum of Lyme disease. 201–208.

Arnaboldi, P. M., Seedarnee, R., Sambir, M., Callister, S. M., Imparato, J. A., & Dattwyler, R. J. (2013). Outer Surface Protein C Peptide Derived from Borrelia burgdorferi Sensu Stricto as a Target for Serodiagnosis of Early Lyme Disease. *Clinical and Vaccine Immunology; CVI, 20*(4), 474–481. DOI: 10.1128/CVI.00608-12 PMID: 23365204

Barclay, S. S., Melia, M. T., & Auwaerter, P. G. (2012). Misdiagnosis of Late- Onset Lyme Arthritis by Inappropriate Use of Borrelia burgdorferi Immunoblot Testing with Synovial Fluid. *Clinical and Vaccine Immunology; CVI, 19*(11), 1806–1809. DOI: 10.1128/CVI.00383-12 PMID: 22971779

Bremell, D., Mattsson, N., Edsbagge, M., Blennow, K., Andreasson, U., Wikkelsö, C., Zetterberg, H., & Hagberg, L. (2013). Cerebrospinal fluid CXCL13 in Lyme neuroborreliosis and asymptomatic HIV infection. *BMC Neurology, 13*(1), 2. DOI: 10.1186/1471-2377-13-2 PMID: 23294475

Burbelo, P. D., Issa, A. T., Ching, K. H., Cohen, J. I., Iadarola, M. J., & Marques, A. (2010). Rapid, Simple, Quantitative, and Highly Sensitive Antibody Detection for Lyme Disease. *Clinical and Vaccine Immunology; CVI, 17*(6), 904–909. DOI: 10.1128/CVI.00476-09 PMID: 20392886

Gomes-Solecki, M. J. C., Dunn, J. J., Luft, B. J., Castillo, J., Dykhuizen, D. E., Yang, X., Glass, J. D., & Dattwyler, R. J. (2000). Recombinant Chimeric Borrelia Proteins for Diagnosis of Lyme Disease. *Journal of Clinical Microbiology, 38*(7), 2530–2535. DOI: 10.1128/JCM.38.7.2530-2535.2000 PMID: 10878038

Hinckley, A. F., Connally, N. P., Meek, J. I., Johnson, B. J., Kemperman, M. M., Feldman, K. A., White, J. L., & Mead, P. S. (2014). Lyme Disease Testing by Large Commercial Laboratories in the United States. *Clinical Infectious Diseases, 59*(5), 676–681. DOI: 10.1093/cid/ciu397 PMID: 24879782

Klempner, M. S., Schmid, C. H., Hu, L., Steere, A. C., Johnson, G., McCloud, B., Noring, R., & Weinstein, A. (2001). Intralaboratory reliability of serologic and urine testing for Lyme disease. *The American Journal of Medicine, 110*(3), 217–219. DOI: 10.1016/S0002-9343(00)00701-4 PMID: 11182109

Lelovas, P., Dontas, I., Bassiakou, E., & Xanthos, T. (2008). Cardiac implications of Lyme disease, diagnosis and therapeutic approach. *International Journal of Cardiology, 129*(1), 15–21. DOI: 10.1016/j.ijcard.2008.01.044 PMID: 18508142

Li, X., McHugh, G. A., Damle, N., Sikand, V. K., Glickstein, L., & Steere, A. C. (2011). Burden and viability of Borrelia burgdorferi in skin and joints of patients with erythema migrans or lyme arthritis. *Arthritis and Rheumatism*, *63*(8), 2238–2247. DOI: 10.1002/art.30384 PMID: 21590753

Liveris, D., Schwartz, I., McKenna, D., Nowakowski, J., Nadelman, R., DeMarco, J., Iyer, R., Bittker, S., Cooper, D., Holmgren, D., & Wormser, G. P. (2012). Comparison of five diagnostic modalities for direct detection of Borrelia burgdorferi in patients with early Lyme disease. *Diagnostic Microbiology and Infectious Disease*, *73*(3), 243–245. DOI: 10.1016/j.diagmicrobio.2012.03.026 PMID: 22571973

Lyme disease. A rigorous review of diagnostic criteria and treatment. (n.d.). https://doi.org/https://doi.org/10.1016/j.jaut.2014.09.004

Maraspin, V., Ogrinc, K., Ružić-Sabljić, E., Lotrič-Furlan, S., & Strle, F. (2011). Isolation of Borrelia burgdorferi sensu lato from blood of adult patients with borrelial lymphocytoma, Lyme neuroborreliosis, Lyme arthritis and acrodermatitis chronica atrophicans. *Infection*, *39*(1), 35–40. DOI: 10.1007/s15010-010-0062-8 PMID: 21153429

Marques, A., Brown, M. R., & Fleisher, T. A. (2009). Natural Killer Cell Counts Are Not Different between Patients with Post-Lyme Disease Syndrome and Controls. *Clinical and Vaccine Immunology; CVI*, *16*(8), 1249–1250. DOI: 10.1128/CVI.00167-09 PMID: 19515868

Müllegger, R. R., & Glatz, M. (2008). Skin Manifestations of Lyme Borreliosis. *American Journal of Clinical Dermatology*, *9*(6), 355–368. DOI: 10.2165/0128071-200809060-00002 PMID: 18973402

Mygland, Å., Ljøstad, U., Fingerle, V., Rupprecht, T., Schmutzhard, E., & Steiner, I. (2010). EFNS guidelines on the diagnosis and management of European Lyme neuroborreliosis. *European Journal of Neurology*, *17*(1), 8. DOI: 10.1111/j.1468-1331.2009.02862.x PMID: 19930447

Ogrinc, K., Lotrič-Furlan, S., Maraspin, V., Lusa, L., Cerar, T., Ružič-Sabljič, E., & Strle, F. (2013). Suspected Early Lyme Neuroborreliosis in Patients With Erythema Migrans. *Clinical Infectious Diseases*, *57*(4), 501–509. DOI: 10.1093/cid/cit317 PMID: 23667259

Philipp, M. T., Wormser, G. P., Marques, A. R., Bittker, S., Martin, D. S., Nowakowski, J., & Dally, L. G. (2005). A Decline in C 6 Antibody Titer Occurs in Successfully Treated Patients with Culture-Confirmed Early Localized or Early Disseminated Lyme Borreliosis. *Clinical and Vaccine Immunology; CVI*, *12*(9), 1069–1074. DOI: 10.1128/CDLI.12.9.1069-1074.2005 PMID: 16148173

Radesich, C., Del Mestre, E., Medo, K., Vitrella, G., Manca, P., Chiatto, M., Castrichini, M., & Sinagra, G. (2022). Lyme Carditis: From Pathophysiology to Clinical Management. *Pathogens (Basel, Switzerland)*, *11*(5), 582. Advance online publication. DOI: 10.3390/pathogens11050582 PMID: 35631104

Roos, B. K. L. (2021).. . *Neurologic Complications of Lyme Disease.*, (August), 1040–1050.

Roos, K. L. (2021). Neurologic complications of Lyme disease. *CONTINUUM: Lifelong Learning in Neurology*, *27*(4), 1040–1050. PMID: 34623103

Schoen, R. T. (2020). Challenges in the diagnosis and treatment of Lyme disease. *Current Rheumatology Reports*, *22*(1), 1–11. DOI: 10.1007/s11926-019-0857-2 PMID: 31912251

Smith, B. G., Cruz, A. I.Jr, Milewski, M. D., & Shapiro, E. D. (2011). Lyme disease and the orthopaedic implications of Lyme arthritis. *The Journal of the American Academy of Orthopaedic Surgeons*, *19*(2), 91–100. DOI: 10.5435/00124635-201102000-00004 PMID: 21292932

Steere, A. C., Berardi, V. P., Weeks, K. E., Logigian, E. L., & Ackermann, R. (1990). Evaluation of the Intrathecal Antibody Response to Borrelia burgdorferi as a Diagnostic Test for Lyme Neuroborreliosis. *The Journal of Infectious Diseases*, *161*(6), 1203–1209. DOI: 10.1093/infdis/161.6.1203 PMID: 2345301

Steere, A. C., Strle, F., Wormser, G. P., Hu, L. T., Branda, J. A., Hovius, J. W., Li, X., & Mead, P. S. (2016). Lyme borreliosis. *Nature Reviews. Disease Primers*, *2*(1), 1–19. DOI: 10.1038/nrdp.2016.90 PMID: 27976670

The Impact of Lyme Disease on Mental Health. Understanding the Connection and Seeking Support. (n.d.). https://projectlyme.org/the-impact-of-lyme-disease-on -mental-health-understanding-t he-connection-and-seeking-support/

Wang, G., Van Dam, A. P., Schwartz, I., & Dankert, J. (1999). Molecular typing of Borrelia burgdorferi sensu lato: Taxonomic, epidemiological, and clinical implications. *Clinical Microbiology Reviews*, *12*(4), 633–653. DOI: 10.1128/CMR.12.4.633 PMID: 10515907

What are some unusual symptoms of Lyme disease? (n.d.). https://www .medicalnewstoday.com/articles/unusual-symptoms-of-lyme- disease#com plications

# Chapter 14
# Lassa Fever

**Esraa M Halawa**
*Faculty of Science, Cairo University, Egypt*

**Dina Shaaban**
*Faculty of Agriculture, Mansura University, Egypt*

**Menna A El-Khouly**
*Faculty of Medicine, Portsaid University, Egypt*

**Yomna A Lashean**
*Faculty of Medicine, Portsaid University, Egypt*

**Yusuf Aly Mahmoud**
*Faculty of Science, Ain Shams University, Egypt*

## ABSTRACT

*Lassa virus (LASV), which is commonly found among rodent populations in West African countries such as Sierra Leone and Nigeria, frequently transmits to humans, leading to the development of Lassa fever, a viral hemorrhagic fever characterized by a high fatality rate. Despite making certain advancements, there are still significant gaps in our comprehension of the immunology, epidemiology, ecology, and pathogenesis of Lassa fever. Several factors, including recurrent outbreaks, the potential dissemination of rodent reservoirs like Mastomys natalensis, the relative ease of acquiring and potentially weaponizing LASV, the importation of LASV to North America and Europe, and the emergence of new strains in densely populated West Africa, have spurred renewed efforts to develop countermeasures against LASV. Although several promising candidates are presently undergoing evaluation, there are currently no approved vaccines or treatments for human use. This chapter comprehensively examines the epidemiology and prevalence of Lassa fever in both*

DOI: 10.4018/979-8-3693-1990-1.ch014

*developing and developed nations.*

## INTRODUCTION

Lassa fever, a highly lethal viral hemorrhagic fever (VHF) caused by Lassa virus (LASV), has been identified as a result of zoonotic transfers of LASV to humans that have been occurring for centuries, according to genetic dating studies (Andersen et al., 2015). However, it was not until 1969 that the first recorded case of Lassa fever was documented. The patient in question was a missionary nurse who contracted the infection while working at a rural clinic near Lassa, Nigeria (Pinneo & Pinneo, 1971). Despite being transported over 600 km to a hospital in Jos, she tragically succumbed to the illness. In Jos, two additional nurses became infected and also succumbed to the disease. However, a third nurse named Lily (Penny) Pinneo survived the infection after being transported to New York City (Watts, 2013). Blood samples obtained from the infected nurses were subsequently analyzed at Yale University, where LASV was first isolated. The strain isolated from Pinneo was designated as the type strain. During these initial studies, two researchers from Yale contracted LASV, and unfortunately, one of them died. The surviving virologist, Dr. Jordi Casals, received blood donated by Pinneo as a form of passive immunotherapy (Leifer et al., 1970; Buckley et al., 1970; Buckley & Casals, 1970). These early encounters with LASV provided the impetus for the development of improved measures to investigate emerging pathogens, including the establishment of high-biocontainment laboratories operating under strict regulations and oversight. Further investigation into a Lassa fever outbreak in the Eastern Province of Sierra Leone in 1972 revealed that the peri-domestic rodent Mastomys natalensis serves as the primary reservoir for LASV (Monath et al., 1974). LASV is transmitted vertically to the offspring of infected rodents and horizontally to humans and other rodents (Fichet-Calvet et al., 2014; Fichet-Calvet et al., 2008). Lassa fever is endemic among Mastomys populations in Nigeria, Sierra Leone, Guinea, and Liberia. There have been reports of infected rodents or sporadic human cases in other West African countries, including Mali, Togo, and Benin (Kakaī et al., 2020; Patassi et al., 2017). The endemic range of LASV appears to be expanding (Sogoba et al., 2012). Here, in the current chapter, we discuss the epidemiology and prevalence of Lassa fever in both developing and developed nations, the pathogenesis, symptoms, and diagnosis of the disease, available treatment options, challenges faced by each country, and novel strategies for controlling its spread.

## DEFINITION OF LASSA FEVER

Lassa fever is a distinctive type of viral hemorrhagic fever that is prevalent in certain regions of West Africa, particularly Sierra Leone, Guinea, Liberia, and Nigeria. The causative agent of this disease is the Lassa virus, which belongs to the Old World arenavirus family. The primary reservoir host for this virus is the multimammate rodent Mastomys nataliensis, which commonly resides in close proximity to human populations. Recent estimates indicate that Lassa fever results in approximately two million cases and 5,000 to 10,000 deaths on an annual basis, primarily occurring in West Africa (Happi et al., 2019).

## EPIDEMIOLOGY AND PREVALENCE OF LASSA FEVER IN DEVELOPING AND DEVELOPED NATIONS

Lassa fever is characterized by a systemic primary viral infection caused by a single-stranded RNA virus (Healing & Gopal, 2001; Johnson et al., 1987). A prominent characteristic of the fatal form of the disease involves compromised or delayed cellular immunity, which results in rapid and severe viremia (Chen & Cosgriff, 2000). In terms of seroprevalence, the presence of antibodies against the Lassa virus has been detected in varying proportions in different populations. Specifically, in Sierra Leone, the prevalence ranges from 8% to 52% (McCormick et al., 1987), while in Guinea, it varies from 4% to 55% (Lukashevich et al., 1993). In Nigeria, the seropositivity rate is reported to be 21% (Tomori et al., 1988). Additionally, seropositivity has been identified in regions such as the Central African Republic, the Democratic Republic of the Congo, Mali, and Senegal (Andersen et al., 2015). Tragically, individuals from organizations such as the UK Department for International Development, the International Committee of the Red Cross, and the United Nations Mission in Sierra Leone have succumbed to the disease. Furthermore, sporadic cases have been documented in travelers returning to the United Kingdom, the Netherlands, and Germany.

### The Current Epidemiology of Lassa Fever

Between epidemiological weeks 1 and 15 of 2023 (ending on 16 April), Nigeria has been grappling with a significant outbreak of Lassa fever, encompassing 4702 suspected cases, five probable cases, and 877 confirmed cases. Among the confirmed cases, there have been 152 deaths, resulting in a case fatality rate (CFR) of 17%. This represents a 20% increase in the number of confirmed cases compared to the corresponding period in 2022, which reported 733 cases. The outbreak has been observed across 101 local government areas (LGAs) in 26 out of the 36 states, including the Federal Capital Territory (FCT). The majority of the confirmed cases (72%) are concentrated in three states: Ondo (32%), Edo (29%), and Bauchi (11%). Additionally, laboratory-confirmed cases have been identified in states bordering Cameroon (Adamawa, Benue, Cross Rivers, and Taraba) as well as states bordering Benin (Oyo and Niger) (World Health Organization, 2023a).

### Nation Has Lately Been Affected by Lassa Fever

Lassa fever is considered endemic in several West African nations, including Benin, Ghana, Guinea, Liberia, Mali, Sierra Leone, and Nigeria, and it is probable that the disease is also present in other countries within the region. In Guinea, the first diagnosis of Lassa fever occurred in October 2011, and subsequent outbreaks and sporadic cases have been documented in the country (World Health Organization, 2022).

## RISK FACTORS ESPECIALLY IN THESE NATIONS

Lassa fever is primarily contracted through exposure to contaminated rat excrement (feces) or urine, which can contaminate surfaces or food sources. Additionally, transmission can occur through contact with the bodily fluids of individuals infected with the Lassa virus (LASV), including exposure to their feces, urine, or blood. It is important to note that LASV can persist in urine for an extended period of time following infection in both humans and animals. Inadequate sanitation practices or the absence or improper use of personal protective equipment (PPE) can facilitate the transmission of Lassa fever within healthcare facilities (Cleveland Clinic, 2022).

The risk of acquiring Lassa fever is particularly high for individuals residing in or traveling to regions of West Africa where the disease is prevalent. These areas encompass Nigeria, Benin, Guinea, Liberia, Mali, and Sierra Leone. Pregnant individuals face an elevated risk of experiencing complications and mortality associated with Lassa fever (Cleveland Clinic, 2022).

## PATHOGENESIS OF LASSA FEVER

Lassa virus (LASV) can infect multiple types of host cells at initial entry sites. It then disseminates through the bloodstream and can eventually reach the lymph nodes, liver, and spleen, where it can successfully replicate inside (Torriani et al., 2016). As a result of the virus's successful accessibility to host tissues, it starts a close conflict between the spread and replication of the virus and the host's innate immune system (Torriani et al., 2016; McCormick et al., 1987). Immune cells like dendritic cells (DCs) and macrophages (MPs) are the first cells infected by LASV. These cells do not become activated and secrete low amounts of proinflammatory cytokines, leading to a failure in the stimulation of costimulatory molecules and T-cell activation (Pannetier et al., 2014; Raabe et al., 2022). The reason that enables the virus to circumvent the innate immune response is inherent in its genetic composition. The LASV genome is constituted by two genomic RNA segments known as the large (L) segment and the small (S) segment (Loureiro et al., 2018). Each segment encodes two viral proteins, using an ambisense coding strategy, which means that the L segment encodes both the L and Z proteins (Auperin et al., 1984; Murphy & Ly, 2022). The L protein is an RNA-dependent RNA polymerase that promotes the transcription and replication of viral RNA. The Z protein, which contains a matrix protein with zinc-finger motifs, can obstruct the detection of viral double-stranded RNA (dsRNA) in the cytoplasm of an infected cell by inhibiting viral dsRNA receptors, such as retinoic acid-inducible gene I (RIG-I) and melanoma differentiation-associated gene 5 (MDA-5) (Raabe et al., 2022; Murphy & Ly, 2022; Hastie et al., 2012; Huang et al., 2020). Meanwhile, the S segment encodes the nucleoprotein (NP) and the precursor of the envelope glycoprotein complex (GPC). The LASV nucleoprotein plays a crucial role in the replication and transcription of the virus by forming ribonucleoprotein complexes, which are necessary for the synthesis of viral RNA (Murphy & Ly, 2022). Furthermore, NP blocks the translocation of interferon regulatory factor 3 (IRF-3) from the cytoplasm to the nucleus, which would otherwise suppress the host's innate immune response (Raabe et al., 2022; Mateer et al., 2020). The LASV glycoprotein, which studs the virus envelope, directly interacts with the host plasma membrane via alpha-dystroglycan, acting as a cellular entry receptor and thereby facilitating the internalization of the viral particle into the host cell (Murphy & Ly, 2022). Infection with LASV starts as flu-like symptoms, including fever, headache, sore throat, myalgia, and nausea, then progresses to facial edema, pleural effusion, renal failure, pericardial effusion, mucosal bleeding, sensorineural deafness, and encephalopathy in severe cases, ultimately leading to death (McLay et al., 2014; Brosh-Nissimov, 2016).

## SYMPTOMS AND SIGNS

The symptoms of Lassa fever can be challenging to differentiate from malaria and typhoid, so it's important to consider other potentially serious illnesses in individuals. In a study conducted at a hospital in Sierra Leone, all 441 patients admitted with Lassa fever exhibited fever. Additionally, more than 70% of these patients experienced chest pain, diarrhea, vomiting, and headache. An interesting and unique diagnostic sign is hearing loss or impairment, which was observed in approximately 29% of 49 acutely febrile patients diagnosed with Lassa fever in Sierra Leone (Houlihan & Behrens, 2017).

Classic skin rash is not a characteristic symptom of Lassa fever, and subcutaneous bleeding (ecchymoses or petechiae) is not commonly observed. However, cases of facial, neck, and jaw edema have been reported. A reduced Glasgow Coma Scale score or seizures may indicate Lassa fever encephalopathy. In cases of late presentation or deterioration, bleeding (17%) and effusions (3%) have been documented, with the latter being associated with proteinuria (McCormick & Fisher-Hoch, 2002).

Lassa fever typically starts gradually, after an incubation period of 7-18 days. It presents with fever, weakness, malaise, severe frontal headache, and a highly painful sore throat. More than half of the patients subsequently develop joint and lumbar pain, while 60% experience a nonproductive cough. A significant number also suffer from severe retrosternal chest pain, and about half of the patients exhibit symptoms of nausea, vomiting, diarrhea, and abdominal pain. Bleeding occurs in only 15%-20% of patients, primarily limited to mucosal surfaces, or occasionally manifesting as conjunctival hemorrhages, gastrointestinal bleeding, or vaginal bleeding. Fatal cases often involve severe pulmonary edema and adult respiratory distress syndrome, characterized by pronounced edema in the head and neck, pharyngeal stridor, and hypovolemic shock.

In summary, Lassa fever manifests with various symptoms that overlap with other illnesses, making accurate diagnosis challenging. However, certain indicators such as hearing loss and specific clinical manifestations can aid in identifying the disease.

## DIAGNOSIS OF LASSA FEVER

Diagnosing Lassa fever poses challenges due to its clinical similarities with other prevalent African illnesses like malaria, typhoid fever, influenza, and rickettsia infections (Brosh-Nissimov, 2016). Complicating matters, the Federal Drug Administration (FDA) has not endorsed any validated laboratory tests for the virus (World Health Organization, 2016). However, there are several diagnostic methods available that combine clinical observations, serological testing, and molecular diagnostic assays, including viral cultures, enzyme-linked immunosorbent serologic assay (ELISA), immunofluorescence, plaque neutralization, and polymerase chain reaction (PCR) (Oti, 2018).

PCR, in particular, exhibits high sensitivity to the virus, making it the most effective technique for diagnosis (Brosh-Nissimov, 2016). Additionally, laboratory findings associated with Lassa fever often reveal lymphopenia, thrombocytopenia, and increased blood levels of aspartate aminotransferase (Oti, 2018; Raabe & Koehler, 2017; Russier et al., 2012). It's worth noting that viremia does not occur (Ezeomah et al., 2019).

In summary, diagnosing Lassa fever presents challenges due to its resemblance to other African illnesses, and the lack of FDA-approved laboratory tests adds to the complexity. However, a combination of clinical observations, serological testing, and molecular diagnostic assays, with PCR being the most sensitive, can aid in accurate diagnosis. Laboratory results often show characteristic abnormalities such as lymphopenia, thrombocytopenia, and elevated levels of aspartate aminotransferase, while viremia is not observed.

## TREATMENT

1. Ribavirin (1-[(2R,3R,4S,5R)-3,4-dihydroxy-5-(hydroxymethyl)oxolan-2-yl]-1,2,4-triazole-3-carboxamide) is a drug that potentially exerts its effects by inhibiting macrophage activation, cytokine production, and lymphocyte proliferation (Hansen et al., 2021).
2. Favipiravir (T-705, 6-fluoro-3-hydroxypyrazine-2-carboxamide) has demonstrated antiviral activity against various RNA viruses, including orthomyxoviruses, arenaviruses, bunyaviruses, filoviruses, flaviviruses, and coronaviruses such as SARS-CoV-2. In 2014, favipiravir was approved in Japan for emergency influenza infections, and stockpiles of the drug were established. Currently, favipiravir is being investigated in multiple clinical trials for the treatment of COVID-19 (Hansen et al., 2021).
3. Stampidine (methyl 2-[[(4-bromophenoxy)-[[(2S,5R)-5-(5-methyl-2,4-dioxopyrimidin-1-yl)-2,5-dihydrofuran-2-yl]methoxy]phosphoryl]amino] propanoate) is a nucleoside analog derived from d4T, a potent inhibitor of retroviral reverse transcriptase. In a semi-lethal CBA mouse model, stampidine demonstrated increased survival against LASV challenge compared to vehicle controls when administered in two different dose regimens (Khan et al., 2008).
4. ST-193 (1-(4-methoxyphenyl)-N-[(4-propan-2-ylphenyl)methyl]benzimidazol-5-amine) (Khan et al., 2008).
5. Immune Plasma: The use of convalescent plasma treatment in human Lassa fever cases predates animal studies and was first employed to treat a virologist in Connecticut shortly after the disease's discovery in 1969. Convalescent plasma therapy has since been utilized in various Lassa fever patient settings (Khan et al., 2008).

6. Monoclonal Antibodies: Monoclonal antibody (MAb) treatments have been developed for numerous diseases and several viruses, including Synagis. Due to advancements in technology, such as high specificity and targeting of specific single epitopes, MAb humanization, predictable consistency in manufacturing, and improved safety compared to polyclonal antibody/convalescent plasma treatments, MAbs have significant potential for the treatment of virus-induced illnesses, including Lassa fever (Khan et al., 2008).

## CHALLENGES OF LASSA VIRUS MANAGEMENT AND CONTROL

### High Rates of Virulence, Fatality, and Contagiousness

The symptoms of LV are non-specific and variable, especially at the early stages of the infection. Therefore, it is difficult to be distinguished from other fevers such as the Ebola virus or malaria. This exaggerates the rates of virulence, fatality, and contagiousness and makes the investigations and diagnosis more difficult (Ibekwe, 2012; Aloke et al., 2023).

- **Route of transmission.**

Its fomite and aerosol route of transmission threaten all who deal with the patient such as healthcare workers or his relatives, (Ibekwe, 2012; Aloke et al., 2023).

- **Vector control is difficult.**

The vector is the infected Mastomys rat which lives around farms and homes. Although its biological and chemical controls show some potential, they can destroy the ecosystem in the long term because these cannot eliminate the rats alone, (Ibekwe, 2012; Aloke et al., 2023)

- **It can be used as a biological weapon.**

Lassa fever became a worldwide issue because some accidentally imported cases to other countries. So, its lethal characteristics make it a suitable biological weapon, (Ibekwe, 2012).

- **Lack of safe vaccination and efficient diagnoses rapid kits,** (Ibekwe, 2012).

- **The complications for survivors and those who did not exhibit any symptoms.**

Survivors with sensorineural hearing losses suffer from distinguished inadequate speech differentiation and cannot be managed by hearing devices. Also, using anti-oxidants and higher pressure of oxygen for hearing loss and neurological conditions is still speculative, (Ibekwe, 2012; Aloke et al., 2023).

- **Lack of standard personal protective materials (PPM).**

The availability of PPM such as gloves, goggles, and masks is essential to protect healthcare workers and the public from this virulent infection, especially during outbreaks, (Aloke et al., 2023).

- **Lack of awareness.**

Lack of healthcare workers and people's knowledge leads to the fear of infection and the tension between healthcare workers involved in patients' management, (Aloke et al., 2023).

- **Determining the disease origin and contact with the missing patients,** (Aloke et al., 2023).

## NOVEL RESEARCH STRATEGIES TO LIMIT THE SPREAD OF LASSA FEVER

### Vaccine Efforts

Vaccine Efforts According to a research study conducted in 2019, there was no vaccine that protects against the Lassa fever virus (LASV). The World Health Organization finalized a Lassa fever vaccine Target Product Profile (TPP) in June 2017. In response, LASV was made one of the priorities for vaccine development funding by the multiagency Coalition for Epidemic Preparedness Innovations (CEPI), using a multisector partnership approach to finance and develop vaccines for infections of epidemic potential (Mazzola & Kelly-Cirino, 2019). A number of different platform technologies have been evaluated as potential Lassa fever vaccines, including virus-like particles, DNA vaccines, and non-replicating (inactivated) viruses such as Lassa and Yellow Fever. For the vaccine platforms, recombinant VSV/LASV and reassortant ML29 are considered the most advanced vaccine candidates in clinical development. Despite promising preclinical evaluation, none of these vaccine candidates have advanced to human clinical trials till 2019 (Mazzola & Kelly-Cirino, 2019). A scoping review of vaccine clinical trials published in April 2023 found that four Lassa fever vaccine candidates (INO-4500, MV-LASV, rVSVΔG-LASV-GPC, and EBS-LASV) have entered the clinical stage of assessment. Five phase 1 trials (all focused on healthy adults) and one phase 2 trial (involving a broader age group from 18 months to 70 years) evaluating one of these vaccines have been registered to date. Though Lassa fever vaccine development is still in the early stages, current progress towards a safe and effective vaccine is encouraging (Sulis et al., 2023).

## Mano River Union Lassa Fever Network (MRU LFN)

The Ministries of Health of Guinea, Liberia, and Sierra Leone, WHO, the Office of United States Foreign Disaster Assistance, the United Nations, and other partners have worked together to establish the Mano River Union Lassa Fever Network. Rather than start completely de novo, the MRU LFN builds on four pre-existing laboratories in the MRU countries: the KGH Lassa Laboratory in Kenema; the Central Public Health Laboratory Service in Monrovia, Liberia; the Program on Hemorrhagic Fevers in Conakry, Guinea; and the International Center for Research on Tropical Infections in Guinea. Training in laboratory diagnosis, clinical management, and environmental control is also included (World Health Organization, n.d.; Khan et al., 2008).

The cornerstone of the MRU LFN is the enhancement of laboratory capacity. The emphasis on the laboratory was a conscious decision taking into account the very non-specific clinical presentation of LF that continually undermines efforts to establish surveillance and control programs and the extreme difficulty of sending diagnostic specimens for testing at laboratories outside the MRU region (Khan et al., 2008).

## Research Priorities for Treatment and Pathogenesis:

1. A better understanding of disease pathogenesis and determinants of severity.
2. Efficacy of general supportive measures.
3. Optimization of ribavirin therapy.
4. Testing of new anti-arenavirus drugs.
5. Testing of non-arenavirus-specific drugs, (Khan et al., 2008).

## REFERENCES


Aloke, C., Obasi, N. A., Aja, P. M., Emelike, C. U., Egwu, C. O., Jeje, O., Edeogu, C. O., Onisuru, O. O., Orji, O. U., & Achilonu, I. (2023, January 3). Combating Lassa Fever in West African Sub-Region: Progress, Challenges, and Future Perspectives. *Viruses*, *15*(1), 146. DOI: 10.3390/v15010146 PMID: 36680186

Andersen, K. G., Shapiro, B. J., Matranga, C. B., Sealfon, R., Lin, A. E., Moses, L. M., Folarin, O. A., Goba, A., Odia, I., Ehiane, P. E., Momoh, M., England, E. M., Winnicki, S., Branco, L. M., Gire, S. K., Phelan, E., Tariyal, R., Tewhey, R., Omoniwa, O., & Sabeti, P. C. (2015). Clinical sequencing uncovers origins and evolution of Lassa virus. *Cell*, *162*(4), 738–750. DOI: 10.1016/j.cell.2015.07.020 PMID: 26276630

Auperin, D. D., Romanowski, V., Galinski, M. R., & Bishop, D. H. (1984). Sequencing studies of pichinde arenavirus S RNA indicate a novel coding strategy, an ambisense viral S RNA. *Journal of Virology*, *52*(3), 897–904. DOI: 10.1128/jvi.52.3.897-904.1984 PMID: 6492264

Brosh-Nissimov, T. (2016). Lassa fever: Another threat from West Africa. *Disaster and Military Medicine*, *2*(1), 2. DOI: 10.1186/s40696-016-0018-3 PMID: 28265442

Buckley, S. M., & Casals, J. (1970). Lassa fever, a new virus disease of man from West Africa. 3. Isolation and characterization of the virus. *The American Journal of Tropical Medicine and Hygiene*, *19*(4), 680–691. DOI: 10.4269/ajtmh.1970.19.680 PMID: 4987547

Buckley, S. M., Casals, J., & Downs, W. G. (1970). Isolation and antigenic characterization of Lassa virus. [This work reports the initial isolation and characterization of Lassa virus.]. *Nature*, *227*(5254), 174. DOI: 10.1038/227174a0 PMID: 5428406

Chen, J. P., & Cosgriff, T. M. (2000). Hemorrhagic fever virus-induced changes in hemostasis and vascular biology. *Blood Coagulation & Fibrinolysis*, *11*(5), 461–483. DOI: 10.1097/00001721-200007000-00010 PMID: 10937808

Ezeomah, C., Adoga, A. A., Ihekweazu, C., Paessler, S., Cisneros, I. L., Tomori, O., & Walker, D. H. (2019). Sequelae of Lassa Fever: Postviral Cerebellar Ataxia. *Open Forum Infectious Diseases*, *6*(12), 6. DOI: 10.1093/ofid/ofz512 PMID: 31879673

Hansen, F., Jarvis, M. A., Feldmann, H., & Rosenke, K. (2021). Lassa virus treatment options. *Microorganisms*, *9*(4), 772.

Fichet-Calvet, E., Becker-Ziaja, B., Koivogui, L., & Gunther, S. (2014). Lassa serology in natural populations of rodents and horizontal transmission. *Vector Borne and Zoonotic Diseases (Larchmont, N.Y.)*, *14*(9), 665–674. DOI: 10.1089/vbz.2013.1484 PMID: 25229705

Fichet-Calvet, E., Lecompte, E., Koivogui, L., Daffis, S., & ter Meulen, J. (2008). Reproductive characteristics of Mastomys natalensis and Lassa virus prevalence in Guinea, West Africa. *Vector Borne and Zoonotic Diseases (Larchmont, N.Y.)*, *8*(1), 41–48. DOI: 10.1089/vbz.2007.0118 PMID: 18237265

Happi, A. N., Happi, C. T., & Schoepp, R. J. (2019, August). Lassa fever diagnostics: Past, present, and future. *Current Opinion in Virology*, *37*, 132–138. DOI: 10.1016/j.coviro.2019.08.002 PMID: 31518896

Hastie, K. M., Bale, S., Kimberlin, C. R., & Saphire, E. O. (2012). Hiding the evidence: Two strategies for innate immune evasion by hemorrhagic fever viruses. *Current Opinion in Virology*, *2*(2), 151–156. DOI: 10.1016/j.coviro.2012.01.003 PMID: 22482712

Healing, T., & Gopal, R. Report on an assessment visit to Sierra Leone, April 12th-30th 2001. London: Merlin, 2001.

Houlihan, C., & Behrens, R. (2017). Lassa fever. *BMJ (Clinical Research Ed.)*, *358*, j2986. DOI: 10.1136/bmj.j2986 PMID: 28701331

Huang, Q., Liu, X., Brisse, M., Ly, H., & Liang, Y. (2020). Effect of strain variations on Lassa virus Z protein-mediated human RIG-I inhibition. *Viruses*, *12*(9), 907. DOI: 10.3390/v12090907 PMID: 32824946

Ibekwe, T. (2012). Lassa fever: The challenges of curtailing a deadly disease. [Internet]. *The Pan African Medical Journal*, *11*, 55. https://www.ncbi.nlm.nih.gov/pmc/articles/PMC3343683/ PMID: 22593791

Johnson, K. M., McCormick, J. B., Webb, P. A., Smith, E. S., Elliott, L. H., & King, I. J. (1987). Clinical virology of Lassa fever in hospitalized patients. *The Journal of Infectious Diseases*, *155*(3), 456–464. DOI: 10.1093/infdis/155.3.456 PMID: 3805773

Kakaī, C. G., Okunromade, O. F., Dan-Nwafor, C. C., Chabi, A. I. B., Martial, G. T. P., Dalhat, M. M., Ward, S., Tante, O., Nguku, P. M., Hamadi, A., Ilori, E., Lokossou, V., Brito, C., Ojo, O. E., Kone, I., Agbeko, T. T., Ihekweazu, C., & Merrill, R. D. (2020). Improving cross-border preparedness and response: Lessons learned from 3 lassa fever outbreaks across Benin, Nigeria, and Togo, 2017–2019. *Health Security*, *18*(S1), S105–S112. DOI: 10.1089/hs.2019.0080 PMID: 32004125

Khan, S. H., Goba, A., Chu, M., Roth, C., Healing, T., Marx, A., Fair, J., Guttieri, M. C., Ferro, P., Imes, T., Monagin, C., Garry, R. F., & Bausch, D. G. (2008). New opportunities for field research on the pathogenesis and treatment of Lassa fever. *Antiviral Research, 78*(1), 103–115. DOI: 10.1016/j.antiviral.2007.11.003 PMID: 18241935


Khan, S. H., Goba, A., Chu, M., Roth, C., Healing, T., Marx, A., Fair, J., Guttieri, M. C., Ferro, P., Imes, T., Monagin, C., Garry, R. F., & Bausch, D. G. (2008). New opportunities for field research on the pathogenesis and treatment of Lassa fever. *Antiviral Research, 78*(1), 103–115. DOI: 10.1016/j.antiviral.2007.11.003 PMID: 18241935


Lassa fever - guinea. World Health Organization. Available from: https://www.who.int/emergencies/disease-outbreak-news/item/2022-DON382

Lassa fever - nigeria. World Health Organization. Available from: https://www.who.int/emergencies/disease-outbreak-news/item/2023-DON463

Leifer, E., Gocke, D. J., & Bourne, H. (1970). Lassa fever, a new virus disease of man from West Africa. II. Report of a laboratory-acquired infection treated with plasma from a person recently recovered from the disease. *The American Journal of Tropical Medicine and Hygiene, 19*(4), 677–679. DOI: 10.4269/ajtmh.1970.19.677 PMID: 4987546

Loureiro, M. E., Zorzetto-Fernandes, A. L., Radoshitzky, S., Chi, X., Dallari, S., Marooki, N., Lèger, P., Foscaldi, S., Harjono, V., Sharma, S., Zid, B. M., López, N., de la Torre, J. C., Bavari, S., & Zúñiga, E. (2018). DDX3 suppresses type I interferons and favors viral replication during Arenavirus infection. *PLoS Pathogens, 14*(7), e1007125. DOI: 10.1371/journal.ppat.1007125 PMID: 30001425

Lukashevich, L. S., Clegg, J. C., & Sidibe, K. (1993). Lassa virus activity in Guinea: Distribution of human antiviral antibody defined using enzyme-linked immunosorbent assay with recombinant antigen. *Journal of Medical Virology, 40*(3), 210–217. DOI: 10.1002/jmv.1890400308 PMID: 8355019

Mateer, E. J., Maruyama, J., Card, G. E., Paessler, S., & Huang, C. (2020). Lassa virus, but not highly pathogenic New World arenaviruses, restricts immunostimulatory double-stranded RNA accumulation during infection. *Journal of Virology, 94*(9), 10–1128. DOI: 10.1128/JVI.02006-19 PMID: 32051278

Mazzola, L. T., & Kelly-Cirino, C. (2019). Diagnostics for Lassa fever virus: A genetically diverse pathogen found in low-resource settings. *BMJ Global Health, 4*(Suppl 2), e001116. DOI: 10.1136/bmjgh-2018-001116 PMID: 30899575

McCormick, J. B., & Fisher-Hoch, S. P. (2002). *"Lassa fever." Arenaviruses I: the Epidemiology*. Molecular and Cell Biology of Arenaviruses.

McCormick, J. B., King, I. J., Webb, P. A., Johnson, K. M., O'Sullivan, R., Smith, E. S., Trippel, S., Trippel, S., & Tong, T. C. (1987). A case-control study of the clinical diagnosis and course of Lassa fever. *The Journal of Infectious Diseases*, *155*(3), 445–455. DOI: 10.1093/infdis/155.3.445 PMID: 3805772

McCormick, J. B., Webb, P. A., Krebs, J. W., Johnson, K. M., & Smith, E. S. (1987). A prospective study of the epidemiology and ecology of Lassa fever. *The Journal of Infectious Diseases*, *155*(3), 437–444. DOI: 10.1093/infdis/155.3.437 PMID: 3805771

McLay, L., Liang, Y., & Ly, H. (2014). Comparative analysis of disease pathogenesis and molecular mechanisms of New World and Old World arenavirus infections. *The Journal of General Virology*, *95*(Pt 1), 1–15. DOI: 10.1099/vir.0.057000-0 PMID: 24068704

Monath, T. P., Newhouse, V. F., Kemp, G. E., Setzer, H. W., & Cacciapuoti, A. (1974). Lassa virus isolation from Mastomys natalensis rodents during an epidemic in Sierra Leone. [This work is the first demonstration that Lassa virus is rodent-borne.]. *Science*, *185*(4147), 263–265. DOI: 10.1126/science.185.4147.263 PMID: 4833828

Murphy, H., & Ly, H. (2022). Understanding Immune Responses to Lassa Virus Infection and to Its Candidate Vaccines. *Vaccines*, *10*(10), 10. DOI: 10.3390/vaccines10101668 PMID: 36298533

Oti, V. B. (2018). *A Reemerging Lassa Virus: Aspects of Its Structure, Replication, Pathogenicity and Diagnosis*. Current Topics in Tropical Emerging Diseases and Travel Medicine.

Pannetier, D., Reynard, S., Russier, M., Carnec, X., & Baize, S. (2014). Production of CXC and CC Chemokines by Human Antigen-Presenting Cells in Response to Lassa Virus or Closely Related Immunogenic Viruses, and in Cynomolgus Monkeys with Lassa Fever. *PLoS Neglected Tropical Diseases*, *8*(1), 8. DOI: 10.1371/journal.pntd.0002637 PMID: 24421914

Patassi, A. A., Landoh, D. E., Mebiny-Essoh Tchalla, A., Halatoko, W. A., Assane, H., Saka, B., Naba, M. A., Yaya, I., Edou, K. A., Tamekloe, T. A., Banla, A. K., Davi, K. M., Manga, M., Kassankogno, Y., & Salmon-Ceron, D. (2017). Emergence of lassa fever disease in northern Togo: Report of two cases in Oti district in 2016. *Case Reports in Infectious Diseases*, *2017*, 8242313. DOI: 10.1155/2017/8242313 PMID: 29391958

Pinneo, L., & Pinneo, R. (1971). Mystery virus from Lassa. *The American Journal of Nursing*, *71*, 1352–1355. PMID: 4996954

professional CC medical. Lassa fever. Available from: https://my.clevelandclinic.org/health/diseases/25095-lassa-fever

Raabe, V. N., & Koehler, J. W. (2017). Laboratory Diagnosis of Lassa Fever. *Journal of Clinical Microbiology*, *55*(6), 1629–1637. DOI: 10.1128/JCM.00170-17 PMID: 28404674

Raabe, V.N., Mehta, A.K., & Evans, J.D. (2022). Lassa Virus Infection: a Summary for Clinicians. *International journal of infectious diseases: IJID: official publication of the International Society for Infectious Diseases.*

Russier, M., Pannetier, D., & Baize, S. (2012). Immune Responses and Lassa Virus Infection. *Viruses*, *4*(11), 2766–2785. DOI: 10.3390/v4112766 PMID: 23202504

Sogoba, N., Feldmann, H., & Safronetz, D. (2012). Lassa fever in West Africa: Evidence for an expanded region of endemicity. *Zoonoses and Public Health*, *59*(s2), 43–47. DOI: 10.1111/j.1863-2378.2012.01469.x PMID: 22958249

Sulis, G., Peebles, A., & Basta, N. E. (2023). Lassa fever vaccine candidates: A scoping review of vaccine clinical trials. *Tropical Medicine & International Health*, *28*(6), 420–431. DOI: 10.1111/tmi.13876 PMID: 37095630

Tomori, O., Fabiyi, A., Sorungbe, A., Smith, A., & McCormick, J. B. (1988). Viral hemorrhagic fever antibodies in Nigerian populations. *The American Journal of Tropical Medicine and Hygiene*, *38*(2), 407–410. DOI: 10.4269/ajtmh.1988.38.407 PMID: 3128130

Torriani, G., Galan-Navarro, C., & Kunz, S. (2016). Lassa Virus Cell Entry Reveals New Aspects of Virus-Host Cell Interaction. *Journal of Virology*, *91*(4), e01902-16. Advance online publication. DOI: 10.1128/JVI.01902-16 PMID: 27928003

Watts, G. M. (2013). Lily Lyman Pinneo. *Lancet*, *380*(9853), 1552. DOI: 10.1016/S0140-6736(12)61871-6

World Health Organization. (2016). *WHO Calls for Early Diagnostic Tests for Lassa Fever.* World Health Organization.

World Health Organization. (n.d.). Lassa fever. World Health Organization. https://www.who.int/news-room/fact-sheets/detail/lassa-fever

# Chapter 15
# Dengue and Dengue Hemorrhagic Fever

**Sharjeel Chaudhry**
https://orcid.org/0000-0002-7070-1326
*Dow University of Health Sciences, Pakistan*

**Zarmina Ehtesham**
https://orcid.org/0000-0002-8094-476X
*Hamdard University, Pakistan*

## ABSTRACT

*Emphasizing the worldwide significance of tropical diseases, the chapter addresses Dengue and Dengue Hemorrhagic Fever. The distribution, prevalence, and challenges that developed and developing nations confront are analyzed. Prevention strategies are studied simultaneously with clinical signs, diagnosis, and treatment alternatives. The requirement for specialized solutions is underlined when disparities between developed and developing nations are addressed. Difficulties include socioeconomic reasons, poor sanitation, and a limited healthcare system. The chapter stresses the significance of future plans, research strategies, and international collaboration in the struggle against infectious diseases. In order to develop a health-conscious global population, it ends by emphasizing the relationship between socioeconomic difficulties, healthcare systems, and infectious diseases.*

## INTRODUCTION

Infectious diseases provide a persistent threat to global public health due to their impact on individuals in both affluent and impoverished countries. The chapter currently mostly focuses on tropical diseases, specifically Dengue and Dengue

DOI: 10.4018/979-8-3693-1990-1.ch015

Haemorrhagic Fever. The impact of tropical diseases is shaped by the convergence of climatic, environmental, and socioeconomic factors. Discussions pertaining to global health sometimes overlook them. The Aedes mosquito, which serves as the main carrier of the dengue virus, is predominantly found in tropical locations. This geographical advantage shields these areas from the colder portions of the planet. Tropical diseases are a collection of contagious ailments that mostly impact individuals residing in tropical and subtropical areas. Various pathogens, including microorganisms, viruses, parasites, and fungus, can be responsible for causing various disorders. Tropical diseases can propagate through several means, such as sexual transmission, consumption of infected food or water, and mosquito bites.

Tropical diseases present a significant risk to the overall well-being of the population in underdeveloped nations. According to the World Health Organization (WHO), around 1 billion individuals are afflicted with tropical diseases annually, resulting in the deaths of millions, (World Health Organization, 2023). Tropical diseases exert a significant financial impact on developing nations, resulting in billions of dollars being spent annually on healthcare expenses and productivity losses. This chapter aims to offer a thorough overview of these illnesses by examining their prevalence, causes, symptoms, risk factors, diagnostic complexities, lack of awareness regarding antibiotic usage, treatment strategies, and future research objectives.

Throughout this chapter centered around tropical diseases, specifically dengue and dengue hemorrhagic fever, it is imperative to emphasize the importance of comprehending, responding to, and cooperating on an international level. Infectious diseases, especially those common in tropical locations, provide a complicated set of challenges that go beyond national boundaries and affect both developed and developing countries. The discrepancies in the incidence and impact of dengue fever across developed and developing nations underscore the necessity for tailored interventions. In developed nations, even with advanced healthcare systems and infrastructure, uncommon incidents that are commonly linked to overseas travel can quickly escalate if not properly monitored. The two major challenges are addressing early detection and providing training to healthcare staff who may not have experience in treating these diseases.

## DISTRIBUTION AND PREVALENCE

Dengue and dengue hemorrhagic fever (DHF) are prevalent tropical diseases worldwide. Dengue fever, a contagious disease transmitted by mosquitoes, is caused by one of four distinct serotypes of the dengue virus. The DHF strain is more lethal than the other strain, (Centers for Disease Control and Prevention, 2023). Dengue and DHF are prevalent in around 120 countries located in tropical and subtropical regions worldwide. Dengue and DHF are prevalent in Southeast Asia, South Asia, and Latin America.

## Dengue in Developing Countries

The high incidence of dengue in developing countries can be ascribed to factors such as dense population, insufficient sanitation, and an inadequate healthcare system, (Weaver, 2018). The Aedes mosquito, which flourishes in such circumstances, is responsible for recurrent instances of the infection.

## Dengue in Developed Countries

In developed nations with advanced sanitation and healthcare systems, occurrences of dengue are infrequent and mostly associated with international travel. However, it is essential to engage in vigilant surveillance as there is a potential for transmission within the local community, (Rothman, 2011).

*Figure 1. Map*

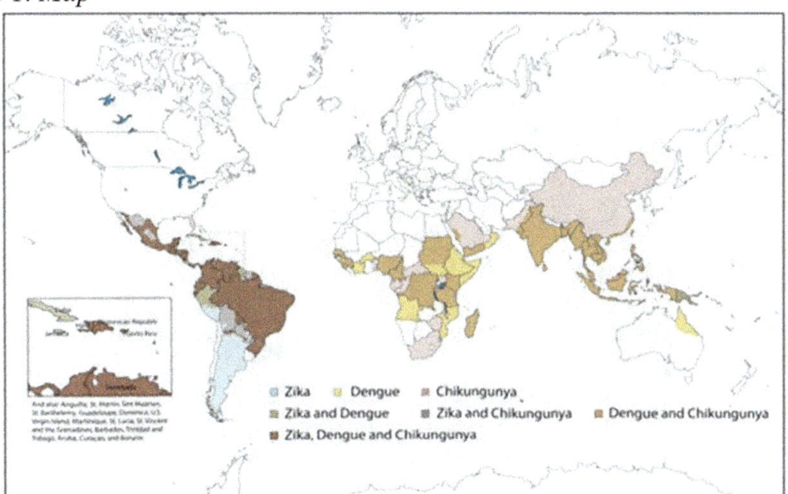


Disparities exist in the allocation of dengue cases between developed and developing nations. Developed countries see sporadic instances that are often associated with travel or imported cases, whereas developing countries face significant epidemics. This world map displays the geographical distribution of dengue and DHF. The proper determination of the prevalence of dengue and DHF is hindered by a significant number of untreated cases. According to estimates from the World

Health Organization (WHO), more than 390 million individuals contract dengue fever year. Additionally, over 500,000 people are hospitalized, and more than 20,000 individuals succumb to dengue hemorrhagic fever (DHF) each year, (World Health Organization, 2023).

## EPIDEMIOLOGY AND PATHOPHYSIOLOGY

Dengue and DHF can be caused in humans by the bite of an Aedes mosquito that is infected. The diurnal biting Aedes mosquito is most active during the early morning and late afternoon, (Centers for Disease Control and Prevention, 2023). Upon infiltration into the bloodstream by a mosquito bite, the dengue virus undergoes replication in multiple organs, including the liver. Following a brief period, the virus is released back into the bloodstream and has the potential to invade more cells, (Weaver, 2018). The dengue virus can infect various types of cells, including endothelial cells that form the inner lining of blood vessels. When a person is infected with the dengue virus, the presence of leaky dengue endothelial cells can lead to bleeding and the loss of plasma, (Rothman, 2011).

*Figure 2. Image of Aedes aegypti mosquito*

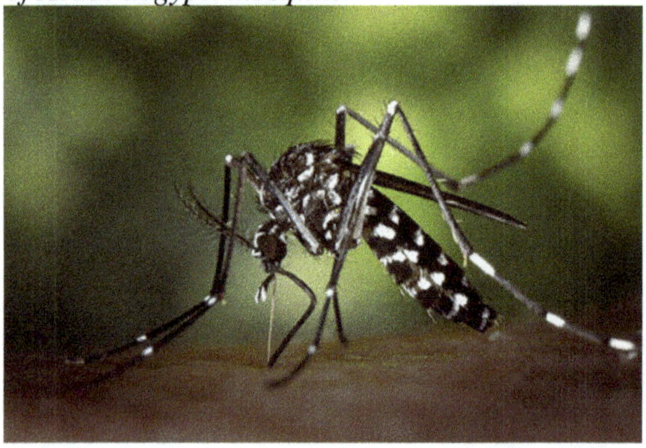

Comprehending the pathophysiology of dengue and dengue hemorrhagic fever is essential, (Horstick & Göbel, 2013). The presence of the hemorrhagic virus variant poses extra difficulties in treatment as it has the ability to invade immune cells and induce significant vascular permeability, (Al-Saad, Al-Wabel, & Khan, 2020). The pathophysiology of DHF is believed to be influenced by various factors, but it is thought to be caused by a combination of factors, including:

- The virulence of the dengue virus serotype.
- The host immune response.
- The presence of other co-infections, (Guzman, Vazquez, & Martinez, 2014).

## CLINICAL MANIFESTATIONS

The clinical manifestations of dengue and DHF exhibit variability according on the severity of the disease. Dengue typically manifests with an abrupt onset of fever, accompanied by symptoms such as headache, muscle and joint pain, nausea, vomiting, and rash. The standard duration for a severe fever is two to seven days. Usually, the rash appears as maculopapular across the face, trunk, and limbs, (Ahmed & Koo, 2022). Dengue fever initiates with symptoms resembling those of influenza, but it can progress into hemorrhagic fever in more severe instances. Timely identification and implementation of appropriate measures are vital, given the variability of symptoms. Age, viral serotype, and preexisting medical disorders are factors that influence the severity of dengue. Developing nations are at a greater risk since they have inadequate access to healthcare and experience prolonged diagnosis periods.

### Dengue Fever

- Sudden onset of high fever.
- Severe headache.
- Muscle and joint pain.
- Nausea and vomiting.
- Skin rash.

### Dengue Hemorrhagic Fever

- Severe abdominal pain.
- Persistent vomiting.
- Bleeding gums or nose.
- Fatigue and restlessness.
- Blood in vomit or stool.

Bleeding is a common manifestation of DHF. There are two types of bleeding: minor bleeding, which includes petechiae and purpura, and severe bleeding, such as brain hemorrhage or gastrointestinal bleeding, (Bhatt *et al.,* 2013). Shock is a potentially lethal consequence of DHF. Hypotension is the medical term used to describe a hazardous decrease in blood pressure, (Bhatt *et al.*, 2015).

## DIAGNOSIS

An accurate and prompt diagnosis is essential for delivering effective treatment. Molecular methodologies and expedited diagnostic assays are vital; nonetheless, countries with limited resources still encounter obstacles, (Burke *et al.,* 2018). A diagnosis of dengue fever or DHF is established by assessing the patient's symptoms and examining the results of diagnostic tests. Developed nations encounter difficulties in promptly diagnosing Dengue due to healthcare personnel's lack of knowledge with its symptoms, (Cao-Lormeau *et al.,* 2014). The scarcity of resources and diagnostic facilities poses a significant challenge for developing nations.

The following laboratory findings are suggestive of dengue:

*Thrombocytopenia* (low platelet count).

- Normal Range: The platelet count ranges from 150,000 to 450,000 per microliter.
- Findings: An abnormally low platelet count may indicate the presence of dengue fever, (Chen & Wilson, 2020) (World Health Organization, 2009).

Leukopenia (low white blood cell count).

- Normal Range: The range of white blood cells is between 4,000 and 11,000 per microliter.
- Findings: Dengue cases may exhibit a leukopenia, which is a decrease in the number of white blood cells below the expected range.

Elevated liver enzymes.

- Normal Range:
    - * Alanine Transaminase (ALT): 7 to 56 units per liter.
    - * Aspartate Transaminase (AST): 10 to 40 units per liter.
- Findings: Elevated levels of alanine aminotransferase (ALT) and aspartate aminotransferase (AST) can suggest liver damage in cases of Dengue fever.

The following laboratory findings are suggestive of DHF:

Thrombocytopenia (low platelet count).

- Normal Range: The platelet count ranges from 150,000 to 450,000 per microliter.
- Findings: Dengue Hemorrhagic Fever (DHF) is characterized by a reduced number of platelets, similar to Dengue, (Guzman *et al.,* 2011).

Hemoconcentration (increased hematocrit).

- Normal Range:

    * Male: 38.8% to 50%.
    * Female: 34.9% to 44.5%.
- Findings: Increased hematocrit levels may suggest hemoconcentration, which is a hallmark of dengue hemorrhagic fever (DHF).

Plasma leakage (evidence of fluid accumulation in the tissues)

- Normal Range: Lack of substantial fluid buildup.
- Findings: Clinical indications of plasma leakage can be detected by observing elevated hematocrit levels, pleural effusion, or ascites, (World Health Organization, 2023).

## TREATMENT

The over utilization of antibiotics is a worldwide issue. Addressing the misunderstanding surrounding antibiotic usage is crucial in order to prevent antibiotic resistance and enhance illness management, (Gubler, 2020). There is no standardized treatment regimen for dengue or DHF. The approach to providing supportive care encompasses measures such as ensuring adequate rest, administering fluids, and administering analgesic medication. Hospitalization may be necessary for people with severe cases, requiring intravenous fluids and blood transfusions, (Chen & Wilson, 2020). Managed in distinct ways by developed and developing nations. To mitigate dengue epidemics, it is essential to establish and maintain a robust healthcare infrastructure and engage the community in developing countries. This approach differs from developed countries, where the focus is on early detection and providing supportive care.

## PREVENTION

There are a number of ways to prevent dengue and DHF, (Huang *et al.,* 2019):

### Vector Control

- Source reduction: Eradicate Mosquito Breeding Sites.
- Larviciding: Larvicides are utilized to hinder the maturation of mosquito larvae.
- Insecticide spraying: Concentrated on fully developed mosquitoes.
- Environmental management: Creating an inhospitable environment for mosquitoes.

- Environmental management: Creating an inhospitable environment for mosquitoes, (Rothman, 2019).

*Figure 3. Person spraying insecticide on a wall*

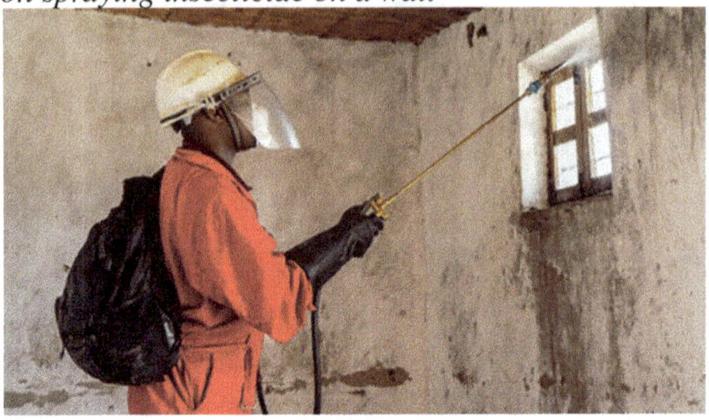

## Personal Protection

- Using insect repellent: Mosquito repellents containing DEET or picaridin are effective in repelling mosquitoes.
- Wearing long-sleeved clothing and pants: Wearing clothing that covers the skin can decrease the likelihood of mosquito bites, (Liew *et al.,* 2020).
- Using bed nets: Sleeping under bed nets treated with pesticides adds an additional degree of protection.

## Vaccination

A safe and efficacious dengue vaccine is currently accessible in some countries. Nevertheless, concerns over cost-effectiveness and limited availability persist. Dengvaxia (CYD-TDV): Dengvaxia, created by Sanofi Pasteur, was one of the initial dengue vaccines to receive approval for use in several countries. The tetravalent vaccine provides protection against all four serotypes of the Dengue virus, (Messina *et al.,* 2020) (Rothman, 2019).

## CHALLENGES

Dengue and dengue hemorrhagic fever (DHF) provide a substantial menace to worldwide well-being, impacting both individuals and healthcare systems in both advanced and emerging countries. Although the underlying condition persists, the challenges and therapeutic approaches in these two patients vary dramatically, (Schneider, Sundararajan, & de Azavedo, 2019) (World Health Organization, 2020). Understanding these subtle distinctions is crucial for successful control and prevention endeavors. The distinct difficulties associated with the management and prevention of dengue and DHF continue to exist in both developed and developing countries, despite increased awareness and research endeavors. These challenges can be broadly categorized into:

### Challenges in Developing Nations

- Limited healthcare infrastructure: The absence of adequate healthcare infrastructure in most developing countries is a challenge in effectively diagnosing and treating Dengue and DHF, (Aguiar, Stollenwerk, & Dotta, 2023). Illustrative instances comprise insufficient hospital infrastructure, a scarcity of proficient healthcare practitioners, and limited availability of diagnostic tools and treatments.
- Poor sanitation and hygiene: Inadequate sanitation and hygiene standards facilitate the proliferation of Aedes mosquitoes, which are the principal vectors of the Dengue virus. The issue is worsened in densely populated regions since there is restricted availability of clean water and sanitation amenities.
- Lack of awareness and education: The lack of public education about dengue and DHF could exacerbate the disease if diagnosis and treatment are delayed, (Aguiar, Stollenwerk, & Dotta, 2023). The presence of disinformation and prevailing cultural attitudes may provide challenges in the successful implementation of effective preventive measures.
- Poverty and socioeconomic factors: Discrepancies in socioeconomic status, namely in terms of income and poverty, serve as robust indicators of the likelihood of dengue and DHF.Individuals residing in poverty may face restricted availability of insecticides, mosquito nets, and other preventive measures. Inadequate housing conditions and road congestion are additional factors that contribute to the proliferation of mosquitoes.

## Challenges in Developed Nations

- Travel and trade: The rise in dengue travel and trade has facilitated the dissemination of dengue and DHF to formerly unaffected regions around the globe, (Araújo *et al.,* 2020). Returning travelers from regions with a high prevalence of the virus can transmit it, resulting in the occurrence of localized epidemics.
- Climate change: Climate change, characterized by elevated temperatures and modified rainfall patterns, is likely causing a surge in mosquito reproduction, perhaps resulting in an upsurge in Dengue transmission in developed countries, (Harris, Vespignani, & Bhatt, 2022).
- Complacency: The vigilance and preparedness of developed nations with a low historical incidence of Dengue fever may decrease, resulting in difficulties in preventing outbreaks, (Bhatt *et al.,* 2022).
- Cost and access to new technologies: Some advanced countries with limited resources may not have easy access to or the financial means to purchase sophisticated treatments such as vaccines and mosquito control devices.

# MANAGEMENT STRATEGIES

A comprehensive and flexible strategy is necessary to effectively handle dengue and dengue hemorrhagic fever (DHF), considering the distinct difficulties encountered by both developed and developing countries. In developed countries, where occasional outbreaks of Dengue present an ongoing danger, it is crucial to have robust surveillance systems, prompt identification, and a resilient healthcare infrastructure, (Blaney & Bloom, 2020). It is imperative to provide education to both the general public and healthcare professionals, debunk erroneous information about vaccines, and exert relentless efforts to combat vaccine skepticism. Concurrently, prioritizing pandemic preparedness guarantees swift reactions to future outbreaks. Developing nations face the challenge of overcoming their constrained resources, which requires investments in healthcare infrastructure, extensive community involvement, and enduring programs to control disease carriers. To address socioeconomic variables, poverty, and access to clean water, a comprehensive approach is necessary, integrating both preventive measures and treatment strategies. International cooperation, joint research endeavors, and fair vaccine allocation are essential for establishing a robust dengue health system that can mitigate the impact of dengue and DHF in many contexts, (Brady *et al.,* 2021). In order for this approach to achieve success, it is crucial to foster cohesion, facilitate the exchange of information, and demonstrate a strong dedication to overcoming obstacles in the goal of global health equity. Efficiently addressing dengue and DHF necessitates employing a varied strategy that considers the distinct obstacles encountered by each nation. Here are some key strategies:

## Developing Nations

- Strengthening healthcare infrastructure: Enhancing the availability of medications, therapies, and healthcare practitioners. In order to mitigate the proliferation of mosquitoes and enhance public health, it is imperative to establish sustainable initiatives focused on cleanliness and sanitation, (Guzmán & Kouri, 2020).
- Improving sanitation and hygiene: Methods to increase awareness about dengue and DHF encompass dispelling misconceptions, disseminating focused educational resources, and engaging the community in prevention endeavors.
- Integrated vector management: Integrated vector control programs encompass the implementation of larviciding, source reduction, and personal protective measures.
- Research and development: Assisting with research endeavors focused on creating novel vaccines, diagnostic tools, and treatments specifically designed for the need of developing countries.

## Developed Nations

- Surveillance and rapid response: Strengthening surveillance systems to facilitate prompt response to potential early detection and outbreaks.
- Vector control programs: Efficiently managing mosquito populations and other disease carriers through the implementation of adaptable programs tailored to local conditions.
- Travel advisories and education: Travelers visiting regions where Dengue is prevalent should receive prompt and precise travel advisories, together with guidance on preventive measures against Dengue, (Gubler, 2020).
- Investing in research and development: Promoting research focused on the development of cost-effective and readily accessible techniques for early identification, treatment, and prevention.
- International collaboration: Strengthening global collaboration and coordination to address dengue epidemics.

## RESEARCH STRATEGIES AND FUTURE PLANS

Global collaboration is essential for addressing the challenges posed by infectious diseases, especially in the context of future plans and research strategies. Developed nations have a vital role in driving technical progress, while developing nations provide valuable perspectives on the distinct challenges they encounter. The collaboration generated by this coordinated endeavor fosters a comprehensive, worldwide approach to combatting infectious diseases. Various strategies can be employed in future plans to eliminate infectious diseases. Strengthening healthcare systems is crucial as it improves overall preparedness and response capabilities, (Johansson *et al.,* 2021). An effective approach to enhance surveillance systems is the use of proactive measures for early detection and containment. Ensuring equal access to vaccines is vital for ensuring that both developed and developing nations may benefit from advancements in preventive measures.

In order to halt the transmission of contagious illnesses, it is imperative to prioritize the advancement of novel antiviral medications and therapeutic approaches within the realm of scientific investigation. The timely and precise identification of diseases such as dengue is crucial for effective intervention, necessitating the advancement of novel diagnostic instruments. The development of genetically modified mosquitoes and innovative pesticides is contributing to the mitigation of disease transmission by mosquitoes. Continuous research is necessary to further our understanding of the biology and immune response to diseases such as dengue. This knowledge significantly influences the advancement of specific therapies and strategies for treatment. Enhancing surveillance systems increases our capacity to monitor disease patterns by supplying vital data to guide control measures and allocate resources effectively, (Bhatt *et al.,* 2013) (Cao-Lormeau *et al.,* 2014) (World Health Organization, 2020) (Araújo e*t al., 2020*). Ultimately, in order to achieve the worldwide elimination of infectious diseases, it is imperative to implement future strategies that focus on enhancing the healthcare system, increasing accessibility, and ensuring fair distribution of vaccines. Collaboration on a global scale in research is vital. The ongoing research and development endeavors that concentrate on antiviral medications, diagnostics, mosquito control, and disease dynamics contribute to a comprehensive strategy for protecting global health, which is feasible.

## CONCLUSION

It is imperative to emphasize the importance of acknowledging, addressing, and collaborating on a worldwide level as we complete this chapter on tropical diseases, specifically focusing on dengue and dengue haemorrhagic fever. Infectious diseases, especially those common in tropical areas, present a complicated set of difficulties that go beyond national boundaries and affect both developed and developing countries. The need for customized approaches is emphasized by variations in dengue occurrence and consequences between developed and developing nations. Even in developed nations with modern healthcare systems and infrastructure, uncommon incidents that are commonly linked to overseas travel can quickly escalate if not properly monitored. One of the challenges is providing education to healthcare staff who may not have experience in treating these diseases, in addition to ensuring early diagnosis. Developing nations bear an unequal share of the burden when it comes to dengue and other tropical diseases. The difficulties are increased by poverty, an inadequate healthcare infrastructure, and restricted availability of clean water and sanitation. To effectively manage infectious diseases in these areas, it is vital to use a comprehensive approach that considers socioeconomic variables, rather than merely relying on symptomatic treatment. Irrespective of their developmental stage, it is imperative for all nations to adopt a comprehensive approach towards dengue management. Developed nations prioritize early diagnosis, supportive infrastructure, and prevention of local transmission more than developing nations on the creation of sustainable healthcare infrastructure, community engagement, and access to essential resources.

The topic of infectious diseases and the worldwide problem of antibiotic resistance highlights the interconnectedness of antibiotic utilization. To improve ethical antibiotic stewardship, global collaboration is necessary to tackle the shared problem of insufficient comprehension regarding the proper utilization of antibiotics. International collaboration is crucial for future endeavours aimed at eliminating infectious diseases such as Dengue. Developed countries should aggressively engage in research collaborations with developing countries, leveraging their distinct viewpoints and experiences, in light of their technical advancements. The future plans prioritize a dedication to global healthcare systems, research customized to the specific requirements of diverse individuals, and ensuring equitable availability of healthcare.

This chapter provides a concise overview of the primary discussion surrounding infectious diseases in both developed and developing countries. A coordinated global response that takes into account the distinct challenges faced by each region is strongly highlighted. Aside from scientific progress, the disparity needs to be addressed by means of diplomacy, socioeconomic factors, and a dedication to addressing health disparities. On the occasion of the one-year anniversary of our goal to investigate the dissemination and management of contagious illnesses, we anticipate that this phase will enhance our comprehension of the worldwide circumstances. The deep interconnections between socioeconomic conditions, healthcare infrastructure, and infectious diseases underscore the necessity of ongoing dialogue, research, and collaboration. By undertaking this activity, we establish the foundation for a stronger and more health-conscious worldwide population that is equipped to confront the difficulties presented by contagious illnesses in the future.

## REFERENCES


Aguiar, R. S., Stollenwerk, N., & Dotta, G. (2023). Dengue virus infection: A review of recent advances in therapeutic interventions and vaccine development. *Drugs*, *83*(1), 29–53.

Ahmed, N. A., & Koo, J. R. (2022). Dengue virus: Viral entry, replication, and transmission. *Antiviral Research*, *207*, 105582.

Al-Saad, K. M., Al-Wabel, A. A., & Khan, A. A. (2020). Dengue fever: Epidemiology, clinical manifestations, diagnosis, and treatment. *Cureus*, *12*(11), e11380. PMID: 33251077

Araújo, E. V., Martins, L. C., Silva, L. F., Araújo, F. R., Fernandes, T. R., & Queiroz, A. S. (2020). Dengue fever: A review of the current knowledge. *Journal of Infection and Public Health*, *13*(10), 1521–1528.

Bhatt, S., Cameron, E., Bharti, N., Grenfell, B. T., Vespignani, A., & Hay, S. I. (2022). Dengue fever: Global burden and spatiotemporal dynamics, 2000-2020. *The Lancet. Infectious Diseases*, *22*(9), e155–e163.

Bhatt, S., Gething, P. W., Brady, O. J., Messina, J. P., Farlow, A. W., Moyes, C. L., & Hay, S. I. (2013). The global distribution of Zika virus: Modelling past, present, and future. *Nature*, *496*(7446), 533–537. PMID: 23542591

Bhatt, S., Katzelnick, L., Messina, J. P., Funk, S., Tatem, A. J., Clements, A. C., & Hay, S. I. (2015). The effect of temperature on dengue disease. *Nature*, *520*(7546), 64–67.

Blaney, J. E., & Bloom, B. R. (2020). The dengue virus nonstructural protein 1: A multi-functional protein essential for viral replication. *Viruses*, *12*(3), 350. PMID: 32235750

Brady, O. J., Messina, J. P., Perkins, T. A., Huang, C. Y., Le Menach, A., Sun, W., & Hay, S. I. (2021). Global seroprevalence of dengue virus infection and risk factors for seropositivity: A systematic review and meta-analysis. *The Lancet. Infectious Diseases*, *21*(12), e342–e351.

Burke, D. S., Monath, T. P., Guirakhoo, F., Phillips, N. B., & Blair, C. D. (2018). Dengue fever and Zika virus: Two mosquito-borne flaviviruses causing outbreaks in the Americas. *Current Opinion in Virology*, *30*, 10–15.

Cao-Lormeau, V. M., Blake, A., Mons, S., Lastère, S., Roche, C., Vanhomwegen, J., & Ghawché, F. (2014). Guillain-Barre syndrome outbreak associated with Zika virus infection in French Polynesia: A case-control study. *Lancet, 383*(9919), 1915–1920. PMID: 26948433

Centers for Disease Control and Prevention. (2023, April 13). Dengue. https://www.cdc.gov/dengue/index.html

Chen, L. H., & Wilson, M. E. (2020). Dengue and Zika: Emerging arboviruses of public health concern. *The American Journal of the Medical Sciences, 359*(6), 509–519. PMID: 32245566

Dengue and severe dengue (2023). World Health Organization. https://www.who.int/news-room/fact-sheets/detail/dengue-and-severe-dengue

Dengue Haemorrhagic Fever. (2009). *Diagnosis, Treatment, Prevention and Control: New Edition*. World Health Organization.

Gubler, D. J. (2020). The global pandemic of dengue/severe dengue: Current status and prospects for control. *Human Vaccines & Immunotherapeutics, 16*(1), 1–14. PMID: 32022652

Gubler, D. J. (2020). Dengue and Zika viruses: Insights into the emergence, global spread, and control of two major vector-borne flaviviruses. *Annual Review of Virology, 7*(1), 193–210.

Guzman, M. G., Halstead, S. B., Artsob, H., Buchy, P., Farrar, J., & Gubler, D. J. & World Health Organization. (2011). Dengue: A continuing global threat. *Nature Reviews. Microbiology, 9*(7), 564–572. PMID: 21079655

Guzmán, M. G., & Kouri, G. (2020). Dengue: History, classification, and clinical features. *The American Journal of Tropical Medicine and Hygiene, 102*(6), 1155–1161.

Guzman, M. G., Vazquez, S., & Martinez, E. (2014). Dengue: Current situation and perspectives for control. *The Lancet. Infectious Diseases.*

Harris, E., Vespignani, A., & Bhatt, S. (2022). Climate change and dengue: A critical and systematic review of quantitative projections. *The Lancet. Planetary Health, 6*(4), e362–e371.

. Horstick, O., & Göbel, U. B. (2013). Dengue virus type 1: Pathogenesis and clinical presentation. Dengue virus infection, 1-20.

Huang, Y. H., Yang, C. M., Chang, L. H., Lin, Y. S., Lai, C. C., Chiu, C. Y., & Tsai, W. P. (2019). Dengue fever and the risk of subsequent severe dengue: A nationwide population-based study. *International Journal of Epidemiology, 48*(2), 521–532.

Johansson, M. A., Aguiar, R. S., Vasilakis, N., & Weaver, S. C. (2021). Dengue virus capsid protein: Structure, function, and role in viral pathogenesis. *Viruses*, *13*(6), 1033. PMID: 34070947

Liew, C. W., Mohd-Noor, N. A., Yusof, R., & Zaini, Z. (2020). Dengue fever: A comprehensive review. *Tropical Biomedicine*, *37*(4), 1355–1374.

Messina, J. P., Brady, O. J., Pigott, D. M., Bhatt, S., Battle, K. E., Myers, M. F., & Hay, S. I. (2020). Global data on the distribution and abundance of Aedes mosquitoes. *Nature Ecology & Evolution*, *4*(1), 157–162.

Rothman, A. L. (2011). Dengue: A vascular disease. *Advances in Virus Research*, *81*, 1–70.

Rothman, A. L. (2019). Dengue: The importance of surveillance and vector control. *Microorganisms*, *7*(12), 619. PMID: 31783517

Schneider, J. R., Sundararajan, S. A., & de Azavedo, J. C. (2019). Dengue: A complex and evolving disease. *The American Journal of Tropical Medicine and Hygiene*, *100*(6), 1299–1304. PMID: 31190683

Weaver, S. C. (2018). Dengue virus pathogenesis: An update. *Viruses*, *10*(2), 75. PMID: 29439402

Weaver, S. C., Reisen, W. K., & Scott, T. W. (2019). Dengue virus: Evolution, transmission, and pathogenesis. *Cold Spring Harbor Perspectives in Biology*, •••, 036902.

World Health Organization. (2020). *A handbook for integrated vector management*. World Health Organization.

World Health Organization. (2023, September 13). Dengue. https://www.who.int/news-room/fact-sheets/detail/dengue-and-severe-dengue

# Chapter 16
# Hepatic Encephalopathy

**Aya Mansour**
*Lebanese University, Lebanon*

**Sawsane Ghaddar**
https://orcid.org/0000-0002-1003-1500
*Lebanese University, Lebanon*

**Youssef Kteiche**
https://orcid.org/0009-0007-0493-8142
*Lebanese University, Lebanon*

**Ayman Bahsoun**
*Lebanese University, Lebanon*

**Jamil Nasrallah**
*Lebanese University, Lebanon*

**Fatima Ahmad Mroueh**
*Lebanese University, Lebanon*

## ABSTRACT

*Hepatic encephalopathy (HE) is a diverse neuropsychiatric disease caused by reduced liver function, which is generally associated with cirrhosis. While cirrhosis is the most common risk factor, there are additional risks that can either cause or worsen the development of HE. The pathophysiology of HE is complex and involves numerous factors. When HE is detected, it poses a considerable danger, resulting in poor clinical results and increased mortality rates. As a result, it is critical to concentrate on prevention and therapy to improve the general quality of life for those impacted. The complex interaction of components in HE necessitates an integrated approach to its care, taking into account underlying liver disease and addressing triggering events. The importance of HE management arises from its ability to substantially impair mental abilities and daily living activities. Timely therapies, such as dietary changes, drugs, and, in serious cases, liver transplantation, are critical in slowing the progression of HE.*

DOI: 10.4018/979-8-3693-1990-1.ch016

## INTRODUCTION

Hepatic encephalopathy (HE) is defined as a neurological impairment resulting from liver insufficiency or portosystemic shunting (PSS), (Hepatic Encephalopathy in Chronic Liver Disease, 2014). It produces a diverse array of neurological and psychiatric manifestations, spanning from subtle subclinical changes to a state of coma, (Hepatic Encephalopathy in Chronic Liver Disease, 2014) (Ferenci *et al.,* 2002). It can be a complication of either acute or chronic liver insufficiency, (Weissenborn, 2019). This HE definition overlooks the root cause of liver disease. Nevertheless, various factors associated with chronic liver diseases (CLDs), such as alcohol-related liver disease, non-alcoholic fatty liver disease, viral hepatitis, and primary biliary cholangitis, can affect the brain independently of the mechanisms triggered by liver failure or dysfunction, (Rose *et al.,* 2020).

At its mildest form, hepatic encephalopathy (HE) affects primarily psychometric tests. As HE advances, discernible shifts in personality, consciousness, and motor function become apparent, (Hepatic Encephalopathy in Chronic Liver Disease, 2014) (Wiley Online Library, n.d.). According to the latest consensus from the International Society for Hepatic Encephalopathy and Nitrogen Metabolism (ISHEN), the onset of overt hepatic encephalopathy is marked by disorientation or asterixis, (Ferenci *et al.,* 2002).

Recently, It has demonstrated its irreversibility, primarily attributed to its neuroinflammatory and neuronal cell death characteristics, (Rose *et al.,* 2020). HE affects up to 40% of cirrhosis patients. After being diagnosed with HE, the average survival for individuals with cirrhosis is significantly reduced, with a median of 2 years, and only 1 year for those aged over 65. Therefore, the onset of HE is considered a turning point in the course of cirrhosis, (Louissaint, Deutsch-Link, & Tapper, 2022). HE is defined by the presence of either hepatocellular failure, portosystemic shunting (PSS), or a combination of both, (Elsaid & Rustgi, 2020). HE is the most frequent initial decompensation event among individuals with nonalcoholic fatty liver disease (NAFLD). Although, it's more prevalent in alcohol-related liver disease (AFLD) and portal hypertension, (Louissaint, Deutsch-Link, & Tapper, 2022).

## EPIDEMIOLOGY

The incidence of HE is influenced by the type and severity of primary hepatic insufficiencies, as demonstrated in several analyses. Studies conducted in both developed and developing countries have reported the overall incidence of HE among cirrhotic patients, (Elsaid & Rustgi, 2020).

In the United States, an analysis of 186,481 patients with cirrhosis from 2008 to 2014 revealed an overall HE incidence of 26%, (Tapper *et al.,* 2019). During the same period, there was a notable 30% increase in hospitalizations related to hepatic failure, (Rose *et al.,* 2020). Similarly, in a cohort analysis of 1,317 Swedish cirrhotic patients from 2001 to 2017, the overall HE incidence was 33%, (Nilsson *et al.,* 2019). The relationship between viral hepatitis and HE incidence in cirrhosis was explored in two Italian studies. In a cohort of 312 Italian patients with compensated cirrhosis due to hepatitis B or C, the overall HE incidence was found to be 1.9%, (Benvegnù *et al.,* 2004).

Meanwhile, in cases of subclinical HE, the overall 48-month incidence of covert HE among cirrhotic patients in Mexico stood at 18.6%, (Ruiz- Margáin *et al.,* 2016). These findings closely mirrored the 17.5% overall minimal hepatic encephalopathy (MHE) incidence reported in a study involving 196 cirrhotic patients in northern India, (Goyal, Sidhu, & Kishore, 2016).

## RISK FACTORS FOR HEPATIC ENCEPHALOPATHY

One of the pivotal risk factors contributing to HE is the accumulation of neurotoxic substances within the body, particularly ammonia and manganese, (Vidal-Cevallos, Chávez-Tapia, & Uribe, 2022). In individuals with liver dysfunction, the impaired detoxification mechanisms allow these toxic compounds to reach the brain, where they inflict damage on neuronal cells, impairing motor functions and cognitive abilities, (Butterworth, 2003). Chronic liver diseases, particularly cirrhosis, are primary precursors to hepatic encephalopathy (HE), (Tapper *et al.,* 2018). Patients afflicted by chronic liver diseases face an increased risk due to the prolonged dysfunction of their liver, which can lead to the accumulation of harmful substances in the bloodstream, thus increasing the likelihood of HE, (Osna, Donohue, & Kharbanda, 2017; Tripathi & Mousa, 2023). The continuous exposure to elevated levels of these neurotoxic substances intensifies the risk of HE, posing a significant challenge in managing patients with chronic liver diseases, (Butterworth, 2003); Fallahzadeh & Rahimi, 2020).

Sarcopenia can result from cirrhosis due to inadequate nutrient intake and malabsorption, (Gairing *et al.,* 2023). According to a recent meta-analysis, approximately 37.5% of all patients are affected, (Tantai *et al.,* 2022). Sacropenia reduces ammonia breakdown by limiting its detoxification in the mitochondria of muscles, (Gairing *et al.,* 2023). This complication is more frequent with low protein intake advanced age and a low BMI, (Park *et al.,* 2021).

HE can be precipitated by variceal bleeding. The occurrence of development of HE in these patients ranges between 16.9% and 40%. This condition is associated with increased morbidity and mortality, (Faccioli *et al.,* 2023).

Another precipitrating factor is portal systemic shunt. Portal-systemic shunts play a role in lowering portal pressure; however, through this, normal liver flow is bypasses, resulting in increased blood concentrations without detoxification or metabolization of various toxic substances Its incidence ranges between 35% and 50%, (Faccioli *et al.,* 2023).

Additionally, certain medications, including opioids, benzodiazepines, and proton pump inhibitors, despite their therapeutic benefits, paradoxically increase the likelihood of incident HE in individuals with compromised liver function. Managing these factors requires a meticulous approach to prevent exacerbation of the condition and improve patient outcomes. Balancing the need for symptom management with the risk of HE associated with certain medications presents a complex dilemma for healthcare providers. Opioids and benzodiazepines, integral in managing cirrhosis-related symptoms, become double-edged swords, requiring careful evaluation and constant monitoring to mitigate the risk of HE, (Williams *et al.,* 2021).

Furthermore, gut microbiome is altered in cirrhosis. Recent data shows a close relationship between HE and the gut microbiota, (Gairing *et al.,* 2023).

## PATHOPHYSIOLOGY

Several hypotheses have been theorized about the mechanisms through which a liver disease or a portosystemic shunt leads to HE (hepatic encephalopathy).

Hyperammonemia is the major factor accounting for the brain abnormalities, (Ciećko-Michalska *et al.,* 2012). Ammonia is primarily synthesized in the GI tract from protein digestion and the bacterial flora of the gut. Normally, the liver detoxifies the majority of ammonia via the urea cycle. Nevertheless, in the context of liver disease, it gets diverted in high concentrations to the skeletal muscles and to the brain, specifically the astrocytes, where it gets converted into glutamine using glutamine synthetase. Glutamine exerts an osmotic effect, causing astrocyte swelling and cerebral edema, (Vidal-Cevallos, Chávez-Tapia, & Uribe, 2022). The cerebral edema gets even worse with an increase in sarcopenia that might be seen in liver dysfunction, (Jindal & Jagdish, 2019). The intestinal and the brain phosphate-activated enzyme glutaminase (PAG) has also an important role in the development of HE, since PAG generates ammonia by glutamine deamination, (Vidal-Cevallos, Chávez-Tapia, & Uribe, 2022).

Additionally, given the toxic effect of ammonia in the brain, the blood-brain barrier (BBB) gets abnormally more permeable. Hence, the gut-derived GABA crosses the BBB and gets inside the brain where the GABA receptors are increased in number, (Jones *et al.,* 1984). In parallel, there's a reduced expression of glutamatergic receptors, (Ciećko-Michalska *et al.,* 2012). This creates an amplified inhibitory neuronal impulse inducing encephalopathy and coma (26).

Moreover, neurosteroids are produced in the brain primarily by the astrocytes, but also by other brain cells. Neurosteroids synthesis, such as allopregnanolone, is independent of the peripheral steroidal sites, (Ahboucha, 2011). Higher levels of allopregnanolone might induce an increase in the brain sensitivity to GABAergic inhibitory signals. This might justify the parkinsonian symptoms (bradykinesia, muscle rigidity, etc.) seen in some patients having developed HE, (Ciećko-Michalska *et al.,* 2012).

A fourth hypothesis was formulated about the neurotoxic effect of Manganese (Mn). In fact, the reduced protein production by the diseased liver leads to an increase in free manganese level. Thus, it causes neuronal death in the basal ganglia, (Lim, Hahm, & Lee, 2023). The buildup of Mn in these regions might also explain the parkinsonian symptoms, (El Khiat *et al.,* 2022).

The inflammatory process is also believed to have a role in the pathogenesis of HE. Inflammatory cytokines (TNF-α, IL-1β, IL-6, INF-ɤ) originating in the affected liver, can freely traverse the BBB. Together with the ammonia, they increase the reactive oxygen species (ROS) and cause brain edema, (Jayakumar, Rama Rao, & Norenberg, 2015)

Furthermore, in the setting of liver failure, oxidative stress is the result of a decreased synthesis of antioxidants (albumin, etc…) as well as the generation of ROS which in turn is exacerbated by high toxic levels of ammonia, (Bai *et al.,* 2023). Besides the oxidative stress, differences in the gut microbiome have been noticed between cirrhosis patients without cognitive impairment and cirrhosis patients with HE, (Won *et al.,* 2022). The small intestinal bacterial overgrowth in liver failure patients favors an expansion of the pathogenic bacteria, and might even raise the risk of bacterial translocation in patients with ascites, (Ciećko-Michalska *et al.,* 2012; Won *et al.,* 2022).

In addition, given the increase levels of aromatic amino acids (AAA) in liver failure, there is synthesis of false neurotransmitters, such as octopamine and phenylethanolamine accompanied with a decrease in the true neurotransmitters (norepinephrine, dopamine…). This might partially explain the neurological abnormalities in HE, (El Khiat *et al.,* 2022).

Finally, ammonia affects the access of energy substrates, like glucose, into the brain. As a result of decreased glucose supply, reduction in the cerebral cortex was observed in patients with liver cirrhosis, contributing to cognitive impairment, (Ciećko-Michalska *et al.,* 2012).

## SIGNS AND SYMPTOMS

Hepatic encephalopathy manifests as a wide range of neurological and psychiatric symptoms that are often non-specific. Patients may experience personality changes, apathy, irritability, sleep disturbances, and asterixis, (Ferenci, 2017). Other symptoms such as parkinsonism, myelopathy, subcortical cognitive impairment, and vision alterations may also occur, (Lizardi-Cervera *et al.,* 2003). In severe cases, patients may become stuporous or enter a comatose state, (Munoz, 2008).

The World Health Congress of Gastroenterology has classified hepatic encephalopathy into three types based on their cause and associated features. These types are as follows:

- Type A (acute): is associated with liver failure and cerebral edema.
- Type B (bypass): is caused by portal-systemic shunting without intrinsic liver damage.
- Type C (cirrhosis): is found in patients with cirrhosis and is divided into three subclasses: episodic, persistent, and minimal, (Mandiga, Foris, & Bollu, 2023).

The ISHEN criteria classify the disease into two categories: covert and overt. Additionally, the West Haven Classification (WHC) identifies five grades of hepatic encephalopathy based on the patient's clinical features and dependence on therapy. The table below illustrates these two main classifications, (Vilstrup *et al*., 2014).

*Table 1. Classification of hepatic encephalopathy according to WHC and ISHEN criteria*

| WHC including MHE | ISHEN | Presentation | Criteria |
|---|---|---|---|
| unimpaired | | • No present or previous HE | • Normal |
| Minimal | Covert | • psychomotor - neuropsychological impairment<br>• Intact mental status<br>• No clinical manifestations | • Psychomotor – neuropsychological |
| Grade I | Covert | • Anxiety<br>• Altered attention<br>• Sleep disturbance<br>• Trouble doing basic math<br>• Cognitive- behavior decline- | • Cognitive – behavioral decline<br>• Intact spatiotemporal orientation |
| Grade II | Overt | • Lethargy<br>• Lack of interest<br>• Cognitive – behavior decline<br>• Asterixis<br>• Temporal disorientation | • Temporal disorientation<br>• +/- other signs and symptoms |
| Grade III | Overt | • Confusion<br>• Aberrant behavior<br>• Semistuporous state<br>• Spatiotemporal disorientation | • Spatiotemporal disorientation<br>• +/- signs and symptoms |
| Grade IV | Overt | • Coma | • No reason to stimuli |

## DIAGNOSIS AND DIFFERENTIAL DIAGNOSES

The diagnosis of hepatic encephalopathy is typically made through clinical observations. During a physical examination, Babinski's sign may be positive, and some patients may exhibit Parkinsonian symptoms like rigidity and tremors, (Mandiga, Foris, & Bollu, 2023).

While high blood ammonia levels are often observed in patients with liver disease, this test is not considered diagnostic on its own, (Ferenci, 2017). As such, it may produce false positive results in patients with Reye's syndrome, citrullinemia, zinc deficiency, atrophic gastritis, those taking certain medications (such as PPIs or valproic acid), or due to poor testing methods (such as prolonged use of a tourniquet during venous blood sampling), (Dara, Sayyari, & Imanzadeh, 2014).

An EEG may show triphasic waves with high amplitude and low frequency, (Mandiga, Foris, & Bollu, 2023). An MRI T1-weighted image may show hyperintensity of the globus pallidus, (Singhal *et al.,* 2009).

Since it is an exclusion diagnosis, an MRI or CT scan of the brain should be used to rule out any lesions or masses, (Mandiga, Foris, & Bollu, 2023).

There are several differential diagnoses of hepatic encephalopathy, including intracranial lesions, infections like meningitis or encephalitis, toxic encephalopathy related to alcohol use, withdrawal, or Wernicke encephalopathy, organic brain syndrome, (Dasarathy & Mullen, 2001), metabolic encephalopathy due to hypoglycemia or anoxia, post-seizure encephalopathy, and iatrogenic causes related to certain antidepressants, antipsychotics, and sedatives, (Mandiga, Foris, & Bollu, 2023).

## TREATMENT

HE has a high mortality rate. Nearly 40% of patients die within a year. Given the high mortality rate, a multidisciplinary team that carefully monitor and treats the patient is critical to improve clinical outcomes, (Mandiga, Foris, & Bollu, 2023). The patient's life and cognitive abilities must be preserved by prompt and effective therapy of hepatic encephalopathy. When a patient present with overt HE, there is usually an underlying precipitant, such as a medications' side effect, infection, gastrointestinal bleeding, or other causes. To diagnose and treat these appropriately, the acute management depends on a thorough history and examination. Resolving the precipitating issue can be used to treat 90% of patients. It is crucial to understand that some patients will not have any underlying HE precipitant, (Swaminathan, Ellul, & Cross, 2018).

In addition, the first-line of treatment is advised to be the nondigestible disaccharides lactitol and lactulose. By changing ammonia to nonabsorbable ammonium, it limits the formation of ammonia by bacteria, decreases ammoniagenic bacteria, and decreases ammonia absorption. Additionally, the higher osmolality quickens intestinal transit, which has the laxative effect of eliminating extra fecal nitrogen. Zinc absorption is further enhanced by lactose, (Ghosh & Ghosh, 2023)

Moreover, it has been studied that using oral antibiotics to alter gut flora and lower ammonia production can help manage HE. Neomycin is an aminoglycoside antibiotic that functions as a glutaminase inhibitor to lower ammonia levels. It is poorly absorbed and accumulates to large amounts in the intestines. It was the first commonly used antibiotic in HE. Nevertheless, neomycin's side effects and the advent of more effective medications prohibit its usage in modern clinical practice, (Vidal-Cevallos, Chávez-Tapia, & Uribe, 2022). Neomycin, flumazenil, metronidazole, and zinc had no appreciable effect when used as stand-alone treatments for HE, (Bajaj, 2010).

Rifaximin derived from rifamycin, is a nonabsorbable semi-synthetic antibiotic. Rifaximin was found to have less side effects, such as nephrotoxicity and ototoxicity, and to be at least as effective as neomycin in lowering blood ammonia levels. For the secondary prophylaxis of overt HE in patients who have experienced more episodes while receiving lactulose therapy, rifaximin is advised, (Vidal-Cevallos, Chávez-Tapia, & Uribe, 2022).

It's interesting to note that rifaximin with lactulose works better together than lactulose does alone to reverse HE and lower mortality, (Swaminathan, Ellul, & Cross, 2018). In addition, during a 6-month follow-up period, the combination of these two medications avoids the recurrence of episodic HE, (Zhan & Stremmel, 2012)

Furthermore, L-ornithine-L-aspartate reduces ammonia levels and enhances mental health. Furthermore, it is equally efficacious as lactulose in enhancing mental state, promoting asterixis, and lowering ammonia levels, (Swaminathan, Ellul, & Cross, 2018). One function for albumin is as a volume expander. Nevertheless, additional characteristics of albumin have been discovered, including the ability to regulate detoxification and the anti-inflammatory response.

Reversing HE and lowering mortality was more effective with lactulose plus albumin than with lactulose alone, (Vidal-Cevallos, Chávez-Tapia, & Uribe, 2022).

Interestingly, probiotics were beneficial in remission and maintenance of secondary prophylaxis of overt hepatic encephalopathy when taken in conjunction with standard treatment (lactulose), (Rehman *et al.*, 2023).

Regardless of the presence of HE, a daily diet of 35–40 kcal/kg body weight and 1.2–1.5 g/kg protein is recommended. Vegetable and dairy proteins are also more easily tolerated. While proteins can cause HE, it's crucial to remember that protein deficiency causes malnourishment and the depletion of the liver's protein reserves, (Swaminathan, Ellul, & Cross, 2018).

Finally, for HE that is resistant to treatment, liver transplantation is the only effective option. A liver transplant is necessary since, despite multiple therapeutic options, the encephalopathy continued to progress, (Lin *et al.,* 2011).

## PREVENTION

Several studies are underway in the sector to better understand and enrich medical practice with evidence-based recommendations for prevention. The following are the major recommendations for preventing a first OHE episode: primary pharmaceutical prophylaxis and appropriate nutrition, (Gairing *et al.*, 2023).

Inadequate nutrition causes sarcopenia, which can affect ammonia metabolism thereby rendering people more susceptible to HE. Currently, guidelines indicate a daily caloric intake of 35-40 kcal/kg bodyweight and a protein consumption of 1.0-1.5 g/kg bodyweight in non-obese patients with cirrhosis, (Bischoff *et al.,* 2020). Based on these findings, it is reasonable to suppose that improving nutritional status, and hence muscle modifications, can be a main prophylactic method for HE. Data on this issue are currently scarce, (Faccioli *et al.,* 2023).

In the pharmacological approach, The current European Association for the Study of the Liver (EASL) guidelines support lactulose medication for primary and secondary prophylaxis of OHE, as well as reversal of an acute episode of OHE, (Bischoff *et al.,* 2020).

Additionally, Rifaximin is licensed and suggested for secondary prophylaxis following a second episode of OHE when used with lactulose or in the case of lactulose intolerance. In contrast, no study has been conducted mainly to investigate the preventative impact of rifaximin on an initial OHE episode, (Gairing *et al*., 2023).

Furthermore, MHE is an established risk factor for OHE progression and death, (Faccioli *et al.,* 2023). Although there is no strong evidence supporting the reduction of HE incidence after MHE therapy,, it is possible that its resolution may have a favorable effect. As a result, EASL guidelines advise screening for MHE in all cirrhotic individuals as well as treating it with non-absorbable disaccharides, (Bischoff *et al.,* 2020).

MHE detection necessitates the use of sophisticated neuropsychological or neurophysiologic testing. The Portosystemic Hepatic Encephalopathy Score (PHES) is regarded the gold standard in most countries, but most physicians do not utilize it in routine care because it takes more than 15 minutes to administer. Other time-saving tests include the QuickStroop test (10 minutes) and the Animal Naming Test (ANT) (1 minute). Cutoffs were determined to detecting MHE, and therefore this is a limitation for all mentioned tests. As it is important to set cutoff to diagnose patients with increased risk for OHE, (Gairing *et al*., 2023).

In certain conditions, in patients with previous episodes of OHE, it is advisable to provide rifaximin for HE prophylaxis before nonurgent TIPS insertion. In the context of visceral bleeding, rapid removal of blood from GI tract and lactulose are recommended, (Gairing *et al*., 2023).

## CONCLUSION

Hepatic encephalopathy is a challenging complication due to its unspecific clinical presentation and its worse outcomes. The only curative treatment is liver transplantation and it is not available for all patients. Current practices try to alleviate symptoms and improve the quality of life. Ongoing researches are conducted to improve the practice and manage the huge burden of this disease.

## REFERENCES


Ahboucha, S. (2011). Neurosteroids and Hepatic Encephalopathy: An Update on Possible Pathophysiologic Mechanisms. *Current Molecular Pharmacology*, *4*(1), 1–13. DOI: 10.2174/1874467211104010001 PMID: 20825363

Bai, Y., Li, K., Li, X., Chen, X., Zheng, J., Wu, F., Chen, J., Li, Z., Zhang, S., Wu, K., Chen, Y., Wang, Y., & Yang, Y. (2023). Effects of oxidative stress on hepatic encephalopathy pathogenesis in mice. *Nature Communications*, *14*(1), 4456. DOI: 10.1038/s41467-023-40081-8 PMID: 37488119

Bajaj, J. S. (2010). Review article: The modern management of hepatic encephalopathy. *Alimentary Pharmacology & Therapeutics*, *31*(5), 537–547. DOI: 10.1111/j.1365-2036.2009.04211.x PMID: 20002027

Benvegnù, L., Gios, M., Boccato, S., & Alberti, A. (2004). Natural history of compensated viral cirrhosis: A prospective study on the incidence and hierarchy of major complications. *Gut*, *53*(5), 744–749. DOI: 10.1136/gut.2003.020263 PMID: 15082595

Bischoff, S. C., Bernal, W., Dasarathy, S., Merli, M., Plank, L. D., Schütz, T., & Plauth, M. (2020). ESPEN practical guideline: Clinical nutrition in liver disease. *Clinical Nutrition (Edinburgh, Lothian)*, *39*(12), 3533–3562. DOI: 10.1016/j.clnu.2020.09.001 PMID: 33213977

Butterworth, R. F. (2003). Hepatic encephalopathy—A serious complication of alcoholic liver disease. *Alcohol Research & Health : the Journal of the National Institute on Alcohol Abuse and Alcoholism*, *27*(2), 143–145. PMID: 15303624

Ciećko-Michalska, I., Szczepanek, M., Słowik, A., & Mach, T. (2012). Pathogenesis of hepatic encephalopathy. *Gastroenterology Research and Practice*, *642108*, 1–7. Advance online publication. DOI: 10.1155/2012/642108 PMID: 23316223

Dara, N., Sayyari, A.-A., & Imanzadeh, F. (2014). Hepatic encephalopathy: Early diagnosis in pediatric patients with cirrhosis. *Iranian Journal of Child Neurology*, *8*(1), 1–11. PMID: 24665321

Dasarathy, S., & Mullen, K. D. (2001). Hepatic encephalopathy. *Current Treatment Options in Gastroenterology*, *4*(6), 517–526. DOI: 10.1007/s11938-001-0017-3 PMID: 11696278

El Khiat, A., Hiba, O. E., Aimrane, A., Draoui, A., Jayakumar, A. R., Norenberg, M. D., & Gamrani, H. (2022). Hepatic Encephalopathy: An Overview of Basic Concepts and Mechanisms. *Frontiers in Medical Case Reports*, *03*(03). Advance online publication. DOI: 10.47746/FMCR.2022.3302

Elsaid, M. I., & Rustgi, V. K. (2020). Epidemiology of Hepatic Encephalopathy. *Clinics in Liver Disease*, *24*(2), 157–174. DOI: 10.1016/j.cld.2020.01.001 PMID: 32245524

Faccioli, J., Nardelli, S., Gioia, S., Riggio, O., & Ridola, L. (2023). Primary Prophylaxis of Overt Hepatic Encephalopathy: Is It Time to Consider It? *Journal of Clinical Medicine*, *12*(12), 3903. DOI: 10.3390/jcm12123903 PMID: 37373598

Fallahzadeh, M. A., & Rahimi, R. S. (2020). Hepatic Encephalopathy and Nutrition Influences: A Narrative Review. *Nutrition in Clinical Practice*, *35*(1), 36–48. DOI: 10.1002/ncp.10458 PMID: 31872484

Ferenci, P. (2017). Hepatic encephalopathy. *Gastroenterology Report*, *5*(2), 138–147. DOI: 10.1093/gastro/gox013 PMID: 28533911

Ferenci, P., Lockwood, A., Mullen, K., Tarter, R., Weissenborn, K., & Blei, A. T. (2002). Hepatic encephalopathy—Definition, nomenclature, diagnosis, and quantification: Final report of the Working Party at the 11th World Congresses of Gastroenterology, Vienna, 1998. *Hepatology (Baltimore, Md.)*, *35*(3), 716–721. DOI: 10.1053/jhep.2002.31250 PMID: 11870389

Gairing, S. J., Schleicher, E. M., Galle, P. R., & Labenz, C. (2023). Prediction and prevention of the first episode of overt hepatic encephalopathy in patients with cirrhosis. *Hepatology Communications*, *7*(4). Advance online publication. DOI: 10.1097/HC9.0000000000000096 PMID: 36930868

Ghosh, J., & Ghosh, J. (2023). Current Management of Hepatic Encephalopathy: A Review Article. *Journal for Research in Applied Sciences and Biotechnology*, *2*(4), 170–175. DOI: 10.55544/jrasb.2.4.24

Goyal, O., Sidhu, S., & Kishore, H. (2016). Incidence, Prevalence and Natural History of Minimal Hepatic Encephalopathy in Cirrhosis. *Journal of Hepatology*, *64*(2), S279. DOI: 10.1016/S0168-8278(16)00334-2

Hepatic Encephalopathy in Chronic Liver Disease. (2014). Practice Guideline by the European Association for the Study of the Liver and the American Association for the Study of Liver Diseases. (2014). *Journal of Hepatology*, *61*(3), 642–659. DOI: 10.1016/j.jhep.2014.05.042 PMID: 25015420

Jayakumar, A. R., Rama Rao, K. V., & Norenberg, M. D. (2015). Neuroinflammation in Hepatic Encephalopathy: Mechanistic Aspects. *Journal of Clinical and Experimental Hepatology*, *5*, S21–S28. DOI: 10.1016/j.jceh.2014.07.006 PMID: 26041953

Jindal, A., & Jagdish, R. K. (2019). Sarcopenia: Ammonia metabolism and hepatic encephalopathy. *Clinical and Molecular Hepatology*, *25*(3), 270–279. DOI: 10.3350/cmh.2019.0015 PMID: 31006226

Jones, E. A., Schafer, D. F., Ferenci, P., & Pappas, S. C. (1984). The GABA hypothesis of the pathogenesis of hepatic encephalopathy: Current status. *The Yale Journal of Biology and Medicine*, *57*(3), 301–316. PMID: 6093394

Lim, C. G., Hahm, M. H., & Lee, H. J. (2023). Hepatic encephalopathy on magnetic resonance imaging and its uncertain differential diagnoses: A narrative review. *Journal of Yeungnam Medical Science*, *40*(2), 136–145. DOI: 10.12701/jyms.2022.00689 PMID: 36624654

Lin, Y.-N., Chou, J.-W., Cheng, K.-S., Peng, C.-Y., Jeng, L.-B., & Chiang, I.-P. (2011). Treatment of Fulminant Autoimmune Hepatitis: Corticosteroid Therapy or Liver Transplantation? A Case Report and Literature Review. *Gastroenterology Research*, *4*(5), 231–235. DOI: 10.4021/gr323w PMID: 27957021

Lizardi-Cervera, J., Almeda, P., Guevara, L., & Uribe, M. (2003). Hepatic encephalopathy: A review. *Annals of Hepatology*, *2*(3), 122–130. DOI: 10.1016/S1665-2681(19)32137-4 PMID: 15115963

Louissaint, J., Deutsch-Link, S., & Tapper, E. B. (2022). Changing Epidemiology of Cirrhosis and Hepatic Encephalopathy. *Clinical Gastroenterology and Hepatology*, *20*(8, Suppl), S1–S8. DOI: 10.1016/j.cgh.2022.04.036 PMID: 35940729

Mandiga, P., Foris, L. A., & Bollu, P. C. (2023). Hepatic Encephalopathy. In *StatPearls*. StatPearls Publishing., https://www.ncbi.nlm.nih.gov/books/NBK430869/

Munoz, S. J. (2008). Hepatic Encephalopathy. *The Medical Clinics of North America*, *92*(4), 795–812. DOI: 10.1016/j.mcna.2008.03.009 PMID: 18570943

Nilsson, E., Anderson, H., Sargenti, K., Lindgren, S., & Prytz, H. (2019). Clinical course and mortality by etiology of liver cirrhosis in Sweden: A population based, long-term follow-up study of 1317 patients. *Alimentary Pharmacology & Therapeutics*, *49*(11), 1421–1430. DOI: 10.1111/apt.15255 PMID: 30957910

Osna, N. A., Donohue, T. M., & Kharbanda, K. K. (2017). Alcoholic Liver Disease: Pathogenesis and Current Management. *Alcohol Research : Current Reviews*, *38*(2), 147–161. PMID: 28988570

Park, J.-H., Kang, M., Jun, D.-W., Kim, M., Kwak, J.-H., & Kang, B.-K. (2021). Determining Whether Low Protein Intake (<1.0 g/kg) Is a Risk Factor for Malnutrition in Patients with Cirrhosis. *Journal of Clinical Medicine*, *10*(10), 2164. DOI: 10.3390/jcm10102164 PMID: 34067667

Rehman, H. A., Nazar, T., Aziz, B., Farooq, H., Nazar, N., & Abdulraffay, . (2023). Role of Probiotics in Secondary Prophylaxis of Hepatic Encephalopathy. *Pakistan Journal of Medical & Health Sciences*, *17*(6), 18–20. DOI: 10.53350/pjmhs202317618

Rose, C. F., Amodio, P., Bajaj, J. S., Dhiman, R. K., Montagnese, S., Taylor-Robinson, S. D., Vilstrup, H., & Jalan, R. (2020). Hepatic encephalopathy: Novel insights into classification, pathophysiology and therapy. *Journal of Hepatology*, *73*(6), 1526–1547. DOI: 10.1016/j.jhep.2020.07.013 PMID: 33097308

Ruiz-Margáin, A., Macías-Rodríguez, R. U., Ampuero, J., Cubero, F. J., Chi-Cervera, L., Ríos-Torres, S. L., Duarte-Rojo, A., Espinosa-Cuevas, Á., Romero-Gómez, M., & Torre, A. (2016). Low phase angle is associated with the development of hepatic encephalopathy in patients with cirrhosis. *World Journal of Gastroenterology*, *22*(45), 10064–10070. DOI: 10.3748/wjg.v22.i45.10064 PMID: 28018114

Singhal, A., Nagarajan, R., Kumar, R., Huda, A., Gupta, R. K., & Thomas, M. A. (2009). Magnetic resonance $T_2$-relaxometry and 2D L-correlated spectroscopy in patients with minimal hepatic encephalopathy. *Journal of Magnetic Resonance Imaging*, *30*(5), 1034–1041. DOI: 10.1002/jmri.21943 PMID: 19856435

Swaminathan, M., Ellul, M. A., & Cross, T. J. (2018). Hepatic encephalopathy: Current challenges and future prospects. *Hepatic Medicine : Evidence and Research*, *10*, 1–11. DOI: 10.2147/HMER.S118964 PMID: 29606895

Tantai, X., Liu, Y., Yeo, Y. H., Praktiknjo, M., Mauro, E., Hamaguchi, Y., Engelmann, C., Zhang, P., Jeong, J. Y., van Vugt, J. L. A., Xiao, H., Deng, H., Gao, X., Ye, Q., Zhang, J., Yang, L., Cai, Y., Liu, Y., Liu, N., & Nguyen, M. H. (2022). Effect of sarcopenia on survival in patients with cirrhosis: A meta-analysis. *Journal of Hepatology*, *76*(3), 588–599. DOI: 10.1016/j.jhep.2021.11.006 PMID: 34785325

Tapper, E. B., Henderson, J. B., Parikh, N. D., Ioannou, G. N., & Lok, A. S. (2019). Incidence of and Risk Factors for Hepatic Encephalopathy in a Population-Based Cohort of Americans With Cirrhosis. *Hepatology Communications*, *3*(11), 1510–1519. DOI: 10.1002/hep4.1425 PMID: 31701074

Tapper, E. B., Parikh, N. D., Sengupta, N., Mellinger, J., Ratz, D., Lok, A. S.-F., & Su, G. L. (2018). A risk score to predict the development of hepatic encephalopathy in a population-based cohort of patients with cirrhosis. *Hepatology (Baltimore, Md.)*, *68*(4), 1498–1507. DOI: 10.1002/hep.29628 PMID: 29091289

Tripathi, N., & Mousa, O. Y. (2023). Hepatitis B. In *StatPearls*. StatPearls Publishing., https://www.ncbi.nlm.nih.gov/books/NBK555945/

Vidal-Cevallos, P., Chávez-Tapia, N. C., & Uribe, M. (2022). Current approaches to hepatic encephalopathy. *Annals of Hepatology*, *27*(6), 100757. DOI: 10.1016/j.aohep.2022.100757 PMID: 36115576

Vilstrup, H., Amodio, P., Bajaj, J., Cordoba, J., Ferenci, P., Mullen, K. D., Weissenborn, K., & Wong, P. (2014). Hepatic encephalopathy in chronic liver disease: 2014 Practice Guideline by the American Association for the Study of Liver Diseases and the European Association for the Study of the Liver. *Hepatology (Baltimore, Md.)*, *60*(2), 715–735. DOI: 10.1002/hep.27210 PMID: 25042402

Weissenborn, K. (2019). Hepatic Encephalopathy: Definition, Clinical Grading and Diagnostic Principles. *Drugs*, *79*(S1, Suppl 1), 5–9. DOI: 10.1007/s40265-018-1018-z PMID: 30706420

Williams, S., Louissaint, J., Nikirk, S., Bajaj, J. S., & Tapper, E. B. (2021). Deprescribing medications that may increase the risk of hepatic encephalopathy: A qualitative study of patients with cirrhosis and their doctors. *United European Gastroenterology Journal*, *9*(2), 193–202. DOI: 10.1177/2050640620975224 PMID: 33226300

Won, S.-M., Oh, K. K., Gupta, H., Ganesan, R., Sharma, S. P., Jeong, J.-J., Yoon, S. J., Jeong, M. K., Min, B. H., Hyun, J. Y., Park, H. J., Eom, J. A., Lee, S. B., Cha, M. G., Kwon, G. H., Choi, M. R., Kim, D. J., & Suk, K. T. (2022). The Link between Gut Microbiota and Hepatic Encephalopathy. *International Journal of Molecular Sciences*, *23*(16), 8999. DOI: 10.3390/ijms23168999 PMID: 36012266

Zhan, T., & Stremmel, W. (2012). The diagnosis and treatment of minimal hepatic encephalopathy. *Deutsches Ärzteblatt International*, *109*(10), 180–187. DOI: 10.3238/arztebl.2012.0180 PMID: 22470407

# Compilation of References

Acar, J. (1997). Broad- and narrow-spectrum antibiotics: An unhelpful categorization. *Clinical Microbiology and Infection*, *3*(4), 395–396. DOI: 10.1111/j.1469-0691.1997.tb00274.x PMID: 11864148

Acosta, C., Galindo, C., Kimario, J., Senkoro, K., Urassa, H., Casals, C., Corachán, M., Eseko, N., Tanner, M., Mshinda, H., Lwilla, F., Vila, J., & Alonso, P. L. (2001). Cholera outbreak in southern Tanzania: Risk factors and patterns of transmission. *Emerging Infectious Diseases*, *7*(3, Suppl), 583–587. https://ora.ox.ac.uk/objects/uuid:dd75b112-5f7a-41f6-81c6-4ac32a37b1f3. DOI: 10.3201/eid0707.010741 PMID: 11485679

Adams, R. A., Leon, G., Miller, N. M., Reyes, S. P., Thanawastien, A., & Kasting, B. J. (2021). Rifamycin antibiotics and the mechanisms of their failure. *The Journal of Antibiotics*, *74*(11), 11. Advance online publication. DOI: 10.1038/s41429-021-00462-x PMID: 34400805

Adeyemi, B. F., Akinyamoju, A. O., & Kolude, B. (2018). Association of squamous cell carcinoma of the tongue with cigarette and alcohol exposure: A retrospective clinicopathological study. *West African Journal of Medicine*, *35*(2), 117–122. PMID: 30027997

Adzitey, F. (2015). Antibiotic classes and antibiotic susceptibility of bacterial isolates from selected poultry: A mini review. *UDS Space*. http://udsspace.uds.edu.gh/handle/123456789/647

Agrawal, P., Neel, A., Deresse, A. S., Gerber, S., & Alonge, O. (2023). Facilitators and barriers to community engagement in the Global Polio Eradication Initiative–A mixed methods study. *PLOS Global Public Health*, *3*(4), e0001643. DOI: 10.1371/journal.pgph.0001643 PMID: 37027352

Aguiar, R. S., Stollenwerk, N., & Dotta, G. (2023). Dengue virus infection: A review of recent advances in therapeutic interventions and vaccine development. *Drugs*, *83*(1), 29–53.

Ahboucha, S. (2011). Neurosteroids and Hepatic Encephalopathy: An Update on Possible Pathophysiologic Mechanisms. *Current Molecular Pharmacology*, *4*(1), 1–13. DOI: 10.2174/1874467211104010001 PMID: 20825363

Ahmed, N. A., & Koo, J. R. (2022). Dengue virus: Viral entry, replication, and transmission. *Antiviral Research*, *207*, 105582.

Akingbola, A., Abiodun, A., Ojo, O., Jessica, O. U., Alao, U. H., Owolabi, A. O., & Chuku, J. (2025). Cholera outbreak in Nigeria: History, review of socioeconomic and meteorological drivers, diagnostic challenges, and artificial intelligence integration. *Global Health, Epidemiology and Genomics*, *2025*(1), 8898076. Advance online publication. DOI: 10.1155/ghe3/8898076 PMID: 40469257

Akram, M., Munir, N., Daniyal, M., Egbuna, C., Găman, M. A., Onyekere, P. F., & Olatunde, A. (2020). Vitamins and Minerals: Types, sources and their functions. Functional Foods and Nutraceuticals: Bioactive Components, Formulations and Innovations, 149-172.

Albeladi, F. I., Salem, I. M. W., Albandar, A. A., Almusaylim, H. A., & Albandar, A. S. (2022). Electrolyte imbalance in infectious disease patients at King Abdulaziz Hospital, Jeddah. *Journal of Taibah University Medical Sciences*, *17*(2), 256–263. DOI: 10.1016/j.jtumed.2021.09.010 PMID: 35592808

Alexandrova, L., Haque, F., Rodriguez, P., Marrazzo, A. C., Grembi, J. A., Ramachandran, V., Hryckowian, A. J., Adams, C. M., Siddique, M. S. A., Khan, A. I., Qadri, F., Andrews, J. R., Rahman, M., Spormann, A. M., Schoolnik, G. K., Chien, A., & Nelson, E. J. (2019). Identification of widespread antibiotic exposure in patients with cholera correlates with clinically relevant microbiota changes. *The Journal of Infectious Diseases*, *220*(10), 1655–1666. DOI: 10.1093/infdis/jiz299 PMID: 31192364

Allerberger, F. (2017). Eliminating measles and rubella in Europe. *Clinical Microbiology and Infection*, *23*(8), 502–503. DOI: 10.1016/j.cmi.2017.04.008 PMID: 28412385

Aloke, C., Obasi, N. A., Aja, P. M., Emelike, C. U., Egwu, C. O., Jeje, O., Edeogu, C. O., Onisuru, O. O., Orji, O. U., & Achilonu, I. (2023, January 3). Combating Lassa Fever in West African Sub-Region: Progress, Challenges, and Future Perspectives. *Viruses*, *15*(1), 146. DOI: 10.3390/v15010146 PMID: 36680186

Al-Saad, K. M., Al-Wabel, A. A., & Khan, A. A. (2020). Dengue fever: Epidemiology, clinical manifestations, diagnosis, and treatment. *Cureus*, *12*(11), e11380. PMID: 33251077

Alsofrom, D. J., Mettler, F. A.Jr, & Mann, J. M. (1981). Radiographic manifestations of plaque in New Mexico, 1975-1980. A review of 42 proved cases. *Radiology*, *139*(3), 561–565. DOI: 10.1148/radiology.139.3.7232721 PMID: 7232721

Al-Tawfiq, J. A., Kattan, R. F., Almoallem, S. A. S., Altawfiq, K. J., Mohsni, E., & Memish, Z. A. (2023). Worldwide poliomyelitis outbreaks: Should mass gathering organizers be concerned? *Journal of Travel Medicine*, *30*(1), taac128. DOI: 10.1093/jtm/taac128 PMID: 36331257

Aminov, R. (2010). A brief history of the antibiotic era: Lessons learned and challenges for the future. *Frontiers in Microbiology*, *1*, 134. Advance online publication. DOI: 10.3389/fmicb.2010.00134 PMID: 21687759

Anasir, M. I., Zarif, F., & Poh, C. L. (2021). Antivirals blocking entry of enteroviruses and therapeutic potential. *Journal of Biomedical Science*, *28*(1), 10. DOI: 10.1186/s12929-021-00708-8 PMID: 33451326

Andersen, K. G., Shapiro, B. J., Matranga, C. B., Sealfon, R., Lin, A. E., Moses, L. M., Folarin, O. A., Goba, A., Odia, I., Ehiane, P. E., Momoh, M., England, E. M., Winnicki, S., Branco, L. M., Gire, S. K., Phelan, E., Tariyal, R., Tewhey, R., Omoniwa, O., & Sabeti, P. C. (2015). Clinical sequencing uncovers origins and evolution of Lassa virus. *Cell*, *162*(4), 738–750. DOI: 10.1016/j.cell.2015.07.020 PMID: 26276630

Andrade, F. F., Silva, D., Rodrigues, A., & Pina-Vaz, C. (2020). Colistin update on its mechanism of action and resistance, present and future challenges. *Microorganisms*, *8*(11), 1716. Advance online publication. DOI: 10.3390/microorganisms8111716 PMID: 33147701

Andrus, J. K., & de Quadros, C. A. (2013). Perspectives on the role of surveillance in eliminating rubella and congenital rubella syndrome in the Americas. *Expert Review of Vaccines*, *12*(9), 989–993. DOI: 10.1586/14760584.2013.841435 PMID: 24053393

Angrup, A., Kanaujia, R., Ray, P., & Biswal, M. (2020). Healthcare facilities in low- and middle-income countries affected by COVID-19: Time to upgrade basic infection control and prevention practices. *Indian Journal of Medical Microbiology*, *38*(2), 139–143. DOI: 10.4103/ijmm.IJMM_20_125 PMID: 32883925

Anisimov, A. P., & Amoako, K. K. (2006). Treatment of plague: Promising alternatives to antibiotics. *Journal of Medical Microbiology*, *55*(Pt 11), 1461–1475. DOI: 10.1099/jmm.0.46697-0 PMID: 17030904

Araújo, E. V., Martins, L. C., Silva, L. F., Araújo, F. R., Fernandes, T. R., & Queiroz, A. S. (2020). Dengue fever: A review of the current knowledge. *Journal of Infection and Public Health*, *13*(10), 1521–1528.

Arnaboldi, P. M., Seedarnee, R., Sambir, M., Callister, S. M., Imparato, J. A., & Dattwyler, R. J. (2013). Outer Surface Protein C Peptide Derived from Borrelia burgdorferi Sensu Stricto as a Target for Serodiagnosis of Early Lyme Disease. *Clinical and Vaccine Immunology; CVI*, *20*(4), 474–481. DOI: 10.1128/CVI.00608-12 PMID: 23365204

Asantewaa, A. A., Odoom, A., Owusu-Okyere, G., & Donkor, E. S. (2024). Cholera outbreaks in low- and middle-income countries in the last decade: A systematic review and meta-analysis. *Microorganisms*, *12*(12), 2504. Advance online publication. DOI: 10.3390/microorganisms12122504 PMID: 39770707

Ashley, R. E., Dittmore, A., McPherson, S. A., Turnbough, C. L.Jr, Neuman, K. C., & Osheroff, N. (2017). Activities of gyrase and topoisomerase IV on positively supercoiled DNA. *Nucleic Acids Research*, *45*(16), 9611–9624. DOI: 10.1093/nar/gkx649 PMID: 28934496

Asima, R. A. N. I., Akhtar, S., Nawaz, S. K., Irfan, S., Sadia, A. Z. A. M., & Arshad, M. (2015). Electrolyte disturbance and the type of malarial infection. *Iranian Journal of Public Health*, *44*(11), 1492. PMID: 26744706

Auperin, D. D., Romanowski, V., Galinski, M. R., & Bishop, D. H. (1984). Sequencing studies of pichinde arenavirus S RNA indicate a novel coding strategy, an ambisense viral S RNA. *Journal of Virology*, *52*(3), 897–904. DOI: 10.1128/jvi.52.3.897-904.1984 PMID: 6492264

Awotiwon, A. A., Oduwole, O., Sinha, A., & Okwundu, C. I. (2017). Zinc supplementation for the treatment of measles in children. *Cochrane Database of Systematic Reviews*, *2017*(6), 6. DOI: 10.1002/14651858.CD011177.pub3 PMID: 28631310

Ayscue, P., Van Haren, K., Sheriff, H., Waubant, E., Waldron, P., & Yagi, S. (2014). Acute flaccid paralysis with anterior myelitis - California, June 2012-June 2014. *MMWR. Morbidity and Mortality Weekly Report*, *63*(40), 903–906. PMID: 25299608

Azman, A. S., Rudolph, K. E., Cummings, D. A. T., & Lessler, J. (2013). The incubation period of cholera: A systematic review. *The Journal of Infection*, *66*(5), 432–438. DOI: 10.1016/j.jinf.2012.11.013 PMID: 23201968

Bachmann, V., Kostiuk, B., Unterweger, D., Diaz-Satizabal, L., Ogg, S., & Pukatzki, S. (2015). Bile salts modulate the mucin-activated type VI secretion system of pandemic *Vibrio cholerae. PLoS Neglected Tropical Diseases*, *9*(8), e0004031. Advance online publication. DOI: 10.1371/journal.pntd.0004031 PMID: 26317760

Bai, Y., Li, K., Li, X., Chen, X., Zheng, J., Wu, F., Chen, J., Li, Z., Zhang, S., Wu, K., Chen, Y., Wang, Y., & Yang, Y. (2023). Effects of oxidative stress on hepatic encephalopathy pathogenesis in mice. *Nature Communications*, *14*(1), 4456. DOI: 10.1038/s41467-023-40081-8 PMID: 37488119

Bajaj, J. S. (2010). Review article: The modern management of hepatic encephalopathy. *Alimentary Pharmacology & Therapeutics*, *31*(5), 537–547. DOI: 10.1111/j.1365-2036.2009.04211.x PMID: 20002027

Bandyopadhyay, A. S., Burke, R. M., & Hawes, K. M. (2024). Polio Eradication: Status, Struggles and Strategies. *The Pediatric Infectious Disease Journal*, *43*(6), e207–e211. DOI: 10.1097/INF.0000000000004330 PMID: 38564755

Bandyopadhyay, A. S., & Zipursky, S. (2023). A novel tool to eradicate an ancient scourge: The novel oral polio vaccine type 2 story. *The Lancet. Infectious Diseases*, *23*(2), e67–e71. DOI: 10.1016/S1473-3099(22)00582-5 PMID: 36162417

Bankamp, B., Hickman, C., Icenogle, J. P., & Rota, P. A. (2019). Successes and challenges for preventing measles, mumps and rubella by vaccination. *Current Opinion in Virology*, *34*, 110–116. DOI: 10.1016/j.coviro.2019.01.002 PMID: 30852425

Baquero, F., & Levin, B. R. (2021). Proximate and ultimate causes of the bactericidal action of antibiotics. *Nature Reviews. Microbiology*, *19*(2), 2. Advance online publication. DOI: 10.1038/s41579-020-00443-1 PMID: 33024310

Baran, A., Kwiatkowska, A., & Potocki, L. (2023). Antibiotics and bacterial resistance—A short story of an endless arms race. *International Journal of Molecular Sciences*, *24*(6), 5777. Advance online publication. DOI: 10.3390/ijms24065777 PMID: 36982857

Barbieri, R., Signoli, M., Chevé, D., Costedoat, C., Tzortzis, S., Aboudharam, G., Raoult, D., & Drancourt, M. (2020). Yersinia pestis: The Natural History of Plague. *Clinical Microbiology Reviews*, *34*(1), e00044–e19. DOI: 10.1128/CMR.00044-19 PMID: 33298527

Barclay, S. S., Melia, M. T., & Auwaerter, P. G. (2012). Misdiagnosis of Late- Onset Lyme Arthritis by Inappropriate Use of Borrelia burgdorferi Immunoblot Testing with Synovial Fluid. *Clinical and Vaccine Immunology; CVI*, *19*(11), 1806–1809. DOI: 10.1128/CVI.00383-12 PMID: 22971779

Barreto, M. L., Teixeira, M. G., & Carmo, E. H. (2006). Infectious diseases epidemiology. *Journal of Epidemiology and Community Health*, *60*(3), 192–195. DOI: 10.1136/jech.2003.011593 PMID: 16476746

Bartram, J., & Cairncross, S. (2010). Hygiene, sanitation, and water: Forgotten foundations of health. *PLoS Medicine*, *7*(11), e1000367. DOI: 10.1371/journal.pmed.1000367 PMID: 21085694

Bassetti, M., Magnè, F., Giacobbe, D. R., Bini, L., & Vena, A. (2022). New antibiotics for Gram-negative pneumonia. *European Respiratory Review : an Official Journal of the European Respiratory Society*, *31*(166), 220119. Advance online publication. DOI: 10.1183/16000617.0119-2022 PMID: 36543346

Bastos, V., Pacheco, V., Rodrigues, É. D. L., Moraes, C. N. S., Nóbile, A. L., Fonseca, D. L. M., Souza, K. B. S., do Vale, F. Y. N., Filgueiras, I. S., Schimke, L. F., Giil, L. M., Moll, G., Cabral-Miranda, G., Ochs, H. D., Vasconcelos, P. F. da C., de M Bastos, V., Pacheco, V., Rodrigues, É. D. L., Moraes, C. N. S., Nóbile, A. L., Fonseca, D. L. M., Souza, K. B. S., do Vale, F. Y. N., Filgueiras, I. S., Schimke, L. F., Giil, L. M., Moll, G., Cabral-Miranda, G., Ochs, H. D., Vasconcelos, P. F. da C., de Melo, G. D., Bourhy, H., Casseb, L. M. N., & Cabral-Marques, O. (2023). Neuroimmunology of rabies: New insights into an ancient disease. Journal of Medical Virology, 95(10), e29042. [Online]. Available: ,DOI: 10.1002/jmv.29042

Bechini, A., Boccalini, S., Tiscione, E., Pesavento, G., Mannelli, F., Peruzzi, M., Rapi, S., Mercurio, S., & Bonanni, P. (2012). Progress towards measles and rubella elimination in Tuscany, Italy: The role of population seroepidemiological profile. *European Journal of Public Health*, *22*(1), 133–139. DOI: 10.1093/eurpub/ckq134 PMID: 20880991

Beigel, J. H., & Hayden, F. G. (2020). Influenza therapeutics in clinical practice—Challenges and recent advances. *Cold Spring Harbor Perspectives in Medicine*, *11*(4), a038463. Advance online publication. DOI: 10.1101/cshperspect.a038463 PMID: 32041763

Beks, H., King, O., Clapham, R., Alston, L., Glenister, K., McKinstry, C., Quilliam, C., Wellwood, I., Williams, C., & Wong Shee, A. (2022). Community Health Programs Delivered Through Information and Communications Technology in High-Income Countries: Scoping Review. *Journal of Medical Internet Research*, *24*(3), e26515. DOI: 10.2196/26515 PMID: 35262498

Bellini, W. J., & Helfand, R. F. (2003). The challenges and strategies for laboratory diagnosis of measles in an international setting. *The Journal of Infectious Diseases*, *187*(s1, Supplement_1), S283–S290. DOI: 10.1086/368040 PMID: 12721927

Benedictow, O. J. (2019). Epidemiology of Plague: Problems with the Use of Mathematical Epidemiological Models in Plague Research and the Question of Transmission by Human Fleas and Lice. The Canadian Journal of Infectious Diseases & Medical Microbiology =. *The Canadian Journal of Infectious Diseases & Medical Microbiology*, *1542024*, 1–20. Advance online publication. DOI: 10.1155/2019/1542024 PMID: 31531149

Benvegnù, L., Gios, M., Boccato, S., & Alberti, A. (2004). Natural history of compensated viral cirrhosis: A prospective study on the incidence and hierarchy of major complications. *Gut*, *53*(5), 744–749. DOI: 10.1136/gut.2003.020263 PMID: 15082595

Bester, J. (2016). Measles and measles vaccination. *JAMA Pediatrics*, *170*(12), 1209. DOI: 10.1001/jamapediatrics.2016.1787 PMID: 27695849

Best, J. M., & Enders, G. (2006). Laboratory Diagnosis of Rubella and Congenital Rubella. In Banatvala, J., & Peckham, C. (Eds.), *Perspectives in Medical Virology* (Vol. 15, pp. 39–77). Elsevier.

Bhardwaj, S. (2016). The Epidemiology of Poliomyelitis Deconstructed. UC Merced Undergraduate Research Journal, 8(2).

Bharti, N., Tatem, A., Ferrari, M., Grais, R., Djibo, A., & Grenfell, B. (2011). Explaining seasonal fluctuations of measles in niger using nighttime lights imagery. *Science*, *334*(6061), 1424–1427. DOI: 10.1126/science.1210554 PMID: 22158822

Bhatt, S., Cameron, E., Bharti, N., Grenfell, B. T., Vespignani, A., & Hay, S. I. (2022). Dengue fever: Global burden and spatiotemporal dynamics, 2000-2020. *The Lancet. Infectious Diseases*, *22*(9), e155–e163.

Bhatt, S., Gething, P. W., Brady, O. J., Messina, J. P., Farlow, A. W., Moyes, C. L., & Hay, S. I. (2013). The global distribution of Zika virus: Modelling past, present, and future. *Nature*, *496*(7446), 533–537. PMID: 23542591

Bhatt, S., Katzelnick, L., Messina, J. P., Funk, S., Tatem, A. J., Clements, A. C., & Hay, S. I. (2015). The effect of temperature on dengue disease. *Nature*, *520*(7546), 64–67.

Bhorat, A. E., Fong, Y., & Corey, L. (2020). A phase 1, open-label, single-arm study to evaluate the safety and immunogenicity of a trivalent influenza vaccine in adults 18 to <50 years of age in South Africa. *Journal of Clinical Virology*, *124*, 104262. DOI: 10.1016/j.jcv.2020.104262

Bischoff, S. C., Bernal, W., Dasarathy, S., Merli, M., Plank, L. D., Schütz, T., & Plauth, M. (2020). ESPEN practical guideline: Clinical nutrition in liver disease. *Clinical Nutrition (Edinburgh, Lothian)*, *39*(12), 3533–3562. DOI: 10.1016/j.clnu.2020.09.001 PMID: 33213977

Blair, J. M. A., Richmond, G. E., & Piddock, L. J. V. (2014). Multidrug efflux pumps in Gram-negative bacteria and their role in antibiotic resistance. *Future Microbiology*, *9*(10), 1165–1177. DOI: 10.2217/fmb.14.66 PMID: 25405886

Blaney, J. E., & Bloom, B. R. (2020). The dengue virus nonstructural protein 1: A multi-functional protein essential for viral replication. *Viruses*, *12*(3), 350. PMID: 32235750

Blondel, B., Colbere-Garapin, F., Couderc, T., Wirotius, A., & Guivel-Benhassine, F. (2005). Poliovirus, pathogenesis of poliomyelitis, and apoptosis. Role of apoptosis in infection, 25-56.

Boily, M. C., Abu-Raddad, L., Desai, K., Masse, B., Self, S., & Anderson, R. (2008). Measuring the public-health impact of candidate HIV vaccines as part of the licensing process. *The Lancet. Infectious Diseases*, *8*(3), 200–207. DOI: 10.1016/S1473-3099(07)70292-X PMID: 18291341

Bolaños-Martínez, O. C., Govea-Alonso, D. O., Fragoso, G., Sciutto, E., & Rosales-Mendoza, S. (2022). Carrot cells expressing the VP1 and VP2 poliovirus proteins effectively elicited mucosal immunity. [PCTOC]. *Plant Cell, Tissue and Organ Culture*, *148*(3), 545–556. DOI: 10.1007/s11240-021-02205-0

Bonilla, F. A., & Oettgen, H. C. (2010). Adaptive immunity. *The Journal of Allergy and Clinical Immunology*, *125*(2, Suppl 2), S33–S40. DOI: 10.1016/j.jaci.2009.09.017 PMID: 20061006

Bonville, C. (n.d.). Respiratory syncytial virus. In Domachowske, J. (Ed.), *Vaccines* (pp. 89–97).

Bopegamage, S. A., & Petrovicová, A. (1994). In vitro infection of mouse pancreatic islet cells with coxsackie viruses. *Acta Virologica. English Ed.*, *38*(5), 251–255. PMID: 7725998

Boutayeb, A. (2010). The Burden of Communicable and Non-Communicable Diseases in Developing Countries. In Preedy, V. R., & Watson, R. R. (Eds.), *Handbook of Disease Burdens and Quality of Life Measures* (pp. 531–546). Springer New York. DOI: 10.1007/978-0-387-78665-0_32

Brady, O. J., Messina, J. P., Perkins, T. A., Huang, C. Y., Le Menach, A., Sun, W., & Hay, S. I. (2021). Global seroprevalence of dengue virus infection and risk factors for seropositivity: A systematic review and meta-analysis. *The Lancet. Infectious Diseases*, *21*(12), e342–e351.

Branche, A. R., & Falsey, A. R. (2016). Parainfluenza virus infection. *Seminars in Respiratory and Critical Care Medicine*, *37*(4), 538–554. DOI: 10.1055/s-0036-1584798 PMID: 27486735

Brar, R. K., Jyoti, U., Patil, R. K., & Patil, H. C. (2020). Fluoroquinolone antibiotics: An overview. *Adesh University Journal of Medical Sciences & Research*, *2*(1), 26–30. DOI: 10.25259/AUJMSR_12_2020

Bremell, D., Mattsson, N., Edsbagge, M., Blennow, K., Andreasson, U., Wikkelsö, C., Zetterberg, H., & Hagberg, L. (2013). Cerebrospinal fluid CXCL13 in Lyme neuroborreliosis and asymptomatic HIV infection. *BMC Neurology*, *13*(1), 2. DOI: 10.1186/1471-2377-13-2 PMID: 23294475

Brendish, N. J., Malachira, A. K., Armstrong, L., Houghton, R., Aitken, S., Nyimbili, E., & Clark, T. W. (2017). Routine molecular point-of-care testing for respiratory viruses in adults presenting to hospital with acute respiratory illness (ResPOC): A pragmatic, open-label, randomised controlled trial. *The Lancet. Respiratory Medicine*, *5*(5), 401–411.

Bright, T., Felix, L., Kuper, H., & Polack, S. (2017). A systematic review of strategies to increase access to health services among children in low and middle income countries. *BMC Health Services Research*, *17*(1), 252. DOI: 10.1186/s12913-017-2180-9 PMID: 28381276

Brives, C., & Pourraz, J. (2020). Phage therapy as a potential solution in the fight against AMR: Obstacles and possible futures. *Palgrave Communications*, *6*(1), 1. Advance online publication. DOI: 10.1057/s41599-020-0478-4

Brooks, G. F., Carroll, K. C., Butel, J. S., & Morse, S. A. (2019). *Jawetz*. Melnick & Adelberg's Medical Microbiology.

Brosh-Nissimov, T. (2016). Lassa fever: Another threat from West Africa. *Disaster and Military Medicine*, *2*(1), 2. DOI: 10.1186/s40696-016-0018-3 PMID: 28265442

Bruce, M., Zulz, T., & Koch, A. (2016). Surveillance of infectious diseases in the Arctic. *Public Health*, *137*, 5–12. DOI: 10.1016/j.puhe.2016.06.014 PMID: 27473191

Bryce, J., Boschi-Pinto, C., Shibuya, K., & Black, R. E. (2005). WHO estimates of the causes of death in children. *Lancet*, *365*(9465), 1147–1152. DOI: 10.1016/S0140-6736(05)71877-8 PMID: 15794969

Buckee, C., Noor, A., & Sattenspiel, L. (2021). Thinking clearly about social aspects of infectious disease transmission. *Nature*, *595*(7866), 205–213. DOI: 10.1038/s41586-021-03694-x PMID: 34194045

Buckley, S. M., & Casals, J. (1970). Lassa fever, a new virus disease of man from West Africa. 3. Isolation and characterization of the virus. *The American Journal of Tropical Medicine and Hygiene*, *19*(4), 680–691. DOI: 10.4269/ajtmh.1970.19.680 PMID: 4987547

Buckley, S. M., Casals, J., & Downs, W. G. (1970). Isolation and antigenic characterization of Lassa virus. [This work reports the initial isolation and characterization of Lassa virus.]. *Nature*, *227*(5254), 174. DOI: 10.1038/227174a0 PMID: 5428406

Buliva, E., Elnossery, S., Okwarah, P., Tayyab, M., Brennan, R., & Abubakar, A. (2022). Cholera prevention, control strategies, challenges and World Health Organization initiatives in the Eastern Mediterranean Region: A narrative review. SSRN *Electronic Journal*. DOI: 10.2139/ssrn.4268747

Burbelo, P. D., Issa, A. T., Ching, K. H., Cohen, J. I., Iadarola, M. J., & Marques, A. (2010). Rapid, Simple, Quantitative, and Highly Sensitive Antibody Detection for Lyme Disease. *Clinical and Vaccine Immunology; CVI*, *17*(6), 904–909. DOI: 10.1128/CVI.00476-09 PMID: 20392886

Burke, D. S., Monath, T. P., Guirakhoo, F., Phillips, N. B., & Blair, C. D. (2018). Dengue fever and Zika virus: Two mosquito-borne flaviviruses causing outbreaks in the Americas. *Current Opinion in Virology*, *30*, 10–15.

Burrell, C. J., Howard, C. R., & Murphy, F. A. (2017). *Laboratory Diagnosis of Virus Diseases. Fenner and White's Medical Virology*. Academic Press.

Burrill, C. P., Westesson, O., Schulte, M. B., Strings, V. R., Segal, M., & Andino, R. (2013). Global RNA structure analysis of poliovirus identifies a conserved RNA structure involved in viral replication and infectivity. *Journal of Virology*, *87*(21), 11670–11683. DOI: 10.1128/JVI.01560-13 PMID: 23966409

Burrowes, V., Perin, J., Monira, S., Sack, D. A., Rashid, M., Mahamud, T., Rahman, Z., Mustafiz, M., Bhuyian, S. I., Begum, F., Zohura, F., Biswas, S., Parvin, T., Hasan, T., Zhang, X., Sack, B. R., Saif-Ur-Rahman, K. M., Alam, M., & George, C. M. (2017). Risk factors for household transmission of *Vibrio cholerae* in Dhaka, Bangladesh (CHoBI7 Trial). *The American Journal of Tropical Medicine and Hygiene*, *96*(6), 1382–1387. DOI: 10.4269/ajtmh.16-0871 PMID: 28719281

Butler, T. (1994). Yersinia infections: Centennial of the discovery of the plague bacillus. *Clinical Infectious Diseases*, *19*(4), 655–661. DOI: 10.1093/clinids/19.4.655 PMID: 7803628

Butler, T., Bell, W. R., Linh, N. N., Tiep, N. D., & Arnold, K.Clinical and Hematologic Aspects. (1974). Yersinia pestis infection in Vietnam. I. Clinical and hematologic aspects. *The Journal of Infectious Diseases*, *129*(Suppl), S78–S84. DOI: 10.1093/infdis/129.Supplement_1.S78 PMID: 4825250

Butterworth, R. F. (2003). Hepatic encephalopathy—A serious complication of alcoholic liver disease. *Alcohol Research & Health : the Journal of the National Institute on Alcohol Abuse and Alcoholism*, *27*(2), 143–145. PMID: 15303624

Camejo Leonor, M., & Mendez, M. D. (2023). Rubella *StatPearls*. Treasure Island (FL) with ineligible companies. Disclosure: Magda Mendez declares no relevant financial relationships with ineligible companies.: StatPearls Publishing

Campbell, G. L., & Hughes, J. M. (1995). Plague in India: A New Warning from an Old Nemesis. *Annals of Internal Medicine*, *122*(2), 151–153. DOI: 10.7326/0003-4819-122-2-199501150-00014 PMID: 7992992

Candon, S., Perez-Arroyo, A., Marquet, C., Valette, F., Foray, A.-P., Pelletier, B., Milani, C., Ventura, M., Bach, J.-F., Chatenoud, L., & Lemoine, R. (2015). Antibiotics in early life alter the gut microbiome and increase disease incidence in a spontaneous mouse model of autoimmune insulin-dependent diabetes. *PLoS One*, *10*(5), e0125448. Advance online publication. DOI: 10.1371/journal.pone.0125448 PMID: 25970503

Canouï, E., & Launay, O. (2019). Histoire et principes de la vaccination. *Revue des Maladies Respiratoires*, *36*(1), 74–81. DOI: 10.1016/j.rmr.2018.02.015 PMID: 30579659

Cao-Lormeau, V. M., Blake, A., Mons, S., Lastère, S., Roche, C., Vanhomwegen, J., & Ghawché, F. (2014). Guillain-Barre syndrome outbreak associated with Zika virus infection in French Polynesia: A case-control study. *Lancet*, *383*(9919), 1915–1920. PMID: 26948433

Carlson, J. A., Middleton, P. J., Szymanski, M. T., Huber, J., & Petric, M. (1978). Fatal rotavirus gastroenteritis: An analysis of 21 cases. *American Journal of Diseases of Children*, *132*(5), 477–479. DOI: 10.1001/archpedi.1978.02120300037006 PMID: 206132

Carratalà, A., Bachmann, V., Julian, T. R., & Kohn, T. (2020). Adaptation of Human Enterovirus to Warm Environments Leads to Resistance against Chlorine Disinfection. *Environmental Science & Technology*, *54*(18), 11292–11300. DOI: 10.1021/acs.est.0c03199 PMID: 32875801

Carrol, E. D., Beadsworth, M. B., Jenkins, N., Ratcliffe, L., Ashton, I., Crowley, B., Nye, F. J., & Beeching, N. J. (2006). Clinical and diagnostic findings of an echovirus meningitis outbreak in the north west of England. *Postgraduate Medical Journal*, *82*(963), 60–64. DOI: 10.1136/pgmj.2005.036608 PMID: 16397083

Cash, R. A., Music, S. I., Libonati, J. P., Snyder, M. J., Wenzel, R. P., & Hornick, R. B. (1974). Response of man to infection with *Vibrio cholerae*. I. Clinical, serologic, and bacteriologic responses to a known inoculum. *The Journal of Infectious Diseases*, *129*(1), 45–52. DOI: 10.1093/infdis/129.1.45 PMID: 4809112

Cassel, D., & Pfeuffer, T. (1978). Mechanism of cholera toxin action: Covalent modification of the guanyl nucleotide-binding protein of the adenylate cyclase system. *Proceedings of the National Academy of Sciences of the United States of America*, *75*(6), 2669–2673. DOI: 10.1073/pnas.75.6.2669 PMID: 208069

Centers for Disease C. (2022). *Prevention. National Enterovirus Surveillance System (NESS)*. Surveillance Data.

Centers for Disease Control (CDC) (1991). Aseptic meningitis—New York State and United States, weeks 1-36, 1991. *MMWR. Morbidity and Mortality Weekly Report*, *40*(45), 773–775.

Centers for Disease Control and Prevention. (2010). Update: Outbreak of cholera—Haiti, 2010. *MMWR. Morbidity and Mortality Weekly Report*, *59*(48), 1586–1590. PMID: 21150867

Centers for Disease Control and Prevention. (2021). *Preventing the spread of respiratory viruses*. https://www.cdc.gov/flu/prevent/preventing.htm

Centers for Disease Control and Prevention. *(2021, August 18). Pinkbook: Poliomyelitis. Centers for Disease Control and Prevention.* Https://www.cdc.gov/vaccines/pubs/pinkbook/polio.html. (n.d.).

Centers for Disease Control and Prevention. *(2021, September 28). Poliovirus diagnostic methods. Centers for Disease Control and Prevention.* Https://www.cdc.gov/polio/us/lab-testing/diagnostic.html. (n.d.).

Centers for Disease Control and Prevention. *(2022) Chapter 18: Polio; epidemiology and prevention of vaccine-preventable, Available at:* Https://www.cdc.gov/vaccines/pubs/pinkbook/downloads/polio.pdf. (n.d.).

Centers for Disease Control and Prevention. *(2022, August 3). Vaccine-associated paralytic polio. Centers for Disease Control and Prevention.* Https://www.cdc.gov/vaccines/vpd/polio/hcp/vaccine-associated-paralytic-polio-faq.html. (n.d.).

Centers for Disease Control and Prevention. (2023, April 13). Dengue. https://www.cdc.gov/dengue/index.html

Centers for Disease Control and Prevention. *(2023, July 5). Polio: For travelers. Centers for Disease Control and Prevention.* Https://www.cdc.gov/polio/us/travelers.html. (n.d.).

Centers for Disease Control and Prevention. (n.d.). *Laboratory information for parainfluenza viruses.* https://www.cdc.gov/parainfluenza/hcp/lab.htm

Centers for Disease Control and Prevention. (n.d.). *Prevention and treatment of parainfluenza viruses.* https://www.cdc.gov/parainfluenza/prevention-treatment.html

Centers for Disease Control and Prevention. (n.d.). *Symptoms of parainfluenza viruses.* https://www.cdc.gov/parainfluenza/symptoms.html

Centers for Disease Control and Prevention. Epidemiology and Prevention of Vaccine-Preventable Diseases. 12th ed, second printing. Atkinson W, Wolfe C, Hamborsky J, eds. Washington, DC: Public Health Foundation, 2012.

Chaffey, N. (2003). Alberts, B., Johnson, A., Lewis, J., Raff, M., Roberts, K. and Walter, P. Molecular biology of the cell. 4th edn.

Chang, L. Y., Tsao, K. C., Hsia, S. H., Shih, S. R., Huang, C. G., & Chan, W. K. (2004). Transmission and clinical features of enterovirus 71 infections in household contacts in Taiwan. *Journal of the American Medical Association, 291*(2), 222–227. DOI: 10.1001/jama.291.2.222 PMID: 14722149

Chanteau, S., Rahalison, L., Ralafiarisoa, L., Foulon, J., Ratsitorahina, M., Ratsifasoamanana, L., Carniel, É., & Nato, F. (2003). Development and testing of a rapid diagnostic test for bubonic and pneumonic plague. The Lancet. https://www.semanticscholar.org/paper/Development-and-testing-of-a-rapid-diagnostic-test-Chanteau-Rahalison/0ad30482641f56f661161362b49e68f47bea8ee6

Chaplin, D. D. (2010). Overview of the immune response. *The Journal of Allergy and Clinical Immunology, 125*(2, Suppl 2), S3–S23. DOI: 10.1016/j.jaci.2009.12.980 PMID: 20176265

Chaudhary, S. C., Khandelwal, A., Tandon, R., & Sawlani, K. K. (2021). Rabies encephalitis. BMJ case reports, 14(4), e239249., [Online]. Available: .DOI: 10.1136/bcr-2020-239249

Chen, J. P., & Cosgriff, T. M. (2000). Hemorrhagic fever virus-induced changes in hemostasis and vascular biology. *Blood Coagulation & Fibrinolysis, 11*(5), 461–483. DOI: 10.1097/00001721-200007000-00010 PMID: 10937808

Chen, L. H., & Wilson, M. E. (2020). Dengue and Zika: Emerging arboviruses of public health concern. *The American Journal of the Medical Sciences, 359*(6), 509–519. PMID: 32245566

Choi, U., & Lee, C.-R. (2019). Distinct roles of outer membrane porins in antibiotic resistance and membrane integrity in *Escherichia coli. Frontiers in Microbiology, 10*, 953. Advance online publication. DOI: 10.3389/fmicb.2019.00953 PMID: 31114568

Chowdhury, F., Ross, A. G., Islam, M. T., McMillan, N. A. J., & Qadri, F. (2022). Diagnosis, management, and future control of cholera. *Clinical Microbiology Reviews, 35*(3), e0021121. Advance online publication. DOI: 10.1128/cmr.00211-21 PMID: 35726607

Chuang, Y.-Y., & Huang, Y.-C. (2019). Enteroviral infection in neonates. *Journal of Microbiology, Immunology, and Infection, 52*(6), 851–857. DOI: 10.1016/j.jmii.2019.08.018 PMID: 31607572

Chu, E. C. P., & Lam, K. K. W. (2019). Post-poliomyelitis syndrome. *International Medical Case Reports Journal, 12*, 261–264. DOI: 10.2147/IMCRJ.S219481 PMID: 31496835

Chu, E. C.-P., & Zoubi, F. A. (2023). Post-polio syndrome presenting as isolated neck extensor myopathy: A case report. *AME Case Reports, 7*(0), 0. Advance online publication. DOI: 10.21037/acr-22-76 PMID: 37122964

Chu, M., Yuan, W., Wu, S., Wang, Z., Mao, L., Tian, T., Lu, Y., Zhu, B., Yang, Y., Wang, B., Gao, H., Jiang, L., & Zhuang, X. (2016). Quantitative assessment of polymorphisms in H19 lncRNA and cancer risk: A meta-analysis of 13,392 cases and 18,893 controls. [CrossRef] [PubMed]. *Oncotarget, 7*(48), 78631–78639. DOI: 10.18632/oncotarget.12530 PMID: 27732938

Chunda, P., Chisema, M. N., Mwale, A., Kambalame, D., Mapemba, D., & Muula, A. S. (2022). The 2022 Malawi Polio outbreak. *Malawi Medical Journal : the Journal of Medical Association of Malawi, 34*(3), 223–224. DOI: 10.4314/mmj.v34i3.14 PMID: 36406100

Ciapponi, A., Bardach, A., Ares, L. R., Glujovsky, D., Cafferata, M. L., Cesaroni, S., & Bhatti, A. (2019). Sequential inactivated (IPV) and live oral (OPV) poliovirus vaccines for preventing poliomyelitis. [n.d.]. *Cochrane Database of Systematic Reviews, 2019*(12), 12. DOI: 10.1002/14651858.CD011260.pub2 PMID: 31801180

Ciećko-Michalska, I., Szczepanek, M., Słowik, A., & Mach, T. (2012). Pathogenesis of hepatic encephalopathy. *Gastroenterology Research and Practice*, *642108*, 1–7. Advance online publication. DOI: 10.1155/2012/642108 PMID: 23316223

Cierny, G., 3rd, & DiPasquale, D. (2006). Treatment of chronic infection. *J Am Acad Orthop Surg, 14*(10 Spec No.), S105-110. DOI: 10.5435/00124635-200600001-00025

Cloeckaert, A., & Kuchler, K. (2020). Grand Challenges in Infectious Diseases: Are We Prepared for Worst-Case Scenarios? *Frontiers in Microbiology*, *11*, 613383. DOI: 10.3389/fmicb.2020.613383 PMID: 33329504

Codd, A. A., Hale, J. H., Bell, T. M., Sims, D. G., Bacon, C. J., & Gardner, P. S. (1976). Epidemic of echovirus 19 in the north-east of England. *The Journal of Hygiene*, *76*(2), 307–317. DOI: 10.1017/S0022172400055200 PMID: 1063219

Collins, A. S. (2008). Advances in Patient Safety Preventing Health Care–Associated Infections. In Hughes, R. G. (Ed.), *Patient Safety and Quality: An Evidence-Based Handbook for Nurses*. Agency for Healthcare Research and Quality (US).

Cooper, L. T.Jr. (2009). Myocarditis. *The New England Journal of Medicine*, *360*(15), 1526–1538. DOI: 10.1056/NEJMra0800028 PMID: 19357408

Couch, R. B., Douglas, R. G.Jr, Lindgren, K. M., Gerone, P. J., & Knight, V. (1970). Airborne transmission of respiratory infection with coxsackievirus A type 21. *American Journal of Epidemiology*, *91*(1), 78–86. DOI: 10.1093/oxfordjournals.aje.a121115 PMID: 5415578

Coughlin, M. M., Beck, A. S., Bankamp, B., & Rota, P. A. (2017). Perspective on Global Measles Epidemiology and Control and the Role of Novel Vaccination Strategies. *Viruses*, *9*(1), 11. DOI: 10.3390/v9010011 PMID: 28106841

Crook, L. D., & Tempest, B. (1992). Plague. A clinical review of 27 cases. *Archives of Internal Medicine*, *152*(6), 1253–1256. DOI: 10.1001/archinte.1992.00400180107017 PMID: 1599354

Crowcroft, N. S. (1994). Cholera: Current epidemiology. *Communicable Disease Report. CDR Review*, *4*(13), R157–R164. PMID: 7531564

Curtale, F., Perrelli, F., Mantovani, J., Atti, M., Filia, A., Nicoletti, L., & Lallo, D. (2010). Description of two measles outbreaks in the lazio region, italy (2006-2007). importance of pockets of low vaccine coverage in sustaining the infection. *BMC Infectious Diseases*, *10*(1), 62. Advance online publication. DOI: 10.1186/1471-2334-10-62 PMID: 20219143

Dadgostar, P. (2019). Antimicrobial Resistance: Implications and Costs. *Infection and Drug Resistance, 12*, 3903–3910. DOI: 10.2147/IDR.S234610 PMID: 31908502

Daliento L, Calabrese F, Tona F, Caforio AL, Tarsia G, Angelini A, et al. (2003). Successful treatment of enterovirus-induced myocarditis with interferon-alpha. *The Journal of heart and lung transplantation: the official publication of the International Society for Heart Transplantation. 22*(2):214-7.

Dara, N., Sayyari, A.-A., & Imanzadeh, F. (2014). Hepatic encephalopathy: Early diagnosis in pediatric patients with cirrhosis. *Iranian Journal of Child Neurology, 8*(1), 1–11. PMID: 24665321

Dardona, Z., Amane, M., & Boussaa, S. (2024). Polio in Gaza: Another disastrous outcome of the Gaza conflict, 2023-2024. *Asian Pacific Journal of Tropical Medicine, 17*(9), 381–383. DOI: 10.4103/apjtm.apjtm_535_24

Dasarathy, S., & Mullen, K. D. (2001). Hepatic encephalopathy. *Current Treatment Options in Gastroenterology, 4*(6), 517–526. DOI: 10.1007/s11938-001-0017-3 PMID: 11696278

Dattani, S., Spooner, F., Ochmann, S., & Roser, M. *Polio. Our World Data [Internet]. 2023 Nov 10 [cited 2023 Nov 22]; Available from:* Https://ourworldindata .org/polio. (n.d.).

Davies, H. G., Bowman, C., & Luby, S. P. (2017). Cholera—Management and success. *The Journal of Infection, 74*(Suppl 1), S66–S73. DOI: 10.1016/S0163-4453(17)30194-9 PMID: 28646965

Davis, B. M., Rall, G. F., & Schnell, M. J. (2015). Everything You Always Wanted to Know About Rabies Virus (But Were Afraid to Ask). Annual review of virology, 2(1), 451–471., [Online]. Available: .DOI: 10.1146/annurev-virology-100114-055157

de Crom, S. C., Rossen, J. W., van Furth, A. M., & Obihara, C. C. (2016). Enterovirus and parechovirus infection in children: A brief overview. *European Journal of Pediatrics, 175*(8), 1023–1029. DOI: 10.1007/s00431-016-2725-7 PMID: 27156106

De Jong, N. M. C., Aartse, A., Van Gils, M. J., & Eggink, D. (2020). Development of broadly reactive influenza vaccines by targeting the conserved regions of the hemagglutinin stem and head domains. *Expert Review of Vaccines, 19*(6), 563–577. DOI: 10.1080/14760584.2020.1777861 PMID: 32510256

de Swart, R. L. (2008). The pathogenesis of measles revisited. *The Pediatric Infectious Disease Journal, 27*(10), S84–S88. DOI: 10.1097/INF.0b013e31816857fe PMID: 18820585

Del Fiol, F. S., Balcão, V. M., Barberato-Filho, S., Lopes, L. C., & Bergamaschi, C. C. (2018). Obesity: A new adverse effect of antibiotics? *Frontiers in Pharmacology*, *9*, 1408. Advance online publication. DOI: 10.3389/fphar.2018.01408 PMID: 30559670

Delpeut, S., Noyce, R. S., Siu, R. W., & Richardson, C. D. (2012). Host factors and measles virus replication. *Current Opinion in Virology*, *2*(6), 773–783. DOI: 10.1016/j.coviro.2012.10.008 PMID: 23146309

Demeure, C. E., Dussurget, O., Mas Fiol, G., Le Guern, A.-S., Savin, C., & Pizarro-Cerdá, J. (2019). Yersinia pestis and plague: An updated view on evolution, virulence determinants, immune subversion, vaccination, and diagnostics. *Genes and Immunity*, *20*(5), 357–370. DOI: 10.1038/s41435-019-0065-0 PMID: 30940874

Dengue and severe dengue (2023). World Health Organization. https://www.who.int/news-room/fact-sheets/detail/dengue-and-severe-dengue

Dengue Haemorrhagic Fever. (2009). *Diagnosis, Treatment, Prevention and Control: New Edition*. World Health Organization.

Dennis, D. T. (2005). Plague as a Biological Weapon. In Fong, I. W., & Alibek, K. (Eds.), *Bioterrorism and Infectious Agents: A New Dilemma for the 21st Century* (pp. 37–70). Springer US., DOI: 10.1007/0-387-23685-6_2

Denyer, S. P., Hodges, N. A., & Gorman, S. P. (Eds.). (2004). *Hugo and Russell's pharmaceutical microbiology* (7th ed.). Blackwell Science., DOI: 10.1002/9780470988329

Deogaonkar, R., Hutubessy, R., van der Putten, I., Evers, S., & Jit, M. (2012). Systematic review of studies evaluating the broader economic impact of vaccination in low and middle income countries. *BMC Public Health*, *12*(1), 878. DOI: 10.1186/1471-2458-12-878 PMID: 23072714

Devi, S. (2024). Calls for Gaza ceasefire to tackle poliovirus. *Lancet*, *404*(10455), 837. DOI: 10.1016/S0140-6736(24)01776-8 PMID: 39217989

Ding, J., & Liu, Q. (2019). Toll-like receptor 4: A promising therapeutic target for pneumonia caused by Gram-negative bacteria. *Journal of Cellular and Molecular Medicine*, *23*(9), 5868–5875. DOI: 10.1111/jcmm.14529 PMID: 31350813

Donadel, M., Stănescu, A., Pistol, A., Stewart, B., Butu, C., Janković, D., Paunescu, B., & Zimmerman, L. (2021). Risk factors for measles deaths among children during a nationwide measles outbreak – romania, 2016–2018. *BMC Infectious Diseases*, *21*(1), 279. Advance online publication. DOI: 10.1186/s12879-021-05966-3 PMID: 33740895

Drexler, M., & Institute of, M. (2010) *What You Need to Know About Infectious Disease*. Washington (DC): National Academies Press (US) Copyright © National Academy of Sciences.

Dureab, F., Jahn, A., Krisam, J., Dureab, A., Zain, O., Al-Awlaqi, S., & Müller, O. (2019). Risk factors associated with the recent cholera outbreak in Yemen: A case-control study. *Epidemiology and Health*, *41*, e2019015. Advance online publication. DOI: 10.4178/epih.e2019015 PMID: 31010279

Durham, L. K., Longini, I. M., Halloran, M. E., Clemens, J. D., Nizam, A., & Rao, M. (1998). Estimation of vaccine efficacy in the presence of waning: Application to cholera vaccines. *American Journal of Epidemiology*, *147*(10), 948–959. DOI: 10.1093/oxfordjournals.aje.a009385 PMID: 9596473

Dutta, Tarun Kumar. Rabies: An overview. International Journal of Advanced Medical and Health Research 1(2):p 39-44, Jul–Dec 2014., [Online]. Available: .DOI: 10.4103/2349-4220.147998

Dutt, Y., D'Souza, R., & Garg, M. (2022). The association between biofilm formation and antimicrobial resistance with possible ingenious bio-remedial approaches. *Antibiotics (Basel, Switzerland)*, *11*(7), 930. Advance online publication. DOI: 10.3390/antibiotics11070930 PMID: 35884186

Du, Z., & Wang, X. (2016). Pathology and Pathogenesis of Yersinia pestis. *Advances in Experimental Medicine and Biology*, *918*, 193–222. DOI: 10.1007/978-94-024-0890-4_7 PMID: 27722864

Egorova, A., Ekins, S., Schmidtke, M., & Makarov, V. (2019). Back to the future: Advances in development of broad-spectrum capsid-binding inhibitors of enteroviruses. *European Journal of Medicinal Chemistry*, *178*, 606–622. DOI: 10.1016/j.ejmech.2019.06.008 PMID: 31226653

Ehrnst, A., & Eriksson, M. (1996). Echovirus Type 23 Observed as a Nosocomial Infection in Infants. *Scandinavian Journal of Infectious Diseases*, *28*(2), 205–206. DOI: 10.3109/00365549609049079 PMID: 8792494

Eisenberg, M., & Mordechai, L. (2019). The Justinianic Plague: An interdisciplinary review. *Byzantine and Modern Greek Studies*, *43*(2), 156–180. DOI: 10.1017/byz.2019.10

Eisen, R. J., MacMillan, K., Atiku, L. A., Mpanga, J. T., Zielinski-Gutierrez, E., Graham, C. B., Boegler, K. A., Enscore, R. E., & Gage, K. L. (2014). Identification of Risk Factors for Plague in the West Nile Region of Uganda. *The American Journal of Tropical Medicine and Hygiene*, *90*(6), 1047–1058. DOI: 10.4269/ajtmh.14-0035 PMID: 24686743

El Khiat, A., Hiba, O. E., Aimrane, A., Draoui, A., Jayakumar, A. R., Norenberg, M. D., & Gamrani, H. (2022). Hepatic Encephalopathy: An Overview of Basic Concepts and Mechanisms. *Frontiers in Medical Case Reports*, *03*(03). Advance online publication. DOI: 10.47746/FMCR.2022.3302

Ellis, C. N., LaRocque, R. C., Uddin, T., Krastins, B., Mayo-Smith, L. M., Sarracino, D., Karlsson, E. K., Rahman, A., Shirin, T., Bhuiyan, T. R., Chowdhury, F., Khan, A. I., Ryan, E. T., Calderwood, S. B., Qadri, F., & Harris, J. B. (2015). Comparative proteomic analysis reveals activation of mucosal innate immune signaling pathways during cholera. *Infection and Immunity*, *83*(3), 1089–1103. DOI: 10.1128/IAI.02765-14 PMID: 25561705

Elsaid, M. I., & Rustgi, V. K. (2020). Epidemiology of Hepatic Encephalopathy. *Clinics in Liver Disease*, *24*(2), 157–174. DOI: 10.1016/j.cld.2020.01.001 PMID: 32245524

Elsohaby, I., & Villa, L. (2023). Zoonotic diseases: Understanding the risks and mitigating the threats. *BMC Veterinary Research*, *19*(1), 186. DOI: 10.1186/s12917-023-03736-8 PMID: 37789313

English, R. M., Badcock, J. C., Giay, T., Ngu, T., Waters, A. M., & Bennett, S. A. (1997). Effect of nutrition improvement project on morbidity from infectious diseases in preschool children in Vietnam: Comparison with control commune. *BMJ (Clinical Research Ed.)*, *315*(7116), 1122–1125. DOI: 10.1136/bmj.315.7116.1122 PMID: 9374884

Ertl H. C. J. (2018). Human immune responses to traditional and novel rabies vaccines. Human immune responses to traditional and novel rabies vaccines. Revue scientifique et technique (International Office of Epizootics), 37(2), 649–656. [Online]. Available: DOI: 10.20506/rst.37.2.2830

Expert, W. H. O. (1970). Committee on plague. Fourth report. *World Health Organization Technical Report Series*, *447*, 1–25. PMID: 4986823

Ezeomah, C., Adoga, A. A., Ihekweazu, C., Paessler, S., Cisneros, I. L., Tomori, O., & Walker, D. H. (2019). Sequelae of Lassa Fever: Postviral Cerebellar Ataxia. *Open Forum Infectious Diseases*, *6*(12), 6. DOI: 10.1093/ofid/ofz512 PMID: 31879673

Fabiani, M., Ferrante, G., Minardi, V., Giambi, C., Riccardo, F., Declich, S., & Masocco, M. (2017). Comparison of rubella immunization rates in immigrant and Italian women of childbearing age: Results from the Italian behavioral surveillance system PASSI (2011-2015). *PLoS One*, *12*(10), e0178122. DOI: 10.1371/journal.pone.0178122 PMID: 28968403

Faccioli, J., Nardelli, S., Gioia, S., Riggio, O., & Ridola, L. (2023). Primary Prophylaxis of Overt Hepatic Encephalopathy: Is It Time to Consider It? *Journal of Clinical Medicine*, *12*(12), 3903. DOI: 10.3390/jcm12123903 PMID: 37373598

Fairweather, D., Frisancho-Kiss, S., & Rose, N. R. (2005). Viruses as adjuvants for autoimmunity: Evidence from Coxsackievirus-induced myocarditis. *Reviews in Medical Virology*, *15*(1), 17–27. DOI: 10.1002/rmv.445 PMID: 15386590

Fairweather, D., Kaya, Z., Shellam, G. R., Lawson, C. M., & Rose, N. R. (2001). From Infection to Autoimmunity. *Journal of Autoimmunity*, *16*(3), 175–186. DOI: 10.1006/jaut.2000.0492 PMID: 11334481

Fallahzadeh, M. A., & Rahimi, R. S. (2020). Hepatic Encephalopathy and Nutrition Influences: A Narrative Review. *Nutrition in Clinical Practice*, *35*(1), 36–48. DOI: 10.1002/ncp.10458 PMID: 31872484

Falsey, A. R., Formica, M. A., & Walsh, E. E. (2002). Diagnosis of respiratory syncytial virus infection: Comparison of reverse transcription-PCR to viral culture and serology in adults with respiratory illness. *Journal of Clinical Microbiology*, *40*(3), 817–820. DOI: 10.1128/JCM.40.3.817-820.2002 PMID: 11880399

Ferenci, P. (2017). Hepatic encephalopathy. *Gastroenterology Report*, *5*(2), 138–147. DOI: 10.1093/gastro/gox013 PMID: 28533911

Ferenci, P., Lockwood, A., Mullen, K., Tarter, R., Weissenborn, K., & Blei, A. T. (2002). Hepatic encephalopathy—Definition, nomenclature, diagnosis, and quantification: Final report of the Working Party at the 11th World Congresses of Gastroenterology, Vienna, 1998. *Hepatology (Baltimore, Md.)*, *35*(3), 716–721. DOI: 10.1053/jhep.2002.31250 PMID: 11870389

Fernandez-Garcia MD, Garcia-Ibañez N, Camacho J, Gutierrez A, Sánchez García L, Calvo C, et al. (2024). Enhanced echovirus 11 genomic surveillance in neonatal infections in Spain following a European alert reveals new recombinant forms linked to severe cases, 2019 to 2023. *European communicable disease bulletin. 29*(44).

Ferrari, M., Grais, R., Bharti, N., Conlan, A., Bjørnstad, O., Wolfson, L., Guerin, P. J., Djibo, A., & Grenfell, B. (2008). The dynamics of measles in sub-saharan africa. *Nature*, *451*(7179), 679–684. DOI: 10.1038/nature06509 PMID: 18256664

Fichet-Calvet, E., Becker-Ziaja, B., Koivogui, L., & Gunther, S. (2014). Lassa serology in natural populations of rodents and horizontal transmission. *Vector Borne and Zoonotic Diseases (Larchmont, N.Y.), 14*(9), 665–674. DOI: 10.1089/vbz.2013.1484 PMID: 25229705

Fichet-Calvet, E., Lecompte, E., Koivogui, L., Daffis, S., & ter Meulen, J. (2008). Reproductive characteristics of Mastomys natalensis and Lassa virus prevalence in Guinea, West Africa. *Vector Borne and Zoonotic Diseases (Larchmont, N.Y.), 8*(1), 41–48. DOI: 10.1089/vbz.2007.0118 PMID: 18237265

Figuereo, S., Yoon, I., Kaddu, S. S., Lubogo, M., Baruch, J., Hossain, A. A., Mohamed, S. I., Abubakar, A. H. A., Mohamud, K. M., & Malik, S. M. M. R. (2024). Cost of cholera for households and health facilities, Somalia. *Journal of Epidemiology and Global Health, 14*(3), 1219–1230. DOI: 10.1007/s44197-024-00278-6 PMID: 39023718

Filia, A., Bella, A., Manso, M., Baggieri, M., Magurano, F., & Rota, M. (2017). Ongoing outbreak with well over 4,000 measles cases in italy from january to end august 2017 – what is making elimination so difficult? *Eurosurveillance, 22*(37). Advance online publication. DOI: 10.2807/1560-7917.ES.2017.22.37.30614 PMID: 28933342

Fisher, C. R., Streicker, D. G., & Schnell, M. J. (2018). The spread and evolution of rabies virus: conquering new frontiers. Nature reviews. Microbiology, 16(4), 241–255., [Online]. Available: .DOI: 10.1038/nrmicro.2018.11

Florescu, D. F., & Schaenman, J. M. (2019). Adenovirus in solid organ transplant recipients: Guidelines from the American Society of Transplantation Infectious Diseases Community of Practice. *Clinical Transplantation, 33*(9), e13527. DOI: 10.1111/ctr.13527 PMID: 30859626

Fooks, A. R., Banyard, A. C., Horton, D. L., Johnson, N., McElhinney, L. M., & Jackson, A. C. (2014). Current status of rabies and prospects for elimination. Lancet (London, England), 384(9951), 1389–1399., [Online]. Available: .DOI: 10.1016/S0140-6736(13)62707-5

Fooks, A. R., Cliquet, F., Finke, S., Freuling, C., Hemachudha, T., Mani, R. S., Müller, T., Nadin-Davis, S., Picard-Meyer, E., Wilde, H., & Banyard, A. C. (2017). Rabies. Nature Reviews Disease Primers, 3(1), 17091., [Online]. Available: .DOI: 10.1038/nrdp.2017.9

Forbes, J. D. (2020). Clinically Important Toxins in Bacterial Infection: Utility of Laboratory Detection. *Clinical Microbiology Newsletter, 42*(20), 163–170. DOI: 10.1016/j.clinmicnews.2020.09.003 PMID: 33046946

Foti, C., Piperno, A., Scala, A., & Giuffrè, O. (2021). Oxazolidinone antibiotics: Chemical, biological and analytical aspects. *Molecules (Basel, Switzerland)*, *26*(14), 4280. Advance online publication. DOI: 10.3390/molecules26144280 PMID: 34299555

Founou, R. C., Founou, L. L., & Essack, S. Y. (2017). Clinical and economic impact of antibiotic resistance in developing countries: A systematic review and meta-analysis. *PLoS One*, *12*(12), e0189621. Advance online publication. DOI: 10.1371/journal.pone.0189621 PMID: 29267306

Fox, M. (2013). Importance of Sodium. *Living Strong Foundation*. Available from: https://www.livestrong.com/article/499403-importance-of-sodium/

Fredrick, D.R. (2023). Conjunctivitis beyond the neonatal period.

Frenk, J., Gómez-Dantés, O., & Knaul, F. M. (2011). Globalization and infectious diseases. *Infect Dis Clin North Am, 25*(3), 593-599, viii. DOI: 10.1016/j.idc.2011.05.003

Freter, R., O'Brien, P. C., & Macsai, M. S. (1981). Role of chemotaxis in the association of motile bacteria with intestinal mucosa: In vivo studies. *Infection and Immunity*, *34*(1), 234–240. DOI: 10.1128/iai.34.1.234-240.1981 PMID: 7298185

Fu, J., Chu, J., Wang, J., Cai, R., Cheng, W., Lifei, S., & Xing, Y. (2019). A hospital-associated measles outbreak in health workers in beijing: Implications for measles elimination in china, 2018. *International Journal of Infectious Diseases*, *78*, 85–92. DOI: 10.1016/j.ijid.2018.10.023 PMID: 30391419

Furuse, Y., & Oshitani, H. (2017). Global Transmission Dynamics of Measles in the Measles Elimination Era. *Viruses*, *9*(4), 82. DOI: 10.3390/v9040082 PMID: 28420160

Gadre, G., Satishchandra, P., Mahadevan, A., Suja, M. S., Madhusudana, S. N., Sundaram, C., & Shankar, S. K. (2010). Rabies viral encephalitis: clinical determinants in diagnosis with special reference to paralytic form. Journal of neurology, neurosurgery, and psychiatry, 81(7), 812–820., [Online]. Available: DOI: 10.1136/jnnp.2009.185504

Gage, K. L., Dennis, D. T., Orloski, K. A., Ettestad, P., Brown, T. L., Reynolds, P. J., Pape, W. J., Fritz, C. L., Carter, L. G., & Stein, J. D. (2000). Cases of Cat-Associated Human Plague in the Western US, 1977-1998. *Clinical Infectious Diseases*, *30*(6), 893–900. DOI: 10.1086/313804 PMID: 10852811

Gairing, S. J., Schleicher, E. M., Galle, P. R., & Labenz, C. (2023). Prediction and prevention of the first episode of overt hepatic encephalopathy in patients with cirrhosis. *Hepatology Communications*, *7*(4). Advance online publication. DOI: 10.1097/HC9.0000000000000096 PMID: 36930868

Galimand, M., Guiyoule, A., Gerbaud, G., Rasoamanana, B., Chanteau, S., Carniel, E., & Courvalin, P. (1997). Multidrug Resistance in Yersinia pestis Mediated by a Transferable Plasmid. *The New England Journal of Medicine*, *337*(10), 677–681. DOI: 10.1056/NEJM199709043371004 PMID: 9278464

Gamble, D. R. (1962). Isolation of Coxsackie viruses from normal children aged 0-5 years. *British Medical Journal*, *1*(5270), 16–18. DOI: 10.1136/bmj.1.5270.16 PMID: 13896555

Ganasegeran, K., Jamil, M. F. A., Ch'ng, A. S. H., Looi, I., & Peariasamy, K. M. (2021). Influence of Population Density for COVID-19 Spread in Malaysia: An Ecological Study. *International Journal of Environmental Research and Public Health*, *18*(18), 9866. Advance online publication. DOI: 10.3390/ijerph18189866 PMID: 34574790

Garde, S., Chodisetti, P. K., & Reddy, M. (2021). Peptidoglycan: Structure, synthesis, and regulation. *EcoSal Plus*, *9*(2), ecosalplus.ESP-0010-2020. Advance online publication. DOI: 10.1128/ecosalplus.ESP-0010-2020 PMID: 33470191

Gasparrini, A. J., Wang, B., Sun, X., Kennedy, E. A., Hernandez-Leyva, A., Ndao, I. M., Tarr, P. I., Warner, B. B., & Dantas, G. (2019). Persistent metagenomic signatures of early-life hospitalization and antibiotic treatment in the infant gut microbiota and resistome. *Nature Microbiology*, *4*(12), 12. Advance online publication. DOI: 10.1038/s41564-019-0550-2 PMID: 31501537

Gastañaduy, P., Banerjee, E., DeBolt, C., Bravo-Alcántara, P., Samad, S., Pastor, D., Rota, P. A., Patel, M., Crowcroft, N. S., & Durrheim, D. (2018). Public health responses during measles outbreaks in elimination settings: Strategies and challenges. *Human Vaccines & Immunotherapeutics*, *14*(9), 2222–2238. DOI: 10.1080/21645515.2018.1474310 PMID: 29932850

Gelbart D. (2019). Rabies. JAAPA: official journal of the American Academy of Physician Assistants, 32(10), 46–47., [Online]. Available: .DOI: 10.1097/01.JAA.0000580572.87216.17

Gelfand, H. M., Holguin, A. H., Marchetti, G. E., & Feorino, P. M. (1963). A continuing surveillance of enterovirus infections in healthy children in six united states cities. I. Viruses isolated during 1960 and 1961. *American Journal of Hygiene*, *78*, 358–375. PMID: 14071359

Ghai, I., & Ghai, S. (2018). Understanding antibiotic resistance via outer membrane permeability. *Infection and Drug Resistance*, *11*, 523–530. DOI: 10.2147/IDR.S156995 PMID: 29695921

Gherardin, A., & Lau, S. (2007). Intradermal rabies vaccine. The Medical journal of Australia, 187(1), 58–59., [Online]. Available: .DOI: 10.5694/j.1326-5377.2007.tb01128.x

Ghosh, A. (2019). Afghan migration and pakistan's policy response: Dynamics of continuity and change. Public Policy Research in the Global South: A Cross-Country Perspective, 215-230. (n.d.).

Ghosh, J., & Ghosh, J. (2023). Current Management of Hepatic Encephalopathy: A Review Article. *Journal for Research in Applied Sciences and Biotechnology*, *2*(4), 170–175. DOI: 10.55544/jrasb.2.4.24

Giambi, C., Filia, A., Rota, M. C., Del Manso, M., Declich, S., Nacca, G., & Bella, A. (2015). Congenital rubella still a public health problem in Italy: Analysis of national surveillance data from 2005 to 2013. *Eurosurveillance*, *20*(16). Advance online publication. DOI: 10.2807/1560-7917.ES2015.20.16.21103 PMID: 25953272

Gilbert, M., Xiao, X., Domenech, J., Lubroth, J., Martin, V., & Slingenbergh, J. (2006). Anatidae migration in the western Palearctic and spread of highly pathogenic avian influenza H5NI virus. *Emerging Infectious Diseases*, *12*(11), 1650–1656. DOI: 10.3201/eid1211.060223 PMID: 17283613

Glatter, K. A., & Finkelman, P. (2021). History of the Plague: An Ancient Pandemic for the Age of COVID-19. *The American Journal of Medicine*, *134*(2), 176–181. DOI: 10.1016/j.amjmed.2020.08.019 PMID: 32979306

Gomes-Solecki, M. J. C., Dunn, J. J., Luft, B. J., Castillo, J., Dykhuizen, D. E., Yang, X., Glass, J. D., & Dattwyler, R. J. (2000). Recombinant Chimeric Borrelia Proteins for Diagnosis of Lyme Disease. *Journal of Clinical Microbiology*, *38*(7), 2530–2535. DOI: 10.1128/JCM.38.7.2530-2535.2000 PMID: 10878038

Gondo, K., Kusuhara, K., Take, H., & Ueda, K. (1995). Echovirus type 9 epidemic in Kagoshima, southern Japan: Seroepidemiology and clinical observation of aseptic meningitis. *The Pediatric Infectious Disease Journal*, *14*(9), 787–791. DOI: 10.1097/00006454-199509000-00011 PMID: 8559629

Gonzalez, C. F., Finberg, L., & Bluestein, D. D. (1964). Electrolyte concentration during acute infections: Observations in infants and children. *American Journal of Diseases of Children*, *107*(5), 476–482.

Goyal, O., Sidhu, S., & Kishore, H. (2016). Incidence, Prevalence and Natural History of Minimal Hepatic Encephalopathy in Cirrhosis. *Journal of Hepatology*, *64*(2), S279. DOI: 10.1016/S0168-8278(16)00334-2

Grist, N. R., Bell, E. J., & Reid, D. (1975). The epidemiology of enteroviruses. *Scottish Medical Journal*, *20*(1), 27–31. DOI: 10.1177/003693307502000108 PMID: 1111084

Gröndahl, B., Puppe, W., Weigl, J., & Schmitt, H.-J. (2005). Comparison of the BD Directigen Flu A+B Kit and the Abbott TestPack Influenza A/B for rapid detection of influenza viruses. *Clinical Microbiology and Infection*, *11*(2), 120–124. DOI: 10.1111/j.1469-0691.2004.01047.x PMID: 16153263

Gubler, D. J. (2020). Dengue and Zika viruses: Insights into the emergence, global spread, and control of two major vector-borne flaviviruses. *Annual Review of Virology*, *7*(1), 193–210.

Gubler, D. J. (2020). The global pandemic of dengue/severe dengue: Current status and prospects for control. *Human Vaccines & Immunotherapeutics*, *16*(1), 1–14. PMID: 32022652

Guerrant, R. L., Van Gilder, T., Steiner, T. S., Thielman, N. M., Slutsker, L., Tauxe, R. V., Hennessy, T., Griffin, P. M., DuPont, H., Bradley Sack, R., Tarr, P., Neill, M., Nachamkin, I., Reller, L. B., Osterholm, M. T., Bennish, M. L., & Pickering, L. K. (2001). Practice guidelines for the management of infectious diarrhea. *Clinical Infectious Diseases*, *32*(3), 331–351. DOI: 10.1086/318514 PMID: 11170940

Guo, N., Ma, H., Deng, J., Ma, Y., Huang, L., Guo, R., & Zhang, L. (2018). Effect of hand washing and personal hygiene on hand food mouth disease: A community intervention study. *Medicine*, *97*(51), e13144. DOI: 10.1097/MD.0000000000013144 PMID: 30572426

Gusev, E., Sarapultsev, A., Hu, D., & Chereshnev, V. (2021). Problems of pathogenesis and pathogenetic therapy of COVID-19 from the perspective of the general theory of pathological systems (general pathological processes). *International Journal of Molecular Sciences*, *22*(14), 7582. DOI: 10.3390/ijms22147582 PMID: 34299201

Guzman, M. G., Halstead, S. B., Artsob, H., Buchy, P., Farrar, J., & Gubler, D. J. & World Health Organization. (2011). Dengue: A continuing global threat. *Nature Reviews. Microbiology*, *9*(7), 564–572. PMID: 21079655

Guzmán, M. G., & Kouri, G. (2020). Dengue: History, classification, and clinical features. *The American Journal of Tropical Medicine and Hygiene*, *102*(6), 1155–1161.

Guzman, M. G., Vazquez, S., & Martinez, E. (2014). Dengue: Current situation and perspectives for control. *The Lancet. Infectious Diseases.*

Hansen, F., Jarvis, M. A., Feldmann, H., & Rosenke, K. (2021). Lassa virus treatment options. *Microorganisms*, *9*(4), 772.

Happi, A. N., Happi, C. T., & Schoepp, R. J. (2019, August). Lassa fever diagnostics: Past, present, and future. *Current Opinion in Virology*, *37*, 132–138. DOI: 10.1016/j.coviro.2019.08.002 PMID: 31518896

Harris, E., Vespignani, A., & Bhatt, S. (2022). Climate change and dengue: A critical and systematic review of quantitative projections. *The Lancet. Planetary Health*, *6*(4), e362–e371.

Harris, J. B., Ivers, L. C., & Ferraro, M. J. (2011). Case 19-2011: A 4-year-old Haitian boy with vomiting and diarrhea. *The New England Journal of Medicine*, *364*(25), 2452–2461. DOI: 10.1056/NEJMcpc1100927 PMID: 21696312

Harris, J. B., LaRocque, R. C., Chowdhury, F., Khan, A. I., Logvinenko, T., Faruque, A. S. G., Ryan, E. T., Qadri, F., & Calderwood, S. B. (2008). Susceptibility to *Vibrio cholerae* infection in a cohort of household contacts of patients with cholera in Bangladesh. *PLoS Neglected Tropical Diseases*, *2*(4), e221. Advance online publication. DOI: 10.1371/journal.pntd.0000221 PMID: 18398491

Harris, J. B., LaRocque, R. C., Qadri, F., Ryan, E. T., & Calderwood, S. B. (2012). Cholera. *Lancet*, *379*(9835), 2466–2476. DOI: 10.1016/S0140-6736(12)60436-X PMID: 22748592

Hastie, K. M., Bale, S., Kimberlin, C. R., & Saphire, E. O. (2012). Hiding the evidence: Two strategies for innate immune evasion by hemorrhagic fever viruses. *Current Opinion in Virology*, *2*(2), 151–156. DOI: 10.1016/j.coviro.2012.01.003 PMID: 22482712

Healing, T., & Gopal, R. Report on an assessment visit to Sierra Leone, April 12th-30th 2001. London: Merlin, 2001.

Helfand, R. F., Heath, J. L., Anderson, L. J., Maes, E. F., Guris, D., & Bellini, W. J. (1997). Diagnosis of measles with an IgM capture EIA: The optimal timing of specimen collection after rash onset. *The Journal of Infectious Diseases*, *175*(1), 195–199. DOI: 10.1093/infdis/175.1.195 PMID: 8985220

Hemachudha, T., Laothamatas, J., & Rupprecht, C. E. (2002). Human rabies: a disease of complex neuropathogenetic mechanisms and diagnostic challenges. The Lancet. Neurology, 1(2), 101–109., [Online]. Available: .DOI: 10.1016/S1474-4422(02)00041-8

Hemachudha, T., Ugolini, G., Wacharapluesadee, S., Sungkarat, W., Shuangshoti, S., & Laothamatas, J. (2013). Human rabies: Neuropathogenesis, diagnosis, and management. The Lancet Neurology, 12(5), 498–513, [Online]. Available: .DOI: 10.1016/S1474-4422(13)70038-3

Hepatic Encephalopathy in Chronic Liver Disease. (2014). Practice Guideline by the European Association for the Study of the Liver and the American Association for the Study of Liver Diseases. (2014). *Journal of Hepatology*, *61*(3), 642–659. DOI: 10.1016/j.jhep.2014.05.042 PMID: 25015420

Herman, A., & Herman, A. P. (2014). Nanoparticles as antimicrobial agents: Their toxicity and mechanisms of action. *Journal of Nanoscience and Nanotechnology*, *14*(1), 946–957. DOI: 10.1166/jnn.2014.9054 PMID: 24730311

Hermansson, H., Kumar, H., Collado, M. C., Salminen, S., Isolauri, E., & Rautava, S. (2019). Breast milk microbiota is shaped by mode of delivery and intrapartum antibiotic exposure. *Frontiers in Nutrition*, *6*, 4. Advance online publication. DOI: 10.3389/fnut.2019.00004 PMID: 30778389

He, Y., Lin, F., Chipman, P. R., Bator, C. M., Baker, T. S., Shoham, M., Kuhn, R. J., Medof, M. E., & Rossmann, M. G. (2002). Structure of decay-accelerating factor bound to echovirus 7: A virus-receptor complex. *Proceedings of the National Academy of Sciences of the United States of America*, *99*(16), 10325–10329. DOI: 10.1073/pnas.152161599 PMID: 12119400

Higgins, D., Trujillo, C., & Keech, C. (2019). Progress in the development of parainfluenza virus vaccines. *Viruses*, *11*(12), 1122. DOI: 10.3390/v11121122 PMID: 31817188

Hinckley, A. F., Connally, N. P., Meek, J. I., Johnson, B. J., Kemperman, M. M., Feldman, K. A., White, J. L., & Mead, P. S. (2014). Lyme Disease Testing by Large Commercial Laboratories in the United States. *Clinical Infectious Diseases*, *59*(5), 676–681. DOI: 10.1093/cid/ciu397 PMID: 24879782

Hinnebusch, B. J. (2010). Plague in the 21st Century: Global Public Health Challenges and Goals. In V. St. Georgiev (Ed.), *National Institute of Allergy and Infectious Diseases, NIH: Volume 3: Intramural Research* (pp. 87–94). Humana Press. DOI: 10.1007/978-1-60761-512-5_9

Hinnebusch, B. J. (2005). The evolution of flea-borne transmission in Yersinia pestis. *Current Issues in Molecular Biology*, *7*(2), 197–212. PMID: 16053250

Holmberg, S. D., Harris, J. R., & Kay, D. E.. (1984). Foodborne transmission of cholera in Micronesian households. *Lancet*, *1*(8372), 325–328. DOI: 10.1016/S0140-6736(84)90370-2 PMID: 6141390

Holmgren, J., Lönnroth, I., Månsson, J., & Svennerholm, L. (1975). Interaction of cholera toxin and membrane GM1 ganglioside of small intestine. *Proceedings of the National Academy of Sciences of the United States of America*, *72*(7), 2520–2524. DOI: 10.1073/pnas.72.7.2520 PMID: 1058471

Hoque, M. (2023). A Review on Different Dietary Sources of Important Vitamins and Electrolytes. *International Journal of Research Publication and Reviews*, *4*(8), 731–736. DOI: 10.55248/gengpi.4.823.50408

Houlihan, C., & Behrens, R. (2017). Lassa fever. *BMJ (Clinical Research Ed.)*, *358*, j2986. DOI: 10.1136/bmj.j2986 PMID: 28701331

Hsieh, Y.-C., Chen, H.-Y., & Hsu, H.-C. (2017). Molecular epidemiology of human adenovirus infections in Taiwan, 2013–2014. *Journal of Microbiology, Immunology, and Infection*, *50*(6), 784–790. DOI: 10.1016/j.jmii.2017.03.005

Hsueh, B. Y., & Waters, C. M. (2019). Combating cholera. *F1000Research, 8*, Article 589. DOI: 10.12688/f1000research.18093.1

Huang, H. W. (2020). DAPTOMYCIN, its membrane-active mechanism vs. that of other antimicrobial peptides. *Biochimica et Biophysica Acta (BBA) -. Biomembranes*, *1862*(10), 183395. Advance online publication. DOI: 10.1016/j.bbamem.2020.183395 PMID: 32526177

Huang, Q., Liu, X., Brisse, M., Ly, H., & Liang, Y. (2020). Effect of strain variations on Lassa virus Z protein-mediated human RIG-I inhibition. *Viruses*, *12*(9), 907. DOI: 10.3390/v12090907 PMID: 32824946

Huang, Y. H., Yang, C. M., Chang, L. H., Lin, Y. S., Lai, C. C., Chiu, C. Y., & Tsai, W. P. (2019). Dengue fever and the risk of subsequent severe dengue: A nationwide population-based study. *International Journal of Epidemiology*, *48*(2), 521–532.

Hübschen, J. M., Bork, S. M., Brown, K. E., Mankertz, A., Santibanez, S., Ben Mamou, M., Mulders, M. N., & Muller, C. P. (2017). Challenges of measles and rubella laboratory diagnostic in the era of elimination. *Clinical Microbiology and Infection*, *23*(8), 511–515. DOI: 10.1016/j.cmi.2017.04.009 PMID: 28412379

Hull, H. F., Montes, J. M., & Mann, J. M. (1986). Plague masquerading as gastrointestinal illness. *The Western Journal of Medicine*, *145*(4), 485–487. PMID: 3788132

Human Plague—United States. 1993-1994. (n.d.). Retrieved December 15, 2023, from https://www.cdc.gov/mmwr/preview/mmwrhtml/00026077.htm

Hutin, Y., Luby, S., & Paquet, C. (2003). A large cholera outbreak in Kano City, Nigeria: The importance of hand washing with soap and the danger of street-vended water. *Journal of Water and Health*, *1*(1), 45–52. DOI: 10.2166/wh.2003.0006 PMID: 15384272

Hviid, A., Hansen, J. V., Frisch, M., & Melbye, M. (2019). Measles, Mumps, Rubella Vaccination and Autism: A Nationwide Cohort Study. *Annals of Internal Medicine*, *170*(8), 513–520. DOI: 10.7326/M18-2101 PMID: 30831578

Hyypiä, T, & Harvala, H. (2015). Echoviruses. doi.org/10.1016/B978-0-12-801238-3.02562-9.

Ibekwe, T. (2012). Lassa fever: The challenges of curtailing a deadly disease. [Internet]. *The Pan African Medical Journal*, *11*, 55. https://www.ncbi.nlm.nih.gov/pmc/articles/PMC3343683/ PMID: 22593791

Igere, B. E., & Ekundayo, T. C. (2020). Global mapping of cholera *Vibrio* and outbreaks in the Pre-Millennium Development Goals (MDG)/Sustainable Development Goals (SDG) and MDGs/SDGs era of 1990–2019. *Microbial Pathogenesis*, *149*, 104319. Advance online publication. DOI: 10.1016/j.micpath.2020.104319 PMID: 32579993

Ison, M. G., & Hayden, R. T. (2016). Adenovirus. *Microbiology Spectrum*, *4*(4), 4.4.41. Advance online publication. DOI: 10.1128/microbiolspec.DMIH2-0020-2015 PMID: 27726766

Iwu, C. D., & Patrick, S. M. (2021). An insight into the implementation of the global action plan on antimicrobial resistance in the WHO African region: A roadmap for action. *International Journal of Antimicrobial Agents*, *58*(4), 106411. Advance online publication. DOI: 10.1016/j.ijantimicag.2021.106411 PMID: 34371112

Jackson A. C. (2016). Human Rabies: a 2016 Update. Current infectious disease reports, 18(11), 38., [Online]. Available: .DOI: 10.1007/s11908-016-0540-y

Jackson A. C. (2018). Rabies: a medical perspective. Rabies: a medical perspective. Revue scientifique et technique (International Office of Epizootics), 37(2), 569–580., [Online]. Available: .DOI: 10.20506/rst.37.2.2825

Jane Ling, M. Y., Halim, A. F. N. A., Ahmad, D., Ramly, N., Hassan, M. R., Syed Abdul Rahim, S. S., Saffree Jeffree, M., Omar, A., & Hidrus, A. (2023). Rabies in Southeast Asia: a systematic review of its incidence, risk factors and mortality. BMJ open, 13(5), e066587, [Online]. Available: , [Online].DOI: 10.1136/bmjopen-2022-066587

Javelle, E., Colson, P., Parola, P., & Raoult, D. (2019). Measles, the need for a paradigm shift. *European Journal of Epidemiology*, *34*(10), 897–915. DOI: 10.1007/s10654-019-00569-4 PMID: 31624970

Jayakumar, A. R., Rama Rao, K. V., & Norenberg, M. D. (2015). Neuroinflammation in Hepatic Encephalopathy: Mechanistic Aspects. *Journal of Clinical and Experimental Hepatology*, *5*, S21–S28. DOI: 10.1016/j.jceh.2014.07.006 PMID: 26041953

Jednačak, T., Mikulandra, I., & Novak, P. (2020). Advanced methods for studying structure and interactions of macrolide antibiotics. *International Journal of Molecular Sciences*, *21*(20), 7799. Advance online publication. DOI: 10.3390/ijms21207799 PMID: 33096889

Jindal, A., & Jagdish, R. K. (2019). Sarcopenia: Ammonia metabolism and hepatic encephalopathy. *Clinical and Molecular Hepatology*, *25*(3), 270–279. DOI: 10.3350/cmh.2019.0015 PMID: 31006226

Johansson, M. A., Aguiar, R. S., Vasilakis, N., & Weaver, S. C. (2021). Dengue virus capsid protein: Structure, function, and role in viral pathogenesis. *Viruses*, *13*(6), 1033. PMID: 34070947

Johnson, J. A. (2002). Nosocomial infections. *The Veterinary Clinics of North America. Small Animal Practice*, *32*(5), 1101–1126. DOI: 10.1016/S0195-5616(02)00038-4 PMID: 12380168

Johnson, K. M., McCormick, J. B., Webb, P. A., Smith, E. S., Elliott, L. H., & King, I. J. (1987). Clinical virology of Lassa fever in hospitalized patients. *The Journal of Infectious Diseases*, *155*(3), 456–464. DOI: 10.1093/infdis/155.3.456 PMID: 3805773

Jonah, J. H., Samuel, G., Abdullahi, M. I., Emmanuel, E. A., Danladi, S. S., & Ekwuluo, C. E. (2024). Nigeria's public health response to disease outbreaks: A review of strengths and weaknesses. *Journal of Public Health in Africa*, *15*(1), 773. Advance online publication. DOI: 10.4102/jphia.v15i1.773 PMID: 40503462

Jones, E. A., Schafer, D. F., Ferenci, P., & Pappas, S. C. (1984). The GABA hypothesis of the pathogenesis of hepatic encephalopathy: Current status. *The Yale Journal of Biology and Medicine*, *57*(3), 301–316. PMID: 6093394

Jullien, S., & Garner, P. (2019). Web Annex A. Antibiotics for treating plague [executive summary]. *Systematic Reviews.*

Kadambari, S., Abdullahi, F., Celma, C., & Ladhani, S. (2024). Epidemiological trends in viral meningitis in England: Prospective national surveillance, 2013-2023. *The Journal of Infection, 89*(3), 106223. DOI: 10.1016/j.jinf.2024.106223 PMID: 38986749

Kakaī, C. G., Okunromade, O. F., Dan-Nwafor, C. C., Chabi, A. I. B., Martial, G. T. P., Dalhat, M. M., Ward, S., Tante, O., Nguku, P. M., Hamadi, A., Ilori, E., Lokossou, V., Brito, C., Ojo, O. E., Kone, I., Agbeko, T. T., Ihekweazu, C., & Merrill, R. D. (2020). Improving cross-border preparedness and response: Lessons learned from 3 lassa fever outbreaks across Benin, Nigeria, and Togo, 2017–2019. *Health Security, 18*(S1), S105–S112. DOI: 10.1089/hs.2019.0080 PMID: 32004125

Kang, S., Chowdhury, F., Park, J., Ahmed, T., Tadesse, B. T., Islam, M. T., Kim, D. R., Im, J., Aziz, A. B., Hoque, M., Pak, G., Khanam, F., Ahmmed, F., Liu, X., Zaman, K., Khan, A. I., Kim, J. H., Marks, F., Qadri, F., & Clemens, J. D. (2022). Are better existing WASH practices in urban slums associated with a lower long-term risk of severe cholera? A prospective cohort study with 4 years of follow-up in Mirpur, Bangladesh. *BMJ Open, 12*(9), e060858. DOI: 10.1136/bmjopen-2022-060858 PMID: 36130764

Kaper, J. B., Morris, J. G.Jr, & Levine, M. M. (1995). Cholera. *Clinical Microbiology Reviews, 8*(1), 48–86. DOI: 10.1128/CMR.8.1.48 PMID: 7704895

Kaplan, M. H., Klein, S. W., McPhee, J., & Harper, R. G. (1983). Group B coxsackievirus infections in infants younger than three months of age: A serious childhood illness. *Reviews of Infectious Diseases, 5*(6), 1019–1032. DOI: 10.1093/clinids/5.6.1019 PMID: 6318288

Kapoor, G., Saigal, S., & Elongavan, A. (2017). Action and resistance mechanisms of antibiotics: A guide for clinicians. *Journal of Anaesthesiology, Clinical Pharmacology, 33*(3), 300–305. DOI: 10.4103/joacp.JOACP_349_15 PMID: 29109626

Kasai, C., Sugimoto, K., Moritani, I., Tanaka, J., Oya, Y., Inoue, H., Tsumura, M., Takemura, M., Yamauchi, S., Kaneko, M., Kawakami, M., & Yamada, T. (2015). Comparison of the gut microbiota composition between obese and non-obese individuals in a Japanese population, as analyzed by terminal restriction fragment length polymorphism and next-generation sequencing. *BMC Gastroenterology, 15*(1), 100. Advance online publication. DOI: 10.1186/s12876-015-0330-2 PMID: 26261039

Kaslow, R. A., Stanberry, L. R., & Le Duc, J. W. (Eds.). (2014). *Viral infections of humans: epidemiology and control.* Springer.

Kaufman, D. L., Clare-Salzler, M., Tian, J., Forsthuber, T., Ting, G. S., Robinson, P., Atkinson, M. A., Sercarz, E. E., Tobin, A. J., & Lehmann, P. V. (1993). Spontaneous loss of T-cell tolerance to glutamic acid decarboxylase in murine insulin-dependent diabetes. *Nature*, *366*(6450), 69–72. DOI: 10.1038/366069a0 PMID: 7694152

Keilman, L. J. (2019). Seasonal Influenza (Flu). *The Nursing Clinics of North America*, *54*(2), 227–243. DOI: 10.1016/j.cnur.2019.02.009 PMID: 31027663

Keller, J. M., Dela Cruz, C. S., Pasnick, S., Gross, J. E., Carlos, W. G., Maves, R., & Jamil, S. (2019). Measles. *American Journal of Respiratory and Critical Care Medicine*, *200*(1), 1–P2. DOI: 10.1164/rccm.2001P1 PMID: 31259630

Kesson, A. M. (2012). 12 - Rubella. In Jong, E. C., & Stevens, D. L. (Eds.), *Netter's Infectious Diseases* (pp. 51–54). W.B. Saunders. DOI: 10.1016/B978-1-4377-0126-5.00012-4

Khan, A. I., Islam, M. T., Khan, Z. H., Tanvir, N. A., Amin, M. A., Khan, I. I., Bhuiyan, A. T. M. R. H., Hasan, A. S. M. M., Islam, M. S., Bari, T. I. A., Rahman, A., Islam, M. N., & Qadri, F. (2023). Implementation and delivery of oral cholera vaccination campaigns in humanitarian crisis settings among Rohingya Myanmar nationals in Cox's Bazar, Bangladesh. *Vaccines*, *11*(4), 843. Advance online publication. DOI: 10.3390/vaccines11040843 PMID: 37112756

Khan, I. A. (2004). Plague: The dreadful visitation occupying the human mind for centuries. *Transactions of the Royal Society of Tropical Medicine and Hygiene*, *98*(5), 270–277. DOI: 10.1016/S0035-9203(03)00059-2 PMID: 15109549

Khan, S. H., Goba, A., Chu, M., Roth, C., Healing, T., Marx, A., Fair, J., Guttieri, M. C., Ferro, P., Imes, T., Monagin, C., Garry, R. F., & Bausch, D. G. (2008). New opportunities for field research on the pathogenesis and treatment of Lassa fever. *Antiviral Research*, *78*(1), 103–115. DOI: 10.1016/j.antiviral.2007.11.003 PMID: 18241935

Khan, W. A., Bennish, M. L., Seas, C., Khan, E. H., Ronan, A., Dhar, U., Busch, W., & Salam, M. A. (1996). Randomised controlled comparison of single-dose ciprofloxacin and doxycycline for cholera caused by *Vibrio cholerae* 01 or 0139. *Lancet*, *348*(9023), 296–300. DOI: 10.1016/S0140-6736(96)01180-4 PMID: 8709688

Khouja, T., Mitsantisuk, K., Tadrous, M., & Suda, K. J. (2022). Global consumption of antimicrobials: Impact of the WHO Global Action Plan on Antimicrobial Resistance and 2019 coronavirus pandemic (COVID-19). *The Journal of Antimicrobial Chemotherapy*, *77*(5), 1491–1499. DOI: 10.1093/jac/dkac028 PMID: 35178565

Klein, M., Eggers, H. J., & Nelsen-Salz, B. (2000). Echovirus-9 protein 2C binds single-stranded RNA unspecifically. *The Journal of General Virology*, *81*(Pt 10), 2481–2484. DOI: 10.1099/0022-1317-81-10-2481 PMID: 10993936

Klempner, M. S., Schmid, C. H., Hu, L., Steere, A. C., Johnson, G., McCloud, B., Noring, R., & Weinstein, A. (2001). Intralaboratory reliability of serologic and urine testing for Lyme disease. *The American Journal of Medicine*, *110*(3), 217–219. DOI: 10.1016/S0002-9343(00)00701-4 PMID: 11182109

Kline, K. A., & Bowdish, D. M. E. (2016). Infection in an aging population. *Current Opinion in Microbiology*, *29*, 63–67. DOI: 10.1016/j.mib.2015.11.003 PMID: 26673958

Kogon, A., Spigland, I., Frothingham, T. E., Elveback, L., Williams, C., Hall, C. E., & Fox, J. P. (1969). The virus watch program: A continuing surveillance of viral infections in metropolitan New York families. VII. Observations on viral excretion, seroimmunity, intrafamilial spread and illness association in coxsackie and echovirus infections. *American Journal of Epidemiology*, *89*(1), 51–61. DOI: 10.1093/oxfordjournals.aje.a120915 PMID: 5762818

Koh, W. M., Badaruddin, H., La, H., Chen, M. I., & Cook, A. R. (2018). Severity and burden of hand, foot and mouth disease in Asia: A modelling study. *BMJ Global Health*, *3*(1), e000442. DOI: 10.1136/bmjgh-2017-000442 PMID: 29564154

Kotnik, J. H., Cooper, S., Smedinghoff, S., Gade, P., Scherer, K., Maier, M., Juusola, J., Ramirez, E., Naraghi-Arani, P., Lyon, V., Lutz, B., & Thompson, M. (2022). Flu@home: The comparative accuracy of an at-home influenza rapid diagnostic test using a prepositioned test kit, mobile app, mail-in reference sample, and symptom-based testing trigger. *Journal of Clinical Microbiology*, *60*(3), e02070-21. Advance online publication. DOI: 10.1128/jcm.02070-21 PMID: 35107302

Koulenti, D., Lisboa, T., Brun-Buisson, C., Krueger, W., Macor, A., Sole-Violan, J., Diaz, E., Topeli, A., & Rello, J. (2009). Spectrum of practice in the diagnosis of nosocomial pneumonia in patients requiring mechanical ventilation in European intensive care units. *Critical Care Medicine*, *37*(8), 2360–2368. DOI: 10.1097/CCM.0b013e3181a037ac PMID: 19531951

Krieger, S. E., Kim, C., Zhang, L., Marjomaki, V., & Bergelson, J. M. (2013). Echovirus 1 entry into polarized Caco-2 cells depends on dynamin, cholesterol, and cellular factors associated with macropinocytosis. *Journal of Virology*, *87*(16), 8884–8895. DOI: 10.1128/JVI.03415-12 PMID: 23740983

Królicka, A. L., Kruczkowska, A., Krajewska, M., & Kusztal, M. A. (2020). Hyponatremia in infectious diseases—A literature review. *International Journal of Environmental Research and Public Health*, *17*(15), 5320. DOI: 10.3390/ijerph17155320 PMID: 32718076

Kühl, U., Lassner, D., von Schlippenbach, J., Poller, W., & Schultheiss, H.-P. (2012). Interferon-Beta Improves Survival in Enterovirus-Associated Cardiomyopathy. *Journal of the American College of Cardiology*, *60*(14), 1295–1296. DOI: 10.1016/j.jacc.2012.06.026 PMID: 23017536

Kushner, I. (1982). The phenomenon of the acute phase response. *Annals of the New York Academy of Sciences*, *389*(1), 39–48. DOI: 10.1111/j.1749-6632.1982.tb22124.x PMID: 7046585

Lal, A., Akhtar, J., Isaac, S., Mishra, A. K., Khan, M. S., Noreldin, M., & Abraham, G. M. (2018). Unusual cause of chest pain, Bornholm disease, a forgotten entity; case report and review of literature. *Respiratory Medicine Case Reports*, *25*, 270–273. DOI: 10.1016/j.rmcr.2018.10.005 PMID: 30364740

Lambert, N., Strebel, P., Orenstein, W., Icenogle, J., & Poland, G. A. (2015). Rubella. *Lancet*, *385*(9984), 2297–2307. DOI: 10.1016/S0140-6736(14)60539-0 PMID: 25576992

Lam, E., Diaz, M., Maina, A., & Brennan, M. (2016). Displaced populations due to humanitarian emergencies and its impact on global eradication and elimination of vaccine-preventable diseases. *Conflict and Health*, *10*(1), 27. Advance online publication. DOI: 10.1186/s13031-016-0094-5 PMID: 27956938

Lanks, C. W., Musani, A. I., & Hsia, D. W. (2019). Community-acquired pneumonia and hospital-acquired pneumonia. *The Medical Clinics of North America*, *103*(3), 487–501. DOI: 10.1016/j.mcna.2018.12.008 PMID: 30955516

Lassa fever - guinea. World Health Organization. Available from: https://www.who.int/emergencies/disease-outbreak-news/item/2022-DON382

Lassa fever - nigeria. World Health Organization. Available from: https://www.who.int/emergencies/disease-outbreak-news/item/2023-DON463

Lee, S. E., Greene, S. A., Burns, C. C., Tallis, G., Wassilak, S. G., & Bolu, O. (2023). Progress Toward Poliomyelitis Eradication—Worldwide, January 2021–March 2023. *MMWR. Morbidity and Mortality Weekly Report*, *72*(19), 517–522. DOI: 10.15585/mmwr.mm7219a3 PMID: 37167156

Leifer, E., Gocke, D. J., & Bourne, H. (1970). Lassa fever, a new virus disease of man from West Africa. II. Report of a laboratory-acquired infection treated with plasma from a person recently recovered from the disease. *The American Journal of Tropical Medicine and Hygiene*, *19*(4), 677–679. DOI: 10.4269/ajtmh.1970.19.677 PMID: 4987546

Lei, X., Cui, S., Zhao, Z., & Wang, J. (2015). Etiology, pathogenesis, antivirals and vaccines of hand, foot, and mouth disease. *National Science Review*, *2*(3), 268–284. DOI: 10.1093/nsr/nwv038

Lelovas, P., Dontas, I., Bassiakou, E., & Xanthos, T. (2008). Cardiac implications of Lyme disease, diagnosis and therapeutic approach. *International Journal of Cardiology*, *129*(1), 15–21. DOI: 10.1016/j.ijcard.2008.01.044 PMID: 18508142

Lessler, J., & Metcalf, C. J. (2013). Balancing evidence and uncertainty when considering rubella vaccine introduction. *PLoS One*, *8*(7), e67639. DOI: 10.1371/journal.pone.0067639 PMID: 23861777

Leung, A. K. C., Hon, K. L., & Leong, K. F. (2019). Rubella (German measles) revisited. *Hong Kong Medical Journal*, *25*(2), 134–141. DOI: 10.12809/hkmj187785 PMID: 30967519

Liamis, G., Filippatos, T. D., & Elisaf, M. S. (2015). Correction of hypovolemia with crystalloid fluids: Individualizing infusion therapy. *Postgraduate Medicine*, *127*(4), 405–412. DOI: 10.1080/00325481.2015.1029421 PMID: 25812486

Liew, C. W., Mohd-Noor, N. A., Yusof, R., & Zaini, Z. (2020). Dengue fever: A comprehensive review. *Tropical Biomedicine*, *37*(4), 1355–1374.

Lim, C. G., Hahm, M. H., & Lee, H. J. (2023). Hepatic encephalopathy on magnetic resonance imaging and its uncertain differential diagnoses: A narrative review. *Journal of Yeungnam Medical Science*, *40*(2), 136–145. DOI: 10.12701/jyms.2022.00689 PMID: 36624654

Lim, H. J., Saha, T., Tey, B. T., Tan, W. S., & Ooi, C. W. (2020). Quartz Crystal Microbalance-based biosensors as rapid diagnostic devices for infectious diseases. *Biosensors & Bioelectronics*, *168*, 112513. DOI: 10.1016/j.bios.2020.112513 PMID: 32889395

Lindenbaum, J., Greenough, W. B., & Islam, M. R. (1967). Antibiotic therapy of cholera. *Bulletin of the World Health Organization*, *36*(6), 871–883. PMID: 4865453

Lindler, L. E. (2009). Typing methods for the plague pathogen, Yersinia pestis. *Journal of AOAC International*, *92*(4), 1174–1183. DOI: 10.1093/jaoac/92.4.1174 PMID: 19714987

Lin, T. L., Li, Y. S., Huang, C. W., Hsu, C. C., Wu, H. S., Tseng, T. C., & Yang, C.-F. (2008). Rapid and highly sensitive coxsackievirus a indirect immunofluorescence assay typing kit for enterovirus serotyping. *Journal of Clinical Microbiology*, *46*(2), 785–788. DOI: 10.1128/JCM.01114-07 PMID: 18032614

Lin, T. Y., Kao, H. T., Hsieh, S. H., Huang, Y. C., Chiu, C. H., Chou, Y. H., Yang, P.-H., Lin, R.-I., Tsao, K.-C., Hsu, K.-H., & Chang, L.-Y. (2003). Neonatal enterovirus infections: Emphasis on risk factors of severe and fatal infections. *The Pediatric Infectious Disease Journal*, *22*(10), 889–894. DOI: 10.1097/01.inf.0000091294.63706.f3 PMID: 14551490

Lin, Y.-N., Chou, J.-W., Cheng, K.-S., Peng, C.-Y., Jeng, L.-B., & Chiang, I.-P. (2011). Treatment of Fulminant Autoimmune Hepatitis: Corticosteroid Therapy or Liver Transplantation? A Case Report and Literature Review. *Gastroenterology Research*, *4*(5), 231–235. DOI: 10.4021/gr323w PMID: 27957021

Liping, Z. (2015). Relationship between health education plan and hospitalization frequency in the children with respiratory tract infection. *Pakistan Journal of Pharmaceutical Sciences*, *28*(1, Suppl), 393–395. PMID: 25631503

Lippi, G., South, A. M., & Henry, B. M. (2020). Electrolyte imbalances in patients with severe coronavirus disease 2019 (COVID-19). *Annals of Clinical Biochemistry*, *57*(3), 262–265. DOI: 10.1177/0004563220922255 PMID: 32266828

Liu, C., & Cahill, J. D. (2020). Epidemiology of Rabies and Current US Vaccine Guidelines. Rhode Island medical journal (2013), 103(6), 51–53., [Online]. Available: https://pubmed.ncbi.nlm.nih.gov/32752569/

Liu, F., Enanoria, W., Zipprich, J., Blumberg, S., Harriman, K., Ackley, S., Wheaton, W. D., Allpress, J. L., & Porco, T. (2015). The role of vaccination coverage, individual behaviors, and the public health response in the control of measles epidemics: An agent-based simulation for california. *BMC Public Health*, *15*(1), 447. Advance online publication. DOI: 10.1186/s12889-015-1766-6 PMID: 25928152

Liveris, D., Schwartz, I., McKenna, D., Nowakowski, J., Nadelman, R., DeMarco, J., Iyer, R., Bittker, S., Cooper, D., Holmgren, D., & Wormser, G. P. (2012). Comparison of five diagnostic modalities for direct detection of Borrelia burgdorferi in patients with early Lyme disease. *Diagnostic Microbiology and Infectious Disease*, *73*(3), 243–245. DOI: 10.1016/j.diagmicrobio.2012.03.026 PMID: 22571973

Li, W., Separovic, F., O'Brien-Simpson, N. M., & Wade, J. D. (2018). Covalent conjugation of cationic antimicrobial peptides with a β-lactam antibiotic core. *Peptide Science (Hoboken, N.J.)*, *110*(3), e24059. Advance online publication. DOI: 10.1002/pep2.24059

Li, X., McHugh, G. A., Damle, N., Sikand, V. K., Glickstein, L., & Steere, A. C. (2011). Burden and viability of Borrelia burgdorferi in skin and joints of patients with erythema migrans or lyme arthritis. *Arthritis and Rheumatism*, *63*(8), 2238–2247. DOI: 10.1002/art.30384 PMID: 21590753

Li, X., Sun, L., Xi, S., Hu, Y., Yu, Z., Liu, H., Sun, H., Jing, W., Yuan, L., Liu, H., & Li, T. (2024). V-A ECMO for neonatal coxsackievirus B fulminant myocarditis: A case report and literature review. *Frontiers in Cardiovascular Medicine*, *11*, 1364289. DOI: 10.3389/fcvm.2024.1364289 PMID: 38836060

Lizardi-Cervera, J., Almeda, P., Guevara, L., & Uribe, M. (2003). Hepatic encephalopathy: A review. *Annals of Hepatology*, *2*(3), 122–130. DOI: 10.1016/S1665-2681(19)32137-4 PMID: 15115963

Lo, J. K., & Robinson, L. R. (2018). Postpolio syndrome and the late effects of poliomyelitis. Part 1. Pathogenesis, biomechanical considerations, diagnosis, and investigations. *Muscle & Nerve*, *58*(6), 751–759. DOI: 10.1002/mus.26168 PMID: 29752819

Louissaint, J., Deutsch-Link, S., & Tapper, E. B. (2022). Changing Epidemiology of Cirrhosis and Hepatic Encephalopathy. *Clinical Gastroenterology and Hepatology*, *20*(8, Suppl), S1–S8. DOI: 10.1016/j.cgh.2022.04.036 PMID: 35940729

Loureiro, M. E., Zorzetto-Fernandes, A. L., Radoshitzky, S., Chi, X., Dallari, S., Marooki, N., Lèger, P., Foscaldi, S., Harjono, V., Sharma, S., Zid, B. M., López, N., de la Torre, J. C., Bavari, S., & Zúñiga, E. (2018). DDX3 suppresses type I interferons and favors viral replication during Arenavirus infection. *PLoS Pathogens*, *14*(7), e1007125. DOI: 10.1371/journal.ppat.1007125 PMID: 30001425

Lukashevich, L. S., Clegg, J. C., & Sidibe, K. (1993). Lassa virus activity in Guinea: Distribution of human antiviral antibody defined using enzyme-linked immunosorbent assay with recombinant antigen. *Journal of Medical Virology*, *40*(3), 210–217. DOI: 10.1002/jmv.1890400308 PMID: 8355019

Lyme disease. A rigorous review of diagnostic criteria and treatment. (n.d.). https://doi.org/https://doi.org/10.1016/j.jaut.2014.09.004

Macfarlane, S., Racelis, M., & Muli-Musiime, F. (2000). Public health in developing countries. *Lancet*, *356*(9232), 841–846. DOI: 10.1016/S0140-6736(00)02664-7 PMID: 11022943

Macklin, G. R., Peak, C., Eisenhawer, M., Kurji, F., Mach, O., Konz, J., Gast, C., Bachtiar, N. S., Bandyopadhyay, A. S., & Zipursky, S. (2023). Enabling accelerated vaccine roll-out for public health emergencies of international concern (PHEICs): Novel oral polio vaccine type 2 (nOPV2) experience. *Vaccine*, *41*, A122–A127. DOI: 10.1016/j.vaccine.2022.02.050 PMID: 35307230

Madsen, A., & Cox, R. J. (2020). Prospects and challenges in the development of Universal Influenza Vaccines. *Vaccines*, *8*(3), 361. DOI: 10.3390/vaccines8030361 PMID: 32640619

Mahadevan, A., Suja, M. S., Mani, R. S., & Shankar, S. K. (2016). Perspectives in Diagnosis and Treatment of Rabies Viral Encephalitis: InsightsfromPathogenesis. Neurotherapeutics: the journal of the American Society for Experimental NeuroTherapeutics, 13, (3), 477–492., [Online]. Available: DOI: 10.1007/s13311-016-0452-4

Mahase, E. (2024). Gaza: Polio vaccination campaign gets underway as attacks on humanitarian aid continue. *BMJ (Clinical Research Ed.)*, *386*, q1918. DOI: 10.1136/bmj.q1918 PMID: 39271192

Mahmood, R., Gerriets, V., & Tadi, P. (2023). Rubella Vaccine *StatPearls*. Treasure Island (FL) ineligible companies. Disclosure: Valerie Gerriets declares no relevant financial relationships with ineligible companies. Disclosure: Prasanna Tadi declares no relevant financial relationships with ineligible companies.: StatPearls Publishing Copyright © 2023, StatPearls Publishing LLC.

Makoni, A. C., Chemhuru, M., Bangure, D., Gombe, N. T., & Tshimanga, M. (2015). Rubella outbreak investigation, Gokwe North District, Midlands province, Zimbabwe, 2014 - a case control study. *The Pan African Medical Journal*, *22*, 60. DOI: 10.11604/pamj.2015.22.60.5939 PMID: 26834913

Malik, S., Ahmad, T., Muhammad, K., & Waheed, Y. (2023). Respiratory syncytial virus infection: Treatments and clinical management. *Vaccines*, *11*(2), 491. DOI: 10.3390/vaccines11020491 PMID: 36851368

Mandal, S., Mandal, M. D., & Pal, N. K. (2011). Cholera: A great global concern. *Asian Pacific Journal of Tropical Medicine*, *4*(7), 573–580. DOI: 10.1016/S1995-7645(11)60149-1 PMID: 21803312

Mani, R. S., & Madhusudana, S. N. (2013). Laboratory diagnosis of human rabies: recent advances. TheScientificWorldJournal, 2013, 569712., [Online]. Available: .DOI: 10.1155/2013/569712

Manungo, P., Peterson, D. E., Todd, C. H., Mthamo, N., & Pazvakavambwa, B. (1998). Risk factors for contracting plague in Nkayi district, Zimbabwe. *The Central African Journal of Medicine*, *44*(7), 173–176. PMID: 10028191

Maraspin, V., Ogrinc, K., Ružić-Sabljić, E., Lotrič-Furlan, S., & Strle, F. (2011). Isolation of Borrelia burgdorferi sensu lato from blood of adult patients with borrelial lymphocytoma, Lyme neuroborreliosis, Lyme arthritis and acrodermatitis chronica atrophicans. *Infection*, *39*(1), 35–40. DOI: 10.1007/s15010-010-0062-8 PMID: 21153429

Marie, V., & Gordon, M. L. (2023). The (Re-)Emergence and Spread of Viral Zoonotic Disease: A Perfect Storm of Human Ingenuity and Stupidity. *Viruses*, *15*(8), 1638. Advance online publication. DOI: 10.3390/v15081638 PMID: 37631981

Markley, J. L., & Wencewicz, T. A. (2018). Tetracycline-inactivating enzymes. *Frontiers in Microbiology*, *9*, 1058. Advance online publication. DOI: 10.3389/fmicb.2018.01058 PMID: 29899733

Marques, A., Brown, M. R., & Fleisher, T. A. (2009). Natural Killer Cell Counts Are Not Different between Patients with Post-Lyme Disease Syndrome and Controls. *Clinical and Vaccine Immunology; CVI*, *16*(8), 1249–1250. DOI: 10.1128/CVI.00167-09 PMID: 19515868

Marschall, E., Cryle, M. J., & Tailhades, J. (2019). Biological, chemical, and biochemical strategies for modifying glycopeptide antibiotics. *The Journal of Biological Chemistry*, *294*(49), 18769–18783. DOI: 10.1074/jbc.REV119.006349 PMID: 31672921

Marshall, J. S., Warrington, R., Watson, W., & Kim, H. L. (2018). An introduction to immunology and immunopathology. *Allergy, Asthma, and Clinical Immunology : Official Journal of the Canadian Society of Allergy and Clinical Immunology*, *14*(2), 49. DOI: 10.1186/s13223-018-0278-1 PMID: 30263032

Martini, M., & Orsini, D. (2022). The fight against poliomyelitis through the history: Past, present and hopes for the future. Albert Sabin's missing Nobel and his "gift to all the world's children". *Vaccine*, *40*(47), 6802–6805. DOI: 10.1016/j.vaccine.2022.09.088 PMID: 36244880

Maruyama, T., Saida, J., Uchida, T., Imamura, H., Sasaki, T., Toyoda, M., Imoto, N., Sunayama, T., & Minami, S. (2019). A therapeutic strategy for all pneumonia patients: A 3-year prospective multicenter cohort study using risk factors for multidrug-resistant pathogens to select initial empiric therapy. *Clinical Infectious Diseases*, *68*(7), 1080–1088. DOI: 10.1093/cid/ciy631 PMID: 30084884

Marzia, A., & Ali, L. (2024). A short review on poliomyelitis: Types, transmission, diagnosis, prevention, treatment. *Journal of Contemporary Pharmacy*, *8*(1), 1. DOI: 10.56770/jcp2024819

Mateer, E. J., Maruyama, J., Card, G. E., Paessler, S., & Huang, C. (2020). Lassa virus, but not highly pathogenic New World arenaviruses, restricts immunostimulatory double-stranded RNA accumulation during infection. *Journal of Virology*, *94*(9), 10–1128. DOI: 10.1128/JVI.02006-19 PMID: 32051278

Mateos-Angulo, Á., Salazar-Agulló, J. A., Roldán-Jiménez, C., Trinidad-Fernández, M., & Cuesta-Vargas, A. I. (2022). Ultrasonography Assessment Based on Muscle Thickness and Echo Intensity in Post-Polio Patients. *Diagnostics (Basel)*, *12*(11), 2743. DOI: 10.3390/diagnostics12112743 PMID: 36359586

Mathur, H., Field, D., Rea, M. C., Cotter, P. D., Hill, C., & Ross, R. P. (2018). Fighting biofilms with lantibiotics and other groups of bacteriocins. *NPJ Biofilms and Microbiomes*, *4*(1), 1. Advance online publication. DOI: 10.1038/s41522-018-0053-6 PMID: 29707229

Mazzola, L. T., & Kelly-Cirino, C. (2019). Diagnostics for Lassa fever virus: A genetically diverse pathogen found in low-resource settings. *BMJ Global Health*, *4*(Suppl 2), e001116. DOI: 10.1136/bmjgh-2018-001116 PMID: 30899575

Mbani, C. J., Nekoua, M. P., Moukassa, D., & Hober, D. (2023). The Fight against Poliovirus Is Not Over. *Microorganisms*, *11*(5), 1323. DOI: 10.3390/microorganisms11051323 PMID: 37317297

McAllister, D. A., Liu, L., Shi, T., Chu, Y., Reed, C., Burrows, J., Adeloye, D., Rudan, I., Black, R. E., Campbell, H., & Nair, H. (2019). Global, regional, and national estimates of pneumonia morbidity and mortality in children younger than 5 years between 2000 and 2015: A systematic analysis. *The Lancet. Global Health*, *7*(1), e47–e57. DOI: 10.1016/S2214-109X(18)30408-X PMID: 30497986

McCormick, J. B., & Fisher-Hoch, S. P. (2002). *"Lassa fever." Arenaviruses I: the Epidemiology*. Molecular and Cell Biology of Arenaviruses.

McCormick, J. B., King, I. J., Webb, P. A., Johnson, K. M., O'Sullivan, R., Smith, E. S., Trippel, S., Trippel, S., & Tong, T. C. (1987). A case-control study of the clinical diagnosis and course of Lassa fever. *The Journal of Infectious Diseases*, *155*(3), 445–455. DOI: 10.1093/infdis/155.3.445 PMID: 3805772

McCormick, J. B., Webb, P. A., Krebs, J. W., Johnson, K. M., & Smith, E. S. (1987). A prospective study of the epidemiology and ecology of Lassa fever. *The Journal of Infectious Diseases*, *155*(3), 437–444. DOI: 10.1093/infdis/155.3.437 PMID: 3805771

McDonald, L. C. (2017). Effects of short- and long-course antibiotics on the lower intestinal microbiome as they relate to traveller's diarrhea. *Journal of Travel Medicine*, *24*(Suppl. 1), S35–S38. DOI: 10.1093/jtm/taw084 PMID: 28520993

McGinnis, M. R., & Tyring, S. K. (1996). Introduction to Mycology. In S. Baron (Ed.), *Medical Microbiology*. Galveston (TX): University of Texas Medical Branch at Galveston Copyright © 1996, The University of Texas Medical Branch at Galveston.

McKay, N., & Wallis, L. (2005). Rabies: a review of UK management. Emergency medicine journal: EMJ, 22(5), 316–321., [Online]. Available: .DOI: 10.1136/emj.2003.013805

McLay, L., Liang, Y., & Ly, H. (2014). Comparative analysis of disease pathogenesis and molecular mechanisms of New World and Old World arenavirus infections. *The Journal of General Virology*, *95*(Pt 1), 1–15. DOI: 10.1099/vir.0.057000-0 PMID: 24068704

Mehndiratta, M. M., Mehndiratta, P., & Pande, R. (2014). Poliomyelitis: Historical Facts, Epidemiology, and Current Challenges in Eradication. *The Neurohospitalist*, *4*(4), 223–229. DOI: 10.1177/1941874414533352 PMID: 25360208

Mehtar, S., Almhawish, N., Shobak, K., Reingold, A., Guha-Sapir, D., & Haar, R. (2021). Measles in conflict-affected northern syria: Results from an ongoing outbreak surveillance program. *Conflict and Health*, *15*(1), 95. Advance online publication. DOI: 10.1186/s13031-021-00430-0 PMID: 34933672

Mena, I., Perry, C. M., Harkins, S., Rodriguez, F., Gebhard, J., & Whitton, J. L. (1999). The role of B lymphocytes in coxsackievirus B3 infection. *American Journal of Pathology*, *155*(4), 1205–1215. DOI: 10.1016/S0002-9440(10)65223-6 PMID: 10514403

Menon, T. P., Zinszer, K., & Abuzerr, S. (2024). Detection of polio virus in Gaza's sewage demands immediate action. *Frontiers in Public Health*, *12*, 1474554. Advance online publication. DOI: 10.3389/fpubh.2024.1474554 PMID: 39691657

Mercer, A. (2021). Protection against severe infectious disease in the past. *Pathogens and Global Health*, *115*(3), 151–167. DOI: 10.1080/20477724.2021.1878443 PMID: 33573529

Messina, J. P., Brady, O. J., Pigott, D. M., Bhatt, S., Battle, K. E., Myers, M. F., & Hay, S. I. (2020). Global data on the distribution and abundance of Aedes mosquitoes. *Nature Ecology & Evolution*, *4*(1), 157–162.

Metcalfe, S. (2013). History lessons. *Australian Family Physician*, *42*(8), 519. PMID: 24133699

Meyers, D. J., Ozonoff, A., Baruwal, A., Pande, S., Harsha, A., Sharma, R., Schwarz, D., Schwarz, R. K., Bista, D., Halliday, S., & Maru, D. S. (2016). Combining Healthcare-Based and Participatory Approaches to Surveillance: Trends in Diarrheal and Respiratory Conditions Collected by a Mobile Phone System by Community Health Workers in Rural Nepal. *PLoS One*, *11*(4), e0152738. DOI: 10.1371/journal.pone.0152738 PMID: 27111734

Midgley, C. M., Watson, J. T., Nix, W. A., Curns, A. T., Rogers, S. L., Brown, B. A., Conover, C., Dominguez, S. R., Feikin, D. R., Gray, S., Hassan, F., Hoferka, S., Jackson, M. A., Johnson, D., Leshem, E., Miller, L., Nichols, J. B., Nyquist, A.-C., Obringer, E., & Gerber, S. I. (2015). Severe respiratory illness associated with a nationwide outbreak of enterovirus D68 in the USA (2014): A descriptive epidemiological investigation. *The Lancet. Respiratory Medicine*, *3*(11), 879–887. DOI: 10.1016/S2213-2600(15)00335-5 PMID: 26482320

Mikula, K. M., Kolodziejczyk, R., & Goldman, A. (2012). Yersinia infection tools-characterization of structure and function of adhesins. *Frontiers in Cellular and Infection Microbiology*, *2*, 169. DOI: 10.3389/fcimb.2012.00169 PMID: 23316485

Miller, E., Andrews, N., Stellitano, L., Stowe, J., Winstone, A. M., Shneerson, J., & Verity, C. (2013). Risk of narcolepsy in children and young people receiving AS03 adjuvanted pandemic A/H1N1 2009 influenza vaccine: Retrospective analysis. *BMJ (Clinical Research Ed.)*, *346*(feb26 2), f794. DOI: 10.1136/bmj.f794 PMID: 23444425

Millet, Y. A., Alvarez, D., Ringgaard, S., von Andrian, U. H., Davis, B. M., & Waldor, M. K. (2014). Insights into *Vibrio cholerae* intestinal colonization from monitoring fluorescently labeled bacteria. *PLoS Pathogens*, *10*(10), e1004405. Advance online publication. DOI: 10.1371/journal.ppat.1004405 PMID: 25275396

Minakami, H., Kubo, T., & Unno, N. (2014). Causes of a nationwide rubella outbreak in Japan, 2012-2013. *The Journal of Infection*, *68*(1), 99–101. DOI: 10.1016/j.jinf.2013.09.002 PMID: 24029626

Mittal, A. K., Bhardwaj, R., Mishra, P., & Rajput, S. K. (2020). Antimicrobials misuse/overuse: Adverse effect, mechanism, challenges and strategies to combat resistance. *The Open Biotechnology Journal*, *14*(1), 107–112. DOI: 10.2174/1874070702014010107

Miwa, C., Ohtani, M., Watanabe, H., Fujimoto, J., Kinbara, K., & Tanaka, H. (1980). Epidemic of hand, foot and mouth disease in Gifu Prefecture in 1978. *Japanese Journal of Medical Science & Biology*, *33*(3), 167–180. DOI: 10.7883/yoken1952.33.167 PMID: 6259389

Miyoshi, J., Bobe, A. M., Miyoshi, S., Huang, Y., Hubert, N., Delmont, T. O., Eren, A. M., Leone, V., & Chang, E. B. (2017). Peripartum antibiotics promote gut dysbiosis, loss of immune tolerance, and inflammatory bowel disease in genetically prone offspring. *Cell Reports*, *20*(2), 491–504. DOI: 10.1016/j.celrep.2017.06.060 PMID: 28700948

Modlin, J. F. (1986). Perinatal echovirus infection: Insights from a literature review of 61 cases of serious infection and 16 outbreaks in nurseries. *Reviews of Infectious Diseases*, *8*(6), 918–926. DOI: 10.1093/clinids/8.6.918 PMID: 3541126

Mohammed, A., Tomori, O., & Nkengasong, J. N. (2021). Lessons from the elimination of poliomyelitis in Africa. *Nature Reviews. Immunology*, *21*(12), 823–828. DOI: 10.1038/s41577-021-00640-w PMID: 34697501

Mohanty, A., Rohilla, R., Zaman, K., Hada, V., Dhakal, S., Shah, A., & Al-Tawfiq, J. A. (2023). Vaccine Derived Poliovirus (VDPV). *Le Infezioni in Medicina*, *31*(2), 174. PMID: 37283637

Molla, A. M., Ahmed, S. M., & Greenough, W. B. (1985). Rice-based oral rehydration solution decreases the stool volume in acute diarrhoea. *Bulletin of the World Health Organization*, *63*(4), 751–756. PMID: 3910298

Molla, A. M., Rahman, M., Sarker, S. A., Sack, D. A., & Molla, A. (1981). Stool electrolyte content and purging rates in diarrhea caused by rotavirus, enterotoxigenic *E. coli*, and *V. cholerae* in children. *The Journal of Pediatrics*, *98*(5), 835–838. DOI: 10.1016/S0022-3476(81)80863-3 PMID: 6262471

Monath, T. P., Newhouse, V. F., Kemp, G. E., Setzer, H. W., & Cacciapuoti, A. (1974). Lassa virus isolation from Mastomys natalensis rodents during an epidemic in Sierra Leone. [This work is the first demonstration that Lassa virus is rodent-borne.]. *Science*, *185*(4147), 263–265. DOI: 10.1126/science.185.4147.263 PMID: 4833828

Moore, M. (1982). Centers for Disease Control. Enteroviral disease in the United States, 1970-1979. *The Journal of Infectious Diseases*, *146*(1), 103–108. DOI: 10.1093/infdis/146.1.103 PMID: 6282988

Morgenstern, J., & Thoma, B. (2018). Infectious diarrheal disease and dehydration. In Tintinalli, J. E., Ma, O. J., Yealy, D. M., Meckler, G. D., Stapczynski, J., Cline, M., & Thomas, S. (Eds.), *Tintinalli's emergency medicine: A comprehensive study guide* (9th ed.). McGraw-Hill Education.

Moss, W. J. (2017). Measles. *Lancet*, *390*(10111), 2490–2502. DOI: 10.1016/S0140-6736(17)31463-0 PMID: 28673424

Moten, M., Phillips, A., Saliba, V., Harding, N., & Sibal, B. (2018). Measles: Is it still a threat? *The British Journal of General Practice*, *68*(674), 404–405. DOI: 10.3399/bjgp18X697961 PMID: 29970395

Mousavi, S., & Anjomshoa, M. (2020). Covid-19 in yemen: A crisis within crises. *International Journal for Equity in Health*, *19*(1), 120. Advance online publication. DOI: 10.1186/s12939-020-01231-2 PMID: 32652995

Moyazzem Hossain, M., Abdulla, F., & Rahman, A. (2022). Challenges and difficulties faced in low- and middle-income countries during COVID-19. *Health Policy OPEN*, *3*, 100082. DOI: 10.1016/j.hpopen.2022.100082 PMID: 36405972

Mshelbwala, P. P., Weese, J. S., Sanni-Adeniyi, O. A., Chakma, S., Okeme, S. S., Mamun, A. A., Rupprecht, C. E., & Magalhaes, R. J. S. (2021). Rabies epidemiology, prevention and control in Nigeria: Scoping progress towards elimination. PLoS neglected tro tropical diseases, 15(8), e0009617., [Online]. Available: DOI: 10.1371/journal.pntd.0009617

Muckelbauer JK, Kremer M, Minor I, Diana G, Dutko FJ, Groarke J, et al. (1995). The structure of coxsackievirus B3 at 3.5 A resolution.

Mugoša, B., Ceccarelli, G., Begic, S., Vujošević, D., Zekovic, Ž., Ciccozzi, M., & Vratnica, Z. (2021). Measles outbreak, montenegro january–july 2018: Lessons learned. *Journal of Medical Virology*, *94*(2), 514–520. DOI: 10.1002/jmv.27377 PMID: 34617629

Mulchandani, R., Sibal, B., Phillips, A., Suleman, S., Banerjee, A., Teagle, R., Foulkes, S., Spence, K., & Edeghere, O. (2021). A large outbreak of measles in the west midlands, england, 2017–2018: Descriptive epidemiology, control measures and lessons learnt. *Epidemiology and Infection*, *149*, e114. Advance online publication. DOI: 10.1017/S0950268821000868 PMID: 33866992

Müllegger, R. R., & Glatz, M. (2008). Skin Manifestations of Lyme Borreliosis. *American Journal of Clinical Dermatology*, *9*(6), 355–368. DOI: 10.2165/0128071-200809060-00002 PMID: 18973402

Munoz, S. J. (2008). Hepatic Encephalopathy. *The Medical Clinics of North America*, *92*(4), 795–812. DOI: 10.1016/j.mcna.2008.03.009 PMID: 18570943

Munyenyiwa, A., Zimba, M., Nhiwatiwa, T., & Barson, M. (2019). Plague in Zimbabwe from 1974 to 2018: A review article. *PLoS Neglected Tropical Diseases*, *13*(11), e0007761. DOI: 10.1371/journal.pntd.0007761 PMID: 31751348

Murphy, H., & Ly, H. (2022). Understanding Immune Responses to Lassa Virus Infection and to Its Candidate Vaccines. *Vaccines*, *10*(10), 10. DOI: 10.3390/vaccines10101668 PMID: 36298533

Murray, C. J. L., Ikuta, K. S., Sharara, F., Swetschinski, L., Aguilar, G. R., Gray, A., Han, C., Bisignano, C., Rao, P., Wool, E., & Naghavi, M. (2022). Global burden of bacterial antimicrobial resistance in 2019: A systematic analysis. *Lancet*, *399*(10325), 629–655. DOI: 10.1016/S0140-6736(21)02724-0 PMID: 35065702

Murugaiyan, J., Kumar, P. A., Rao, G. S., Iskandar, K., Hawser, S., Hays, J. P., Mohsen, Y., Adukkadukkam, S., Abiola, A. W., & Essack, S. Y. (2022). Progress in alternative strategies to combat antimicrobial resistance: Focus on antibiotics. *Antibiotics (Basel, Switzerland)*, *11*(2), 200. Advance online publication. DOI: 10.3390/antibiotics11020200 PMID: 35203804

Musa, N., Ghoniem, A., Hsu, C. H., Patel, M. K., & Goodson, J. L. (2024). Progress Toward Measles Elimination — Eastern Mediterranean Region, 2019–2022. *MMWR. Morbidity and Mortality Weekly Report*, *73*(7), 141–145. DOI: 10.15585/mmwr.mm7307a1 PMID: 38386606

Muscat, M., Mamou, M., Shefer, A., Jankovic, D., Deshevoy, S., & Butler, R. (2015). Situación del sarampión y la rubéola en la región europea de la oms. *Revista Española de Salud Pública*, *89*(4), 345–351. DOI: 10.4321/S1135-57272015000400002 PMID: 26580789

Musoke, D., Ndejjo, R., Halage, A. A., Kasasa, S., Ssempebwa, J. C., & Carpenter, D. O. (2018). Drinking Water Supply, Sanitation, and Hygiene Promotion Interventions in Two Slum Communities in Central Uganda. *Journal of Environmental and Public Health*, *3710120*, 1–9. Advance online publication. DOI: 10.1155/2018/3710120 PMID: 29623096

Mwabi, J. K., Adeyemo, F. E., Mahlangu, T. O., Mamba, B. B., Brouckaert, B. M., Swartz, C. D., Offringa, G., Mpenyana-Monyatsi, L., & Momba, M. N. B. (2011). Household water treatment systems: A solution to the production of safe drinking water by the low-income communities of Southern Africa. *Physics and Chemistry of the Earth Parts A/B/C*, *36*(14), 1120–1128. DOI: 10.1016/j.pce.2011.07.078

Mwiinde, A. M., Siankwilimba, E., Sakala, M., Banda, F., & Michelo, C. (2022). Climatic and Environmental Factors Influencing COVID-19 Transmission-An African Perspective. *Tropical Medicine and Infectious Disease*, *7*(12), 433. Advance online publication. DOI: 10.3390/tropicalmed7120433 PMID: 36548688

Mygland, Å., Ljøstad, U., Fingerle, V., Rupprecht, T., Schmutzhard, E., & Steiner, I. (2010). EFNS guidelines on the diagnosis and management of European Lyme neuroborreliosis. *European Journal of Neurology*, *17*(1), 8. DOI: 10.1111/j.1468-1331.2009.02862.x PMID: 19930447

Nagashima, K. A., & Mousa, J. J. (2021). Next-generation influenza HA immunogens and adjuvants in pursuit of a broadly protective vaccine. *Viruses*, *13*(4), 546. DOI: 10.3390/v13040546 PMID: 33805245

Naim, H. Y. (2015). Measles virus. *Human Vaccines & Immunotherapeutics*, *11*(1), 21–26. DOI: 10.4161/hv.34298 PMID: 25483511

Nargund, G. (2009). Declining birth rate in Developed Countries: A radical policy re-think is required. *Facts, Views & Vision in ObGyn*, *1*(3), 191–193. PMID: 25489464

Nathanson, N. (2008). The pathogenesis of poliomyelitis: What we don't know. *Advances in Virus Research*, *71*, 1–50. DOI: 10.1016/S0065-3527(08)00001-8 PMID: 18585526

National Collaborating Centre for Women's and Children's Health (UK). (2009). Fluid management. In *Diarrhoea and vomiting caused by gastroenteritis: Diagnosis, assessment and management in children younger than 5 years*. RCOG Press. https://www.ncbi.nlm.nih.gov/books/NBK63837/

Nau, R., & Eiffert, H. (2002). Modulation of Release of Proinflammatory Bacterial Compounds by Antibacterials: Potential Impact on Course of Inflammation and Outcome in Sepsis and Meningitis. *Clinical Microbiology Reviews*, *15*(1), 95–110. DOI: 10.1128/CMR.15.1.95-110.2002 PMID: 11781269

Nelson, E. J., Grembi, J. A., Chao, D. L., Andrews, J. R., Alexandrova, L., Rodriguez, P. H., Ramachandran, V. V., Sayeed, M. A., Wamala, J. F., Debes, A. K., Sack, D. A., Hryckowian, A. J., Haque, F., Khatun, S., Rahman, M., Chien, A., Spormann, A. M., & Schoolnik, G. K. (2020). Gold standard cholera diagnostics are tarnished by lytic bacteriophage and antibiotics. *Journal of Clinical Microbiology*, *58*(9), e00412–e00420. DOI: 10.1128/JCM.00412-20 PMID: 32611794

Nguyen, K. H., Srivastav, A., Lindley, M. C., Fisher, A., Kim, D., Greby, S. M., Lee, J., & Singleton, J. A. (2022). Parental Vaccine Hesitancy and Association With Childhood Diphtheria, Tetanus Toxoid, and Acellular Pertussis; Measles, Mumps, and Rubella; Rotavirus; and Combined 7-Series Vaccination. *American Journal of Preventive Medicine*, *62*(3), 367–376. DOI: 10.1016/j.amepre.2021.08.015 PMID: 35190101

Nhan, L. N. T., Khanh, T. H., Hong, N. T. T., Van, H. M. T., Nhu, L. N. T., Ny, N. T. H., Nguyet, L. A., Thanh, T. T., Anh, N. T., Hang, V. T. T., Qui, P. T., Viet, H. L., Tung, T. H., Ha, D. Q., Tuan, H. M., Thwaites, G., Chau, N. V. V., Thwaites, L., Hung, N. T., & Tan, L. V. (2020). Clinical, etiological and epidemiological investigations of hand, foot and mouth disease in southern Vietnam during 2015 - 2018. *PLoS Neglected Tropical Diseases*, *14*(8), e0008544. DOI: 10.1371/journal.pntd.0008544 PMID: 32804980

Nhan, L. N. T., Turner, H. C., Khanh, T. H., Hung, N. T., Lien, L. B., Hong, N. T. T., Nhu, L. N. T., Ny, N. T. H., Nguyet, L. A., Thanh, T. T., Van, H. M. T., Viet, H. L., Tung, T. H., Phuong, T. T. L., Devine, A., Thwaites, G., Chau, N. V. V., Thwaites, L., van Doorn, H. R., & Tan, L. V. (2019). Economic Burden Attributed to Children Presenting to Hospitals With Hand, Foot, and Mouth Disease in Vietnam. *Open Forum Infectious Diseases*, *6*(7), ofz284. DOI: 10.1093/ofid/ofz284 PMID: 31363772

Nikaido, H., & Pagès, J.-M. (2012). Broad-specificity efflux pumps and their role in multidrug resistance of Gram-negative bacteria. *FEMS Microbiology Reviews*, *36*(2), 340–363. DOI: 10.1111/j.1574-6976.2011.00290.x PMID: 21707670

Nikiforov, V. V., Gao, H., Zhou, L., & Anisimov, A. (2016). Plague: Clinics, Diagnosis and Treatment. In Yang, R., & Anisimov, A. (Eds.), *Yersinia pestis: Retrospective and Perspective* (pp. 293–312). Springer Netherlands., DOI: 10.1007/978-94-024-0890-4_11

Nikonov, O. S., Chernykh, E. S., Garber, M. B., & Nikonova, E. Y. (2017). Enteroviruses: Classification, Diseases They Cause, and Approaches to Development of Antiviral Drugs. *Biochemistry (Moscow)*, *82*(13), 1615–1631. DOI: 10.1134/S0006297917130041 PMID: 29523062

Nilsson, E., Anderson, H., Sargenti, K., Lindgren, S., & Prytz, H. (2019). Clinical course and mortality by etiology of liver cirrhosis in Sweden: A population based, long-term follow-up study of 1317 patients. *Alimentary Pharmacology & Therapeutics*, *49*(11), 1421–1430. DOI: 10.1111/apt.15255 PMID: 30957910

Noori, N., Drake, J. M., & Rohani, P. (2017). Comparative epidemiology of poliovirus transmission. *Scientific Reports*, *7*(1), 17362. DOI: 10.1038/s41598-017-17749-5 PMID: 29234135

Nunes, O. C., Manaia, C. M., Kolvenbach, B. A., & Corvini, P. F.-X. (2020). Living with sulfonamides: A diverse range of mechanisms observed in bacteria. *Applied Microbiology and Biotechnology*, *104*(24), 10389–10408. DOI: 10.1007/s00253-020-10982-5 PMID: 33175245

Nusrat, F., Akanda, A. S., Islam, A., & et al. (2024). Satellite-derived, smartphone-delivered geospatial cholera risk information for vulnerable populations. *GeoHealth, 8*(11), Article e2024GH001039. DOI: 10.1029/2024GH001039

Nyirenda, S. S., Hang'ombe, B. M., Machang'u, R., Mwanza, J., & Kilonzo, B. S. (2017). Identification of Risk Factors Associated with Transmission of Plague Disease in Eastern Zambia. *The American Journal of Tropical Medicine and Hygiene*, *97*(3), 826–830. DOI: 10.4269/ajtmh.16-0990 PMID: 28722614

O'Connor, P., Jankovic, D., Muscat, M., Ben-Mamou, M., Reef, S., Papania, M., Singh, S., Kaloumenos, T., Butler, R., & Datta, S. (2017). Measles and rubella elimination in the WHO Region for Europe: Progress and challenges. *Clinical Microbiology and Infection*, *23*(8), 504–510. DOI: 10.1016/j.cmi.2017.01.003 PMID: 28111293

O'Hanlon, R., & Shaw, M. L. (2019). Baloxavir Marboxil: The new influenza drug on the market. *Current Opinion in Virology*, *35*, 14–18. DOI: 10.1016/j.coviro.2019.01.006 PMID: 30852344

O'Reilly, K. M., Lamoureux, C., Molodecky, N. A., Lyons, H., Grassly, N. C., & Tallis, G. (2017). An assessment of the geographical risks of wild and vaccine-derived poliomyelitis outbreaks in Africa and Asia. *BMC Infectious Diseases*, *17*(1), 1–14. DOI: 10.1186/s12879-017-2443-4 PMID: 28549485

Ogrinc, K., Lotrič-Furlan, S., Maraspin, V., Lusa, L., Cerar, T., Ružič-Sabljič, E., & Strle, F. (2013). Suspected Early Lyme Neuroborreliosis in Patients With Erythema Migrans. *Clinical Infectious Diseases*, *57*(4), 501–509. DOI: 10.1093/cid/cit317 PMID: 23667259

Olivera Mesa, D., Hogan, A. B., Watson, O. J., Charles, G. D., Hauck, K., Ghani, A. C., & Winskill, P. (2022). Modelling the impact of vaccine hesitancy in prolonging the need for Non-Pharmaceutical Interventions to control the COVID-19 pandemic. *Communications Medicine*, *2*(1), 14. DOI: 10.1038/s43856-022-00075-x PMID: 35603311

Oloke, J. K. (2000). Activity pattern of natural and synthetic antibacterial agents among hospital isolates. *Microbios*, *102*(403), 175–181. PMID: 10955832

Onorato, I. M., Morens, D. M., Schonberger, L. B., Hatch, M. H., Kaminski, R. M., & Turner, J. P. (1985). Acute hemorrhagic conjunctivitis caused by enterovirus type 70: An epidemic in American Samoa. *The American Journal of Tropical Medicine and Hygiene*, *34*(5), 984–991. DOI: 10.4269/ajtmh.1985.34.984 PMID: 2994502

Osna, N. A., Donohue, T. M., & Kharbanda, K. K. (2017). Alcoholic Liver Disease: Pathogenesis and Current Management. *Alcohol Research : Current Reviews*, *38*(2), 147–161. PMID: 28988570

Ostrowsky, J., Arpey, M., Moore, K., Osterholm, M., Friede, M., Gordon, J., Higgins, D., Molto-Lopez, J., Seals, J., & Bresee, J. (2020). Tracking progress in Universal Influenza Vaccine Development. *Current Opinion in Virology*, *40*, 28–36. DOI: 10.1016/j.coviro.2020.02.003 PMID: 32279026

Oti, V. B. (2018). *A Reemerging Lassa Virus: Aspects of Its Structure, Replication, Pathogenicity and Diagnosis*. Current Topics in Tropical Emerging Diseases and Travel Medicine.

Ozawa, S., Shankar, R., Leopold, C., & Orubu, S. (2019). Access to medicines through health systems in low- and middle-income countries. *Health Policy and Planning*, *34*(Supplement_3), iii1–iii3. DOI: 10.1093/heapol/czz119 PMID: 31816069

Pancu, D. F., Scurtu, A., Macasoi, I. G., Marti, D., Buzatu, R., Dinu, S., Socoliuc, V., & Dehelean, C. A. (2021). Antibiotics: Conventional therapy and natural compounds with antibacterial activity—A pharmaco-toxicological screening. *Antibiotics (Basel, Switzerland)*, *10*(4), 401. Advance online publication. DOI: 10.3390/antibiotics10040401 PMID: 33917092

Pannetier, D., Reynard, S., Russier, M., Carnec, X., & Baize, S. (2014). Production of CXC and CC Chemokines by Human Antigen-Presenting Cells in Response to Lassa Virus or Closely Related Immunogenic Viruses, and in Cynomolgus Monkeys with Lassa Fever. *PLoS Neglected Tropical Diseases*, *8*(1), 8. DOI: 10.1371/journal.pntd.0002637 PMID: 24421914

Park, J.-H., Kang, M., Jun, D.-W., Kim, M., Kwak, J.-H., & Kang, B.-K. (2021). Determining Whether Low Protein Intake (<1.0 g/kg) Is a Risk Factor for Malnutrition in Patients with Cirrhosis. *Journal of Clinical Medicine*, *10*(10), 2164. DOI: 10.3390/jcm10102164 PMID: 34067667

Parkman, P. D. (1996). Togaviruses: Rubella Virus. In S. Baron (Ed.), *Medical Microbiology*. Galveston (TX): University of Texas Medical Branch at Galveston Copyright © 1996, The University of Texas Medical Branch at Galveston.

Parsi, V. K. (2001). Cholera. *Primary Care Update for Ob/Gyns*, *8*(3), 106–109. DOI: 10.1016/S1068-607X(00)00086-X PMID: 11378428

Patangia, D. V., Ryan, C. A., Dempsey, E., Ross, R. P., & Stanton, C. (2022). Impact of antibiotics on the human microbiome and consequences for host health. *MicrobiologyOpen*, *11*(1), e1260. Advance online publication. DOI: 10.1002/mbo3.1260 PMID: 35212478

Patassi, A. A., Landoh, D. E., Mebiny-Essoh Tchalla, A., Halatoko, W. A., Assane, H., Saka, B., Naba, M. A., Yaya, I., Edou, K. A., Tamekloe, T. A., Banla, A. K., Davi, K. M., Manga, M., Kassankogno, Y., & Salmon-Ceron, D. (2017). Emergence of lassa fever disease in northern Togo: Report of two cases in Oti district in 2016. *Case Reports in Infectious Diseases*, *2017*, 8242313. DOI: 10.1155/2017/8242313 PMID: 29391958

Pates, K. M., Periselneris, J. N., & Brown, J. S. (2023). Pneumonia. *Medicine*, *51*(11), 763–767. DOI: 10.1016/j.mpmed.2023.08.003 PMID: 36775251

Pattanaik, A., & Mani, R. S. (2019). WHO's new rabies recommendations: implications for high incidence countries. Current opinion in infectious diseases, 32(5), 401–406., [Online]. Available: .DOI: 10.1097/QCO.0000000000000578

Pechous, R. D., Sivaraman, V., Stasulli, N. M., & Goldman, W. E. (2016). Pneumonic Plague: The Darker Side of Yersinia pestis. *Trends in Microbiology*, *24*(3), 190–197. DOI: 10.1016/j.tim.2015.11.008 PMID: 26698952

Perry, R. T., & Halsey, N. A. (2004). The clinical significance of measles: A review. *The Journal of Infectious Diseases*, *189*(Supplement_1), S4–S16. DOI: 10.1086/377712 PMID: 15106083

Persson, C., Carballeira, N., Wolf-Watz, H., & Fällman, M. (1997). The PTPase YopH inhibits uptake of Yersinia, tyrosine phosphorylation of p130Cas and FAK, and the associated accumulation of these proteins in peripheral focal adhesions. *The EMBO Journal*, *16*(9), 2307–2318. DOI: 10.1093/emboj/16.9.2307 PMID: 9171345

Peters, D. H., Garg, A., Bloom, G., Walker, D. G., Brieger, W. R., & Rahman, M. H. (2008). Poverty and access to health care in developing countries. *Annals of the New York Academy of Sciences*, *1136*(1), 161–171. DOI: 10.1196/annals.1425.011 PMID: 17954679

Peterson, K. M., & Gellings, P. S. (2018). Multiple intraintestinal signals coordinate the regulation of *Vibrio cholerae* virulence determinants. *Pathogens and Disease*, *76*(1), ftx126. Advance online publication. DOI: 10.1093/femspd/ftx126 PMID: 29315383

Philipp, M. T., Wormser, G. P., Marques, A. R., Bittker, S., Martin, D. S., Nowakowski, J., & Dally, L. G. (2005). A Decline in C 6 Antibody Titer Occurs in Successfully Treated Patients with Culture-Confirmed Early Localized or Early Disseminated Lyme Borreliosis. *Clinical and Vaccine Immunology; CVI*, *12*(9), 1069–1074. DOI: 10.1128/CDLI.12.9.1069-1074.2005 PMID: 16148173

Pillsbury, A., Chiew, M., Bag, S., Hope, K., Norton, S., Conaty, S., Sheppeard, V., & McIntyre, P. (2016). The changing epidemiology of measles in an era of elimination: Lessons from health-care-setting transmissions of measles during an outbreak in new south wales, australia, 2012. *Western Pacific Surveillance and Response Journal : WPSAR*, *7*(4), 12–20. DOI: 10.5365/wpsar.2016.7.1.010 PMID: 28246577

Pinneo, L., & Pinneo, R. (1971). Mystery virus from Lassa. *The American Journal of Nursing*, *71*, 1352–1355. PMID: 4996954

Plotkin, S. A., Reef, S. E., Cooper, L. Z., & Alford, C. A. (2011). CHAPTER 28 - Rubella. In Remington, J. S., Klein, J. O., Wilson, C. B., Nizet, V., & Maldonado, Y. A. (Eds.), *Infectious Diseases of the Fetus and Newborn* (7th ed., pp. 861–898). W.B. Saunders. DOI: 10.1016/B978-1-4160-6400-8.00028-6

*Polio eradication strategy 2022–2026: Delivering on a promise*. (n.d.). Retrieved November 30, 2023, from https://www.who.int/publications-detail-redirect/9789240031937

Polio Factsheet. *(2023, February 23). Health Protection Surveillance Centre.* Https://www.hpsc.ie/a-z/vaccinepreventable/polio/factsheet/. (n.d.).

*Poliomyelitis (polio). (2019, November 18).* Https://www.who.int/health-topics/poliomyelitis. (n.d.).

Pons-Salort, M., Parker, E. P., & Grassly, N. C. (2015). The epidemiology of non-polio enteroviruses: Recent advances and outstanding questions. *Current Opinion in Infectious Diseases*, *28*(5), 479–487. DOI: 10.1097/QCO.0000000000000187 PMID: 26203854

Pragmatic, A. (2017, May). open-label, Randomised Controlled Trial. [PubMed<]. *The Lancet. Respiratory Medicine*, *5*(5), 401–411. DOI: 10.1016/S2213-2600(17)30120-0

Prentice, M. B., & Rahalison, L. (2007). Plague. *Lancet*, *369*(9568), 1196–1207. DOI: 10.1016/S0140-6736(07)60566-2 PMID: 17416264

Priyadharshini, & Jasmine, A. (2019). Coverage survey of Measles-Rubella mass vaccination campaign in a rural area in Tamil Nadu. *J Family Med Prim Care, 8*(6), 1884-1888. DOI: 10.4103/jfmpc.jfmpc_319_19 professional CC medical. Lassa fever. Available from: https://my.clevelandclinic.org/health/diseases/25095-lassa-fever

Pscheidt, V. M., Gregianini, T. S., Martins, L. G., & Veiga, A. B. (2021). Epidemiology of human adenovirus associated with respiratory infection in southern Brazil. *Reviews in Medical Virology*, *31*(4), e2189. DOI: 10.1002/rmv.2189 PMID: 33156553

Pulli, T., Koivunen, E., & Hyypiä, T. (1997). Cell-surface interactions of echovirus 22. *The Journal of Biological Chemistry*, *272*(34), 21176–21180. DOI: 10.1074/jbc.272.34.21176 PMID: 9261123

Qadri, F., Bhuiyan, T. R., & Dutta, K. K.. (2004). Acute dehydrating disease caused by *Vibrio cholerae* serogroups O1 and O139 induce increases in innate cells and inflammatory mediators at the mucosal surface of the gut. *Gut*, *53*(1), 62–69. DOI: 10.1136/gut.53.1.62 PMID: 14684578

Qaserah, A. M., Al Amad, M. A., Al Serouri, A. A., & Khader, Y. S. (2021). Risk factors of cholera transmission in Al Hudaydah, Yemen: Case-control study. *JMIR Public Health and Surveillance*, *7*(7), e27627. Advance online publication. DOI: 10.2196/27627 PMID: 36260393

Quarleri, J. (2023). Poliomyelitis is a current challenge: Long-term sequelae and circulating vaccine-derived poliovirus. *GeroScience*, *45*(2), 707–717. DOI: 10.1007/s11357-022-00672-7 PMID: 36260265

Quinn, S. C., & Kumar, S. (2014). Health inequalities and infectious disease epidemics: A challenge for global health security. *Biosecurity and Bioterrorism*, *12*(5), 263–273. DOI: 10.1089/bsp.2014.0032 PMID: 25254915

Raabe, V.N., Mehta, A.K., & Evans, J.D. (2022). Lassa Virus Infection: a Summary for Clinicians. *International journal of infectious diseases: IJID: official publication of the International Society for Infectious Diseases.*

Raabe, V. N., & Koehler, J. W. (2017). Laboratory Diagnosis of Lassa Fever. *Journal of Clinical Microbiology*, *55*(6), 1629–1637. DOI: 10.1128/JCM.00170-17 PMID: 28404674

Radesich, C., Del Mestre, E., Medo, K., Vitrella, G., Manca, P., Chiatto, M., Castrichini, M., & Sinagra, G. (2022). Lyme Carditis: From Pathophysiology to Clinical Management. *Pathogens (Basel, Switzerland)*, *11*(5), 582. Advance online publication. DOI: 10.3390/pathogens11050582 PMID: 35631104

Rahamat-Langendoen, J., Groenewoud, H., Kuijpers, J., Melchers, W. J. G., & van der Wilt, G. J. (2019). Impact of molecular point-of-care testing on Clinical Management and in-hospital costs of patients suspected of influenza or RSV infection: A modeling study. *Journal of Medical Virology*, *91*(8), 1408–1414. DOI: 10.1002/jmv.25479 PMID: 30950066

Ranade, S. *A. (2022). Poliomyelitis clinical presentation. History and Physical Examination, Postpolio Syndrome, Complications.* Https://emedicine.medscape.com/article/1259213-clinical.

Rasoamanana, B., Rahalison, L., Raharimanana, C., & Chanteau, S. (1996). Comparison of Yersinia CIN agar and mouse inoculation assay for the diagnosis of plague. *Transactions of the Royal Society of Tropical Medicine and Hygiene*, *90*(6), 651. DOI: 10.1016/S0035-9203(96)90420-4 PMID: 9015505

Ratsitorahina, M., Chanteau, S., Rahalison, L., Ratsifasoamanana, L., & Boisier, P. (2000). Epidemiological and diagnostic aspects of the outbreak of pneumonic plague in Madagascar. *Lancet*, *355*(9198), 111–113. DOI: 10.1016/S0140-6736(99)05163-6 PMID: 10675169

Rehman, H. A., Nazar, T., Aziz, B., Farooq, H., Nazar, N., & Abdulraffay, . (2023). Role of Probiotics in Secondary Prophylaxis of Hepatic Encephalopathy. *Pakistan Journal of Medical & Health Sciences*, *17*(6), 18–20. DOI: 10.53350/pjmhs202317618

Reygaert, W. C. (2018). An overview of the antimicrobial resistance mechanisms of bacteria. *AIMS Microbiology*, *4*(3), 482–501. DOI: 10.3934/microbiol.2018.3.482 PMID: 31294229

Rima, M., Rima, M., Fajloun, Z., Sabatier, J.-M., Bechinger, B., & Naas, T. (2021). Antimicrobial peptides: A potent alternative to antibiotics. *Antibiotics (Basel, Switzerland)*, *10*(9), 1095. Advance online publication. DOI: 10.3390/antibiotics10091095 PMID: 34572678

Rodriguez, D. L. (2003). Rubella. In Samuels, M. A., & Feske, S. K. (Eds.), *Office Practice of Neurology* (2nd ed., pp. 493–495). Churchill Livingstone. DOI: 10.1016/B0-44-306557-8/50076-9

Rohde, R. E., & Rupprecht, C. E. (2020). Update on lyssaviruses and rabies: will past progress play as prologue in the near term towards future elimination?. Faculty reviews, 9, 9., [Online]. Available: .DOI: 10.12703/b/9-9

Roivainen, M., Knip, M., Hyöty, H., Kulmala, P., Hiltunen, M., Vähäsalo, P., Hovi, T., & Åkerblom, H. K. (1998). Several different enterovirus serotypes can be associated with prediabetic autoimmune episodes and onset of overt IDDM. Childhood Diabetes in Finland (DiMe) Study Group. *Journal of Medical Virology*, *56*(1), 74–78. DOI: 10.1002/(SICI)1096-9071(199809)56:1<74::AID-JMV12>3.0.CO;2-W PMID: 9700636

Roland, S., Benjamin, E., Patrick, B. V., Juana, M., & Derrick, A. (2022). Seroprevalence and predisposing factors of rabies antibodies in unvaccinated dogs in Sierra Leone. Veterinary medicine and science, 8(6), 2345–2350. https://doi.org/, [Online]. Available: https://doi.org/.DOI: 10.1002/vms3

Roos, B. K. L. (2021).. . *Neurologic Complications of Lyme Disease.*, (August), 1040–1050.

Roos, K. L. (2021). Neurologic complications of Lyme disease. *CONTINUUM: Lifelong Learning in Neurology*, *27*(4), 1040–1050. PMID: 34623103

Rorabaugh, M. L., Berlin, L. E., Heldrich, F., Roberts, K., Rosenberg, L. A., Doran, T., & Modlin, J. F. (1993). Aseptic meningitis in infants younger than 2 years of age: Acute illness and neurologic complications. *Pediatrics*, *92*(2), 206–211. DOI: 10.1542/peds.92.2.206 PMID: 8337018

Rosario-Acevedo, R., Biryukov, S. S., Bozue, J. A., & Cote, C. K. (2021). Plague Prevention and Therapy: Perspectives on Current and Future Strategies. *Biomedicines*, *9*(10), 10. Advance online publication. DOI: 10.3390/biomedicines9101421 PMID: 34680537

Rose, C. F., Amodio, P., Bajaj, J. S., Dhiman, R. K., Montagnese, S., Taylor-Robinson, S. D., Vilstrup, H., & Jalan, R. (2020). Hepatic encephalopathy: Novel insights into classification, pathophysiology and therapy. *Journal of Hepatology*, *73*(6), 1526–1547. DOI: 10.1016/j.jhep.2020.07.013 PMID: 33097308

Rose, N. R. (2008). Autoimmunity in coxsackievirus infection. *Current Topics in Microbiology and Immunology*, *323*, 293–314. DOI: 10.1007/978-3-540-75546-3_14 PMID: 18357776

Rosenberg, D., & Rovito, C. (Eds.). *(2021). Post-Polio Syndrome: Background, Management and Treatment, An Issue of Physical Medicine and Rehabilitation Clinics of North America, E-Book (Vol. 32, No. 3). Elsevier Health Sciences.*

Rosen, L., Melnick, J. L., Schmidt, J., & Wenner, H. A. (1970). Subclassification of enteroviruses and ECHO virus type 34. Brief report. *Archiv fur die Gesamte Virusforschung*, *30*(1), 89–92. DOI: 10.1007/BF01262587 PMID: 4986680

Rote, N. S. (2019). Infection. In McCance, K. L., & Huether, S. E. (Eds.), *Pathophysiology: the Biologic basis for disease in adults and children* (8th ed., pp. 289–322). Elsev-Ier.

Rothman, A. L. (2011). Dengue: A vascular disease. *Advances in Virus Research*, *81*, 1–70.

Rothman, A. L. (2019). Dengue: The importance of surveillance and vector control. *Microorganisms*, *7*(12), 619. PMID: 31783517

Rouard, C., Collet, L., Njamkepo, E., Jenkins, C., Sacheli, R., Benoit-Cattin, T., Figoni, J., & Weill, F.-X. (2024). Long-distance spread of a highly drug-resistant epidemic cholera strain. *The New England Journal of Medicine*, *391*(23), 2271–2273. DOI: 10.1056/NEJMc2408761 PMID: 39665659

Rude, R. K. (2010). Magnesium. In: *Encyclopedia of Dietary Supplements*. Eds, Coates PM, Betz JM, Blackman MR, Cragg GM, Levine M, Moss J, White JD. 2nd ed, NY: Informa Healthcare; New York, pp. 527– 37. [Google Scholar]

Rude, R. K. (2012). Magnesium. In Ross, A. C., Caballero, B., Cousins, R. J., Tusker, K. L., & Ziegler, T. R. (Eds.), *Modern nutrition in health and disease* (11th ed., pp. 159–175). Lippincott Williams & Wilkins. [Google Scholar]

Ruiz-Margáin, A., Macías-Rodríguez, R. U., Ampuero, J., Cubero, F. J., Chi-Cervera, L., Ríos-Torres, S. L., Duarte-Rojo, A., Espinosa-Cuevas, Á., Romero-Gómez, M., & Torre, A. (2016). Low phase angle is associated with the development of hepatic encephalopathy in patients with cirrhosis. *World Journal of Gastroenterology*, *22*(45), 10064–10070. DOI: 10.3748/wjg.v22.i45.10064 PMID: 28018114

Rupprecht, C. E., & Salahuddin, N. (2019). Current status of human rabies prevention: remaining barriers to global biologics accessibility and disease elimination. Expert review of vaccines, 18(6), 629–640., [Online]. Available: .DOI: 10.1080/14760584.2019.1627205

Russier, M., Pannetier, D., & Baize, S. (2012). Immune Responses and Lassa Virus Infection. *Viruses*, *4*(11), 2766–2785. DOI: 10.3390/v4112766 PMID: 23202504

Ryan, E. T., Dhar, U., Khan, W. A., Salam, M. A., Faruque, A. S., Fuchs, G. J., Calderwood, S. B., & Bennish, M. L. (2000). Mortality, morbidity, and microbiology of endemic cholera among hospitalized patients in Dhaka, Bangladesh. *The American Journal of Tropical Medicine and Hygiene*, *63*(1–2), 12–20. DOI: 10.4269/ajtmh.2000.63.12 PMID: 11357989

Sabahelzain, M., Moukhyer, M., Borne, B., & Bosma, H. (2022). Vaccine hesitancy among parents and its association with the uptake of measles vaccine in urban settings in khartoum state, sudan. *Vaccines*, *10*(2), 205. DOI: 10.3390/vaccines10020205 PMID: 35214664

Sabahelzain, M., Moukhyer, M., Dubé, E., Hardan, A., Borne, B., & Bosma, H. (2019). Towards a further understanding of measles vaccine hesitancy in khartoum state, sudan: A qualitative study. *PLoS One*, *14*(6), e0213882. DOI: 10.1371/journal.pone.0213882 PMID: 31220092

Sabogal De La Pava, M. L., & Tucker, E. L. (2022). Drug shortages in low- and middle-income countries: Colombia as a case study. *Journal of Pharmaceutical Policy and Practice*, *15*(1), 42. DOI: 10.1186/s40545-022-00439-7 PMID: 35698240

Sack, D. A., Sack, R. B., Nair, G. B., & Siddique, A. K. (2004). Cholera. *The Lancet, 363*(9404), 223–233. https.//DOI: 10.1016/S0140-6736(03)15328-7

Saepudin, M., Pranaka, R. N., Umboh, H. H., & Wardoyo, S. (2022). Risk factors associated with rabies incidence in rabies endemic areas in West Kalimantan. Germs, 12(4), 472–477., [Online]. Available: .DOI: 10.18683/germs.2022.1353

Saha, M., & Sarkar, A. (2021). Review on multiple facets of drug resistance: A rising challenge in the 21st century. *Journal of Xenobiotics*, *11*(4), 4. Advance online publication. DOI: 10.3390/jox11040013 PMID: 34940513

Sahay, M., & Sahay, R. (2014). Hyponatremia: A practical approach. *Indian Journal of Endocrinology and Metabolism*, *18*(6), 760. DOI: 10.4103/2230-8210.141320 PMID: 25364669

Salmon, D. A., Dudley, M. Z., Glanz, J. M., & Omer, S. B. (2015). Vaccine hesitancy: Causes, consequences, and a call to action. *Vaccine*, *33*, D66–D71. DOI: 10.1016/j.vaccine.2015.09.035 PMID: 26615171

Salomão, C., Nacima, A., Cuamba, L., Gujral, L., Amiel, O., Baltazar, C., Cliff, J., & Gudo, E. S. (2017). Epidemiology, clinical features and risk factors for human rabies and animal bites during an outbreak of rabies in Maputo and Matola cities, Mozambique, 2014: Implications for public health interventions for rabies control. PLoS neglected tropical diseases, 11(7), e0005787., [Online]. Available: DOI: 10.1371/journal.pntd.0005787

Samal, D., Turuk, J., Nayak, S. R., Pany, S., Pal, B. B., & Pati, S. (2025). Genomic insights into the dynamic antibiotic resistance landscape of *Vibrio cholerae* during the cholera outbreak 2022 in Odisha, India. *Scientific Reports*, *15*(1), 1503. Advance online publication. DOI: 10.1038/s41598-024-81596-4 PMID: 39789042

Santibanez, S., Hübschen, J. M., Ben Mamou, M. C., Muscat, M., Brown, K. E., Myers, R., Donoso Mantke, O., Zeichhardt, H., Brockmann, D., Shulga, S. V., Muller, C. P., O'Connor, P. M., Mulders, M. N., & Mankertz, A. (2017). Molecular surveillance of measles and rubella in the WHO European Region: New challenges in the elimination phase. *Clinical Microbiology and Infection*, *23*(8), 516–523. DOI: 10.1016/j.cmi.2017.06.030 PMID: 28712666

Sarwar, S., Ali, A., Pal, M., & Chakrabarti, P. (2017). Zinc oxide nanoparticles provide anti-cholera activity by disrupting the interaction of cholera toxin with the human GM1 receptor. *The Journal of Biological Chemistry*, *292*(44), 18303–18311. DOI: 10.1074/jbc.M117.793240 PMID: 28882894

Sayeed, M. A., Islam, K., Hossain, M., Akter, N. J., Alam, M. N., Sultana, N., Khanam, F., Kelly, M., Charles, R. C., Kováč, P., Xu, P., Andrews, J. R., Calderwood, S. B., Amin, J., Ryan, E. T., & Qadri, F. (2018). Development of a new dipstick (Cholkit) for rapid detection of *Vibrio cholerae* O1 in acute watery diarrheal stools. *PLoS Neglected Tropical Diseases*, *12*(3), e0006286. Advance online publication. DOI: 10.1371/journal.pntd.0006286 PMID: 29538377

Schlegel, H. G., & Zaborosch, C. (1993). *General microbiology*. Cambridge University Press.

Schmidt, M. E., & Varga, S. M. (2021). Cytokines and CD8 T cell effector mechanisms during respiratory syncytial virus infection. *Clinical Infectious Diseases*, *73*(3), e773–e779. DOI: 10.1093/cid/ciaa149 PMID: 33569576

Schmidt, N. J., Lennette, E. H., & Ho, H. H. (1974). An apparently new enterovirus isolated from patients with disease of the central nervous system. *The Journal of Infectious Diseases*, *129*(3), 304–309. DOI: 10.1093/infdis/129.3.304 PMID: 4361245

Schneider, J. R., Sundararajan, S. A., & de Azavedo, J. C. (2019). Dengue: A complex and evolving disease. *The American Journal of Tropical Medicine and Hygiene*, *100*(6), 1299–1304. PMID: 31190683

Schoen, R. T. (2020). Challenges in the diagnosis and treatment of Lyme disease. *Current Rheumatology Reports*, *22*(1), 1–11. DOI: 10.1007/s11926-019-0857-2 PMID: 31912251

Schoini, P., Karampitsakos, T., Avdikou, M., Athanasopoulou, A., Tsoukalas, G., & Tzouvelekis, A. (2019). Measles pneumonitis. *Advances in Respiratory Medicine*, *87*(1), 63–67. DOI: 10.5603/ARM.a2019.0010 PMID: 30830960

Scholand, S. J., Quiambao, B. P., & Rupprecht, C. E. (2022). Time to Revise the WHO Categories for Severe Rabies Virus Exposures-Category IV?. Viruses, 14(5), 1111., [Online]. Available: .DOI: 10.3390/v14051111

Schwarz, S., Kehrenberg, C., Doublet, B., & Cloeckaert, A. (2016). Lincosamides, streptogramins, phenicols, and pleuromutilins: Mode of action and mechanisms of resistance. *Cold Spring Harbor Perspectives in Medicine*, *6*(11), a027037. Advance online publication. DOI: 10.1101/cshperspect.a027037 PMID: 27549310

Schwiertz, A., Taras, D., Schäfer, K., Beijer, S., Bos, N. A., Donus, C., & Hardt, P. D. (2010). Microbiota and SCFA in lean and overweight healthy subjects. *Obesity (Silver Spring, Md.)*, *18*(1), 190–195. DOI: 10.1038/oby.2009.167 PMID: 19498350

Scully, C., Georgakopoulou, E. A., & Hassona, Y. (2017). The Immune System: Basis of so much Health and Disease: 3. Adaptive Immunity. *Dental Update*, *44*(4), 322–324, 327. DOI: 10.12968/denu.2017.44.4.322 PMID: 29172358

Second, J., Velter, C., Calès, S., Truchetet, F., Lipsker, D., & Cribier, B. (2017). Clinicopathologic analysis of atypical hand, foot, and mouth disease in adult patients. *Journal of the American Academy of Dermatology*, *76*(4), 722–729. DOI: 10.1016/j.jaad.2016.10.022 PMID: 28027826

Segura, A. (2023). Epidemics and epidemiology: Back to the future. *Gaceta Sanitaria*, *37*, 102277. Advance online publication. DOI: 10.1016/j.gaceta.2022.102277 PMID: 36508988

Sengupta, S., Chattopadhyay, M., & Grossart, H.-P. (2013). The multifaceted roles of antibiotics and antibiotic resistance in nature. *Frontiers in Microbiology*, *4*, 47. Advance online publication. DOI: 10.3389/fmicb.2013.00047 PMID: 23487476

Sen, R., Nayak, L., & De, R. K. (2016). A review on host-pathogen interactions: Classification and prediction. *European Journal of Clinical Microbiology & Infectious Diseases*, *35*(10), 1581–1599. DOI: 10.1007/s10096-016-2716-7 PMID: 27470504

Seto, J., Aoki, Y., Komabayashi, K., Yamada, K., Ishikawa, H., Ichikawa, T., Ahiko, T., & Mizuta, K. (2023). Measles outbreak response activity in japan, and a discussion for a possible strategy of outbreak response using cycle threshold values of real-time reverse transcription pcr for measles virus in measles elimination settings. *Viruses*, *15*(1), 171. DOI: 10.3390/v15010171 PMID: 36680212

Shabana, M. R., Salamony, A., Elleboudy, N. S., & Aboshanab, K. M. (2024). Vaccine-Derived Poliovirus: Epidemiology, Types, Global Response and Future Prospectives. *Archives of Pharmaceutical Sciences Ain Shams University*. DOI: 10.21608/aps.2024.268453.1159

Shabbir, H., Saeed, S., Farhan, M., Abbas, K., Rehman, M. E., Gul, F., & Basit, J. (2022). Poliomyelitis in Pakistan: Challenges to polio eradication and future prospects. *Annals of Medicine and Surgery (London), 80*, 104274. DOI: 10.1016/j.amsu.2022.104274 PMID: 36045811

Shang, Z., Chan, S. Y., Song, Q., Li, P., & Huang, W. (2020). *The strategies of pathogen-oriented therapy on circumventing antimicrobial resistance*. Research. DOI: 10.34133/2020/2016201

Shang, Z., Tan, S., & Ma, D. (2021). Respiratory syncytial virus: From pathogenesis to potential therapeutic strategies. *International Journal of Biological Sciences, 17*(14), 3903–3918. DOI: 10.7150/ijbs.64762 PMID: 34671221

Sharifi-Mood, B., & Metanat, M. (2014). Diagnosis, clinical management, prevention, and control of cholera: A review study. *International Journal of Infection, 1*(1), Article 18303. Devicehttps://DOI: 10.17795/iji-18303

Sharma, A., & Gilbert, J. A. (2018). Microbial exposure and human health. *Current Opinion in Microbiology, 44*, 79–87. DOI: 10.1016/j.mib.2018.08.003 PMID: 30195150

Sheard, D. E., O'Brien-Simpson, N. M., Wade, J. D., & Separovic, F. (2019). Combating bacterial resistance by combination of antibiotics with antimicrobial peptides. *Pure and Applied Chemistry, 91*(2), 199–209. DOI: 10.1515/pac-2018-0707

Shears, P. (2007). Poverty and infection in the developing world: Healthcare-related infections and infection control in the tropics. *The Journal of Hospital Infection, 67*(3), 217–224. DOI: 10.1016/j.jhin.2007.08.016 PMID: 17945396

Shen, Y., Li, S., Huo, D., Dong, S., Yang, Y., & Jia, L. (2023). Economic Burden of Hand, Foot, and Mouth Disease - Beijing Municipality, China, 2016-2019. *China CDC Weekly, 5*(43), 953–957. PMID: 38025512

Shin, W.-J., & Seong, B. L. (2018). Novel antiviral drug discovery strategies to tackle drug-resistant mutants of influenza virus strains. *Expert Opinion on Drug Discovery, 14*(2), 153–168. DOI: 10.1080/17460441.2019.1560261 PMID: 30585088

Shirai, H., Nishibuchi, M., Ramamurthy, T., Bhattacharya, S. K., Pal, S. C., & Takeda, Y. (1991). Polymerase chain reaction for detection of the cholera enterotoxin operon of *Vibrio cholerae. Journal of Clinical Microbiology, 29*(11), 2517–2521. DOI: 10.1128/jcm.29.11.2517-2521.1991 PMID: 1774258

Shukla, S., & Maraqa, N. F. (2023). Congenital Rubella *StatPearls*. Treasure Island (FL) ineligible companies. Disclosure: Nizar Maraqa declares no relevant financial relationships with ineligible companies.: StatPearls Publishing Copyright © 2023, StatPearls Publishing LLC.

Siddique, A. K., Akram, K., Zaman, K., Laston, S., Salam, A., Majumdar, R. N., Islam, M. S., & Fronczak, N. (1995). Why treatment centres failed to prevent cholera deaths among Rwandan refugees in Goma, Zaire. *Lancet*, *345*(8946), 359–361. DOI: 10.1016/S0140-6736(95)90344-5 PMID: 7646639

Sidiropoulou, K., Mamalis, S., Christoforidi, M., & Exindari, M. (n.d.) Epidemiological data of Coxsackie and Echo viruses in N. Greece. *Acta Microbiol Hellen. 64*(3).

Simons, A., Alhanout, K., & Duval, R. E. (2020). Bacteriocins, antimicrobial peptides from bacterial origin: Overview of their biology and their impact against multidrug-resistant bacteria. *Microorganisms*, *8*(5), 639. Advance online publication. DOI: 10.3390/microorganisms8050639 PMID: 32349409

Sinclair, G., Mphahlele, M. J., Duvenhage, H., Nichol, R., Whitehorn, A., & Küstner, H. (1982). Determination of the mode of transmission of cholera in Lebowa: An epidemiological investigation. *South African Medical Journal*, *62*(21), 753–755. https://www.semanticscholar.org/paper/Determination-of-the-mode-of-transmission-of-in-An-Sinclair-Mphahlele/1a6da890dee4498ec8cfebff884cdb585aaa55e8 PMID: 7135139

Singh, R., Singh, K. P., Cherian, S., Saminathan, M., Kapoor, S., Manjunatha Reddy, G. B., Panda, S., & Dhama, K. (2017). Rabies - epidemiology, pathogenesis, public health concerns and advances in diagnosis and control: A comprehensive review. The Veteri nary Quarterly, 37(1), 212–251., [Online]. Available: DOI: 10.1080/01652176.2017.1343516

Singhal, A., Nagarajan, R., Kumar, R., Huda, A., Gupta, R. K., & Thomas, M. A. (2009). Magnetic resonance $T_2$-relaxometry and 2D L-correlated spectroscopy in patients with minimal hepatic encephalopathy. *Journal of Magnetic Resonance Imaging*, *30*(5), 1034–1041. DOI: 10.1002/jmri.21943 PMID: 19856435

Sklar, V. E., Patriarca, P. A., Onorato, I. M., Langford, M. P., Clark, S. W., Culbertson, W. W., & Forster, R. K. (1983). Clinical findings and results of treatment in an outbreak of acute hemorrhagic conjunctivitis in southern Florida. *American Journal of Ophthalmology*, *95*(1), 45–54. DOI: 10.1016/0002-9394(83)90332-X PMID: 6849368

Smiley, S. T. (2008). Immune defense against pneumonic plague. *Immunological Reviews*, *225*(1), 256–271. DOI: 10.1111/j.1600-065X.2008.00674.x PMID: 18837787

Smith, S. P., Wu, G., Fooks, A. R., Ma, J., & Banyard, A. C. (2019). Trying to treat the untreatable: experimental approaches to clear rabies virus infection from the CNS. The Journal of general virology, 100(8), 1171–1186. [Online]. Available: DOI: 10.1099/jgv.0.001269

Smith, B. G., Cruz, A. I.Jr, Milewski, M. D., & Shapiro, E. D. (2011). Lyme disease and the orthopaedic implications of Lyme arthritis. *The Journal of the American Academy of Orthopaedic Surgeons*, *19*(2), 91–100. DOI: 10.5435/00124635-201102000-00004 PMID: 21292932

Sodha, S. V., & Dietz, V. (2015). Strengthening routine immunization systems to improve global vaccination coverage. *British Medical Bulletin*, *113*(1), 5–14. DOI: 10.1093/bmb/ldv001 PMID: 25649959

Sogoba, N., Feldmann, H., & Safronetz, D. (2012). Lassa fever in West Africa: Evidence for an expanded region of endemicity. *Zoonoses and Public Health*, *59*(s2), 43–47. DOI: 10.1111/j.1863-2378.2012.01469.x PMID: 22958249

Somekh, E., Shohat, T., Handsher, R., & Serour, F. (2001). An outbreak of echovirus 11 in a children's home. *Epidemiology and Infection*, *126*(3), 441–444. DOI: 10.1017/S0950268801005404 PMID: 11467801

Song, H. J. J. M. D., Chia, A. Z. Q., Tan, B. K. J., Teo, C. B., Lim, V., Chua, H. R., Samuel, M., & Kee, A. (2023). Electrolyte imbalances as poor prognostic markers in COVID-19: A systemic review and meta-analysis. *Journal of Endocrinological Investigation*, *46*(2), 235–259. DOI: 10.1007/s40618-022-01877-5 PMID: 36070177

Song, M. Y., Blake-Hepburn, D., Karbasi, A., Fadel, S. A., Allin, S., Ataullahjan, A., & Ruggiero, E. D. (2024). Public health partnerships with faith-based organizations to support vaccination uptake among minoritized communities: A scoping review. *PLOS Global Public Health*, *4*(6), e0002765. DOI: 10.1371/journal.pgph.0002765 PMID: 38837963

Song, N., Gao, Z., Wood, J. G., Hueston, L., Gilbert, G. L., MacIntyre, C. R., Quinn, H. E., Menzies, R., & McIntyre, P. (2012). Current epidemiology of rubella and congenital rubella syndrome in Australia: Progress towards elimination. *Vaccine*, *30*(27), 4073–4078. DOI: 10.1016/j.vaccine.2012.04.025 PMID: 22554644

Song, Y., Zhang, Y., Han, Z., Xu, W., Xiao, J., Wang, X., Wang, J., Yang, J., Yu, Q., Yu, D., Chen, J., Huang, W., Li, J., Xie, T., Lu, H., Ji, T., Yang, Q., Yan, D., Zhu, S., & Xu, W. (2020). Genetic recombination in fast-spreading coxsackievirus A6 variants: A potential role in evolution and pathogenicity. *Virus Evolution*, *6*(2), veaa048. DOI: 10.1093/ve/veaa048 PMID: 34804589

Sonibare, M. A., Moody, J. O., & Adesanya, E. O. (2009). Use of medicinal plants for the treatment of measles in Nigeria. *Journal of Ethnopharmacology*, *122*(2), 268–272. DOI: 10.1016/j.jep.2009.01.004 PMID: 19168120

Spence, T. H. (1999). The Truth about Salt. Available from: http://www.pensgard.com/nutrition/13_Salt_Good.htm

Srivastava, D., & McGuire, A. (2015). Patient access to health care and medicines across low-income countries. *Social Science & Medicine*, *133*, 21–27. DOI: 10.1016/j.socscimed.2015.03.021 PMID: 25829195

Steere, A. C., Berardi, V. P., Weeks, K. E., Logigian, E. L., & Ackermann, R. (1990). Evaluation of the Intrathecal Antibody Response to Borrelia burgdorferi as a Diagnostic Test for Lyme Neuroborreliosis. *The Journal of Infectious Diseases*, *161*(6), 1203–1209. DOI: 10.1093/infdis/161.6.1203 PMID: 2345301

Steere, A. C., Strle, F., Wormser, G. P., Hu, L. T., Branda, J. A., Hovius, J. W., Li, X., & Mead, P. S. (2016). Lyme borreliosis. *Nature Reviews. Disease Primers*, *2*(1), 1–19. DOI: 10.1038/nrdp.2016.90 PMID: 27976670

Steiner, I., & Kennedy, P. G. (1995). Herpes simplex virus latent infection in the nervous system. *Journal of Neurovirology*, *1*(1), 19–29. DOI: 10.3109/13550289509111007 PMID: 9222339

Stewart, C. L., Chu, E. Y., Introcaso, C. E., Schaffer, A., & James, W. D. (2013). Coxsackievirus A6-induced hand-foot-mouth disease. *JAMA Dermatology*, *149*(12), 1419–1421. DOI: 10.1001/jamadermatol.2013.6777 PMID: 24172861

Stokholm, J., Sevelsted, A., Bønnelykke, K., & Bisgaard, H. (2014). Maternal propensity for infections and risk of childhood asthma: A registry-based cohort study. *The Lancet. Respiratory Medicine*, *2*(8), 631–637. DOI: 10.1016/S2213-2600(14)70152-3 PMID: 25066330

Straif-Bourgeois, S., Ratard, R., & Kretzschmar, M. (2014). Infectious Disease Epidemiology. In Ahrens, W., & Pigeot, I. (Eds.), *Handbook of Epidemiology* (pp. 2041–2119). Springer New York. DOI: 10.1007/978-0-387-09834-0_34

Strebel, P. M., & Orenstein, W. A. (2019). Measles. *The New England Journal of Medicine*, *381*(4), 349–357. DOI: 10.1056/NEJMcp1905181 PMID: 31184814

Sulis, G., Peebles, A., & Basta, N. E. (2023). Lassa fever vaccine candidates: A scoping review of vaccine clinical trials. *Tropical Medicine & International Health*, *28*(6), 420–431. DOI: 10.1111/tmi.13876 PMID: 37095630

Sultana, F., Khan, S. M., Rahman, M., Winch, P. J., Luby, S. P., & Unicomb, L. (2023). Sustaining an elementary school-based hygiene intervention in Bangladesh by forming 'hygiene committees': A pilot study. *Journal of Water, Sanitation, and Hygiene for Development : a Journal of the International Water Association, 13*(10), 749–763. DOI: 10.2166/washdev.2023.191

Sun, W. (2016). Chapter 12 Plague vaccines: Status and future. *Advances in Experimental Medicine and Biology, 918*, 313–360. DOI: 10.1007/978-94-024-0890-4_12 PMID: 27722869

Sun, W., Luo, T., Liu, W., & Li, J. (2020). Progress in the development of Universal Influenza Vaccines. *Viruses, 12*(9), 1033. DOI: 10.3390/v12091033 PMID: 32957468

Suresh, S. (2023). The medical significance, epidemiology, pathogenesis, detection, and management of respiratory syncytial virus. *Preprints*. DOI: 10.20944/preprints202307.1733.v1

Swaminathan, M., Ellul, M. A., & Cross, T. J. (2018). Hepatic encephalopathy: Current challenges and future prospects. *Hepatic Medicine : Evidence and Research, 10*, 1–11. DOI: 10.2147/HMER.S118964 PMID: 29606895

Swann, N. H. (1961). Epidemic pleurodynia, orchitis, and myocarditis in an adult due to Coxsackie virus, group B, type 4. *Annals of Internal Medicine, 54*(5), 1008–1013. DOI: 10.7326/0003-4819-54-5-1008 PMID: 13774219

Swerdlow, D. L., Malenga, G., Begkoyian, G., Nyangulu, D., Toole, M., Waldman, R. J., Puhr, D. N. D., & Tauxe, R. V. (1997). Epidemic cholera among refugees in Malawi, Africa: Treatment and transmission. *Epidemiology and Infection, 118*(3), 207–214. DOI: 10.1017/S0950268896007352 PMID: 9207730

Świerczyńska, M., Mirowska-Guzel, D. M., & Pindelska, E. (2022). Antiviral drugs in influenza. *International Journal of Environmental Research and Public Health, 19*(5), 3018. DOI: 10.3390/ijerph19053018 PMID: 35270708

Takahashi, S., Metcalf, C., Ferrari, M., Moss, W., Truelove, S., Tatem, A., Grenfell, B. T., & Lessler, J. (2015). Reduced vaccination and the risk of measles and other childhood infections post-ebola. *Science, 347*(6227), 1240–1242. DOI: 10.1126/science.aaa3438 PMID: 25766232

Tang, X., Yue, H., Zhong, X., & Xu, H. (2022). Molecular epidemiology of human adenovirus, astrovirus, and sapovirus among outpatient children with acute diarrhea in Chongqing, China, 2017–2019. *Frontiers in Pediatrics, 10*, 826604. DOI: 10.3389/fped.2022.826600 PMID: 35311045

Tantai, X., Liu, Y., Yeo, Y. H., Praktiknjo, M., Mauro, E., Hamaguchi, Y., Engelmann, C., Zhang, P., Jeong, J. Y., van Vugt, J. L. A., Xiao, H., Deng, H., Gao, X., Ye, Q., Zhang, J., Yang, L., Cai, Y., Liu, Y., Liu, N., & Nguyen, M. H. (2022). Effect of sarcopenia on survival in patients with cirrhosis: A meta-analysis. *Journal of Hepatology*, *76*(3), 588–599. DOI: 10.1016/j.jhep.2021.11.006 PMID: 34785325

Tapper, E. B., Henderson, J. B., Parikh, N. D., Ioannou, G. N., & Lok, A. S. (2019). Incidence of and Risk Factors for Hepatic Encephalopathy in a Population-Based Cohort of Americans With Cirrhosis. *Hepatology Communications*, *3*(11), 1510–1519. DOI: 10.1002/hep4.1425 PMID: 31701074

Tapper, E. B., Parikh, N. D., Sengupta, N., Mellinger, J., Ratz, D., Lok, A. S.-F., & Su, G. L. (2018). A risk score to predict the development of hepatic encephalopathy in a population-based cohort of patients with cirrhosis. *Hepatology (Baltimore, Md.)*, *68*(4), 1498–1507. DOI: 10.1002/hep.29628 PMID: 29091289

Tassin M, Martinovic J, Mirand A, Peigue-Lafeuille H, Picone O, Benachi A, et al. (2014). A case of congenital Echovirus 11 infection acquired early in pregnancy. *Journal of clinical virology: the official publication of the Pan American Society for Clinical Virology. 59*(1):71-3.

Taylor, L. H., & Nel, L. H. (2015). Global epidemiology of canine rabies: past, present, and future prospects. Veterinary medicine (Auckland, N.Z.), 6, 361–371., [Online]. Available: .DOI: 10.2147/VMRR.S51147

Taylor, M. W. (2021). National implementation of HPV vaccination programs in low-resource countries: Lessons, challenges, and future prospects. *Preventive Medicine*, *144*, 106335. DOI: 10.1016/j.ypmed.2020.106335 PMID: 33678232

Taylor, S. (2023). Poliomyelitis and Child Paralysis. In *The Palgrave Encyclopedia of Global Security Studies* (pp. 1143–1147). Palgrave Macmillan., DOI: 10.1007/978-3-319-74319-6_550

Tembo, T., Simuyandi, M., Chiyenu, K., Sharma, A., Chilyabanyama, O. N., Mbwili-Muleya, C., Mazaba, M. L., & Chilengi, R. (2019). Evaluating the costs of cholera illness and cost-effectiveness of a single dose oral vaccination campaign in Lusaka, Zambia. *PLoS One*, *14*(5), e0215972. Advance online publication. DOI: 10.1371/journal.pone.0215972 PMID: 31150406

Terracciano, E., Amadori, F., Pettinicchio, V., Zaratti, L., & Franco, E. (2020). Strategies for elimination of rubella in pregnancy and of congenital rubella syndrome in high and upper-middle income countries. *Journal of Preventive Medicine and Hygiene*, *61*(1), E98–e108. DOI: 10.15167/2421-4248/jpmh2020.61.1.1310 PMID: 32490275

*The effort to eradicate polio globally faces new challenges. (N.d.). UNICEF.* https://www.unicef.org/stories/the-effort-to-eradicate-polio-globally-faces-new-challenges. (n.d.).

The Impact of Lyme Disease on Mental Health. Understanding the Connection and Seeking Support. (n.d.). https://projectlyme.org/the-impact-of-lyme-disease-on-mental-health-understanding-t he-connection-and-seeking-support/

Thiagarajah, J. R., & Verkman, A. S. (2005). New drug targets for cholera therapy. *Trends in Pharmacological Sciences*, *26*(4), 172–175. DOI: 10.1016/j.tips.2005.02.003 PMID: 15808339

Thompson, K. M., & Kalkowska, D. A. (2021). An Updated Economic Analysis of the Global Polio Eradication Initiative. *Risk Analysis*, *41*(2), 393–406. DOI: 10.1111/risa.13665 PMID: 33590521

Thompson, K. M., & Kalkowska, D. A. (2021). Potential future use, costs, and value of poliovirus vaccines. *Risk Analysis*, *41*(2), 349–363. DOI: 10.1111/risa.13557 PMID: 32645244

Thompson, K., & Tebbens, R. (2014). Framework for optimal global vaccine stockpile design for vaccine-preventable diseases: Application to measles and cholera vaccines as contrasting examples. *Risk Analysis*, *36*(7), 1487–1509. DOI: 10.1111/risa.12265 PMID: 25109229

Thong, B. Y.-H. (2010). Update on the management of antibiotic allergy. *Allergy, Asthma & Immunology Research*, *2*(2), 77–86. DOI: 10.4168/aair.2010.2.2.77 PMID: 20358021

Tiller, E. C., Masters, N. B., Raines, K. L., Mathis, A. D., Crooke, S. N., Zwickl, R. C., French, G. K., Alexy, E. R., Koch, E. M., Tucker, N. E., Wilson, E. M., Krauss, T. S., Leasure, E., Budd, J., Billing, L. M., Dewart, C., Tarter, K., Dickerson, K., Iyer, R., & Roberts, M. W. (2023). Notes from the Field: Measles Outbreak - Central Ohio, 2022-2023. *MMWR. Morbidity and Mortality Weekly Report*, *72*(31), 847–849. DOI: 10.15585/mmwr.mm7231a3 PMID: 37535476

Tinari, A., Pietrantoni, A., Ammendolia, M. G., Valenti, P., & Superti, F. (2005). Inhibitory activity of bovine lactoferrin against echovirus induced programmed cell death in vitro. *International Journal of Antimicrobial Agents*, *25*(5), 433–438. DOI: 10.1016/j.ijantimicag.2005.02.011 PMID: 15848300

Tomori, O., Fabiyi, A., Sorungbe, A., Smith, A., & McCormick, J. B. (1988). Viral hemorrhagic fever antibodies in Nigerian populations. *The American Journal of Tropical Medicine and Hygiene*, *38*(2), 407–410. DOI: 10.4269/ajtmh.1988.38.407 PMID: 3128130

Toole, M. J., Steketee, R. W., Waldman, R. J., & Nieburg, P. (1989). Measles prevention and control in emergency settings. *Bulletin of the World Health Organization*, *67*(4), 381. PMID: 2805216

Torres-Torres, S., Myers, A. L., Klatte, J. M., Rhoden, E. E., Oberste, M. S., Collett, M. S., & McCulloh, R. J. (2015). First use of investigational antiviral drug pocapavir (v-073) for treating neonatal enteroviral sepsis. *The Pediatric Infectious Disease Journal*, *34*(1), 52–54. DOI: 10.1097/INF.0000000000000497 PMID: 25229269

Torriani, G., Galan-Navarro, C., & Kunz, S. (2016). Lassa Virus Cell Entry Reveals New Aspects of Virus-Host Cell Interaction. *Journal of Virology*, *91*(4), e01902-16. Advance online publication. DOI: 10.1128/JVI.01902-16 PMID: 27928003

Trombetta, C. M., & Montomoli, E. (2016). Influenza immunology evaluation and correlates of protection: A focus on vaccines. *Expert Review of Vaccines*, *15*(8), 967–976. DOI: 10.1586/14760584.2016.1164046 PMID: 26954563

Trosky, J. E., Liverman, A. D. B., & Orth, K. (2008). Yersinia outer proteins: Yops. *Cellular Microbiology*, *10*(3), 557–565. DOI: 10.1111/j.1462-5822.2007.01109.x PMID: 18081726

Tulchinsky, T. H. (2018). John Snow, cholera, the Broad Street Pump; Waterborne diseases then and now. In *Case studies in public health* (pp. 77–99). Academic Press., DOI: 10.1016/B978-0-12-804571-8.00017-2

Tuomanen, E. I., Austrian, R., & Masure, H. R. (1995). Pathogenesis of pneumococcal infection. *The New England Journal of Medicine*, *332*(19), 1280–1284. DOI: 10.1056/NEJM199505113321907 PMID: 7708073

Turvey, S. E., & Broide, D. H. (2010). Innate immunity. *The Journal of Allergy and Clinical Immunology*, *125*(2, Suppl 2), S24–S32. DOI: 10.1016/j.jaci.2009.07.016 PMID: 19932920

Tyrrell, D. A. (1963). Clinical clues in virus infections. *British Medical Journal*, *1*(5329), 493–496. DOI: 10.1136/bmj.1.5329.493 PMID: 13995046

UNICEF. (2025, June 16). The hygiene revolution in Haiti: Towards a healthier future through community mobilization. https://www.unicef.org/haiti/en/stories/hygiene-revolution-haiti-towards-healthier-future-through-community-mobilization

Uwishema, O., Elebesunu, E. E., Bouaddi, O., Kapoor, A., Akhtar, S., Effiong, F. B., Chaudhary, A., & Onyeaka, H. (2022). Poliomyelitis amidst the COVID-19 pandemic in Africa: Efforts, challenges and recommendations. *Clinical Epidemiology and Global Health, 16*, 101073. DOI: 10.1016/j.cegh.2022.101073 PMID: 35664665

Vagima, Y., Gur, D., Aftalion, M., Moses, S., Levy, Y., Makovitzki, A., Holtzman, T., Oren, Z., Segula, Y., Fatelevich, E., Tidhar, A., Zauberman, A., Rotem, S., Mamroud, E., & Steinberger-Levy, I. (2022). Phage Therapy Potentiates Second-Line Antibiotic Treatment against Pneumonic Plague. *Viruses, 14*(4), 688. DOI: 10.3390/v14040688 PMID: 35458417

Vallès, X., Stenseth, N. C., Demeure, C., Horby, P., Mead, P. S., Cabanillas, O., Ratsitorahina, M., Rajerison, M., Andrianaivoarimanana, V., Ramasindrazana, B., Pizarro-Cerda, J., Scholz, H. C., Girod, R., Hinnebusch, B. J., Vigan-Womas, I., Fontanet, A., Wagner, D. M., Telfer, S., Yazdanpanah, Y., & Baril, L. (2020). Human plague: An old scourge that needs new answers. *PLoS Neglected Tropical Diseases, 14*(8), e0008251. DOI: 10.1371/journal.pntd.0008251 PMID: 32853251

van Seventer, J. M., & Hochberg, N. S. (2017). Principles of Infectious Diseases: Transmission, Diagnosis, Prevention, and Control. In Quah, S. R. (Ed.), *International Encyclopedia of Public Health* (2nd ed., pp. 22–39). Academic Press. DOI: 10.1016/B978-0-12-803678-5.00516-6

Verma, S. K., & Tuteja, U. (2016). Plague Vaccine Development: Current Research and Future Trends. *Frontiers in Immunology, 7*, 602. DOI: 10.3389/fimmu.2016.00602 PMID: 28018363

Verstrepen, W. A., Kuhn, S., Kockx, M. M., Van De Vyvere, M. E., & Mertens, A. H. (2001). Rapid detection of enterovirus RNA in cerebrospinal fluid specimens with a novel single-tube real-time reverse transcription-PCR assay. *Journal of Clinical Microbiology, 39*(11), 4093–4096. DOI: 10.1128/JCM.39.11.4093-4096.2001 PMID: 11682535

Vidal-Cevallos, P., Chávez-Tapia, N. C., & Uribe, M. (2022). Current approaches to hepatic encephalopathy. *Annals of Hepatology, 27*(6), 100757. DOI: 10.1016/j.aohep.2022.100757 PMID: 36115576

Vilar-Compte, D., Camacho-Ortiz, A., & Ponce-de-León, S. (2017). Infection Control in Limited Resources Countries: Challenges and Priorities. *Current Infectious Disease Reports, 19*(5), 20. DOI: 10.1007/s11908-017-0572-y PMID: 28401447

Vilstrup, H., Amodio, P., Bajaj, J., Cordoba, J., Ferenci, P., Mullen, K. D., Weissenborn, K., & Wong, P. (2014). Hepatic encephalopathy in chronic liver disease: 2014 Practice Guideline by the American Association for the Study of Liver Diseases and the European Association for the Study of the Liver. *Hepatology (Baltimore, Md.), 60*(2), 715–735. DOI: 10.1002/hep.27210 PMID: 25042402

Vogel, O. A., & Manicassamy, B. (2020). Broadly protective strategies against influenza viruses: Universal Vaccines and therapeutics. *Frontiers in Microbiology, 11*, 135. Advance online publication. DOI: 10.3389/fmicb.2020.00135 PMID: 32117155

Waldor, M. K., & Mekalanos, J. J. (1996). Lysogenic conversion by a filamentous phage encoding cholera toxin. *Science, 272*(5270), 1910–1914. DOI: 10.1126/science.272.5270.1910 PMID: 8658163

Walter, K., & Malani, P. N. (2022). What Is Measles? *Journal of the American Medical Association, 328*(23), 2370. DOI: 10.1001/jama.2022.21363 PMID: 36374512

Walter, K., & Malani, P. N. (2022). What Is Polio? *Journal of the American Medical Association, 328*(16), 1652–1652. DOI: 10.1001/jama.2022.17159 PMID: 36112391

Wang, F., Zhou, H., Olademehin, O. P., Kim, S. J., & Tao, P. (2018). Insights into key interactions between vancomycin and bacterial cell wall structures. *ACS Omega, 3*(1), 37–45. DOI: 10.1021/acsomega.7b01483 PMID: 29399648

Wang, G., Van Dam, A. P., Schwartz, I., & Dankert, J. (1999). Molecular typing of Borrelia burgdorferi sensu lato: Taxonomic, epidemiological, and clinical implications. *Clinical Microbiology Reviews, 12*(4), 633–653. DOI: 10.1128/CMR.12.4.633 PMID: 10515907

Wang, H., Cui, Y., Wang, Z., Wang, X., Guo, Z., Yan, Y., Li, C., Cui, B., Xiao, X., Yang, Y., Qi, Z., Wang, G., Wei, B., Yu, S., He, D., Chen, H., Chen, G., Song, Y., & Yang, R. (2011). A Dog-Associated Primary Pneumonic Plague in Qinghai Province, China. *Clinical Infectious Diseases, 52*(2), 185–190. DOI: 10.1093/cid/ciq107 PMID: 21288842

Wang, H., Zhang, Y., Mao, N., Zhu, Z., Cui, A., Xu, S., Song, J., Chen, M., Fang, X., Li, C., Feng, D., Zhou, S., Wang, S., Shi, J., Ji, Y., Cao, L., Ren, L., Gao, L., & Xu, W. (2019). Molecular characterization of measles viruses in china: Circulation dynamics of the endemic h1 genotype from 2011 to 2017. *PLoS One, 14*(6), e0218782. DOI: 10.1371/journal.pone.0218782 PMID: 31220172

Wang, J., Atchison, R. W., Walpusk, J., & Jaffe, R. (2001). Echovirus hepatic failure in infancy: Report of four cases with speculation on the pathogenesis. *Pediatric and Developmental Pathology*, *4*(5), 454–460. DOI: 10.1007/s10024001-0043-0 PMID: 11779047

Wang, X., Zhang, X., Zhou, D., & Yang, R. (2013). Live-attenuated Yersinia pestis vaccines. *Expert Review of Vaccines*, *12*(6), 677–686. DOI: 10.1586/erv.13.42 PMID: 23750796

Warrell M. J. (2018). Developments in human rabies prophylaxis. Developments in human rabies prophylaxis. Revue scientifique et technique (International Office of Epizootics), 37(2), 629–647., [Online]. Available: .DOI: 10.20506/rst.37.2.2829

Warren, R., Lockman, H., Barnewall, R., Krile, R., Blanco, O. B., Vasconcelos, D., Price, J., House, R. V., Bolanowksi, M. A., & Fellows, P. (2011). Cynomolgus macaque model for pneumonic plague. *Microbial Pathogenesis*, *50*(1), 12–22. DOI: 10.1016/j.micpath.2010.10.002 PMID: 21040776

Watts, G. M. (2013). Lily Lyman Pinneo. *Lancet*, *380*(9853), 1552. DOI: 10.1016/S0140-6736(12)61871-6

Wayne, M., & Bolker, B. (2023). *Infectious disease: a very short introduction*. Oxford University Press.

Weant, K. A., & Baker, S. N. (2013). Review of human rabies prophylaxis and treatment. Critical care nursing clinics of North America, 25(2), 225–242., [Online]. Available: .DOI: 10.1016/j.ccell.2013.02.001

Weaver, C. M. (2013). Potassium and health. *Advances in Nutrition*, *4*(3), 368S–377S. DOI: 10.3945/an.112.003533 PMID: 23674806

Weaver, S. C. (2018). Dengue virus pathogenesis: An update. *Viruses*, *10*(2), 75. PMID: 29439402

Weaver, S. C., Reisen, W. K., & Scott, T. W. (2019). Dengue virus: Evolution, transmission, and pathogenesis. *Cold Spring Harbor Perspectives in Biology*, •••, 036902.

Weil, A. A., Becker, R. L., & Harris, J. B. (2019). *Vibrio cholerae* at the intersection of immunity and the microbiome. *MSphere*, *4*(6), e00597–e19. DOI: 10.1128/mSphere.00597-19 PMID: 31776240

Weil, A. A., Khan, A. I., Chowdhury, F., LaRocque, R. C., Faruque, A. S. G., Ryan, E. T., Calderwood, S. B., Qadri, F., & Harris, J. B. (2009). Clinical outcomes in household contacts of patients with cholera in Bangladesh. *Clinical Infectious Diseases*, *49*(10), 1473–1479. DOI: 10.1086/644779 PMID: 19842974

Weissenborn, K. (2019). Hepatic Encephalopathy: Definition, Clinical Grading and Diagnostic Principles. *Drugs*, *79*(S1, Suppl 1), 5–9. DOI: 10.1007/s40265-018-1018-z PMID: 30706420

Wells, A. I., Grimes, K. A., Kim, K., Branche, E., Bakkenist, C. J., DePas, W. H., Shresta, S., & Coyne, C. B. (2021). Human FcRn expression and Type I Interferon signaling control Echovirus 11 pathogenesis in mice. *PLoS Pathogens*, *17*(1), e1009252. DOI: 10.1371/journal.ppat.1009252 PMID: 33513208

Welty, T., Grabman, J., Kompare, E., Wood, G., Welty, E., Duzen, J. V., Rudd, P., & Poland, J. (1985). Nineteen cases of plague in Arizona. A spectrum including ecthyma gangrenosum due to plague and plague in pregnancy. The Western Journal of Medicine. https://www.semanticscholar.org/paper/Nineteen-cases-of-plague-in-Arizona.-A-spectrum-due-Welty-Grabman/e8e04e8f9b02b4e4f735e5637e027c5d36563340

What are some unusual symptoms of Lyme disease? (n.d.). https://www.medicalnewstoday.com/articles/unusual-symptoms-of-lyme-disease#complications

Wierzba, T. F. (2019). Oral cholera vaccines and their impact on the global burden of disease. *Human Vaccines & Immunotherapeutics*, *15*(6), 1294–1301. DOI: 10.1080/21645515.2018.1504155 PMID: 30183486

Wilfert, C. M., Lauer, B. A., Cohen, M., Costenbader, M. L., & Myers, E. (1975). An epidemic of echovirus 18 meningitis. *The Journal of Infectious Diseases*, *131*(1), 75–78. DOI: 10.1093/infdis/131.1.75 PMID: 1167369

Williams, S., Louissaint, J., Nikirk, S., Bajaj, J. S., & Tapper, E. B. (2021). Deprescribing medications that may increase the risk of hepatic encephalopathy: A qualitative study of patients with cirrhosis and their doctors. *United European Gastroenterology Journal*, *9*(2), 193–202. DOI: 10.1177/2050640620975224 PMID: 33226300

Withey, J. H., Nag, D., Plecha, S. C., Sinha, R., & Koley, H. (2015). Conjugated linoleic acid reduces cholera toxin production *in vitro* and *in vivo* by inhibiting *Vibrio cholerae* ToxT activity. *Antimicrobial Agents and Chemotherapy*, *59*(12), 7471–7476. DOI: 10.1128/AAC.01029-15 PMID: 26392502

Wolbert, J. G. *(2022). Poliomyelitis. StatPearls—NCBI Bookshelf.* Https://www.ncbi.nlm.nih.gov/books/NBK558944/?report=reader.

Wolbert, J. G., & Higginbotham, K. (n.d.). *(2021). Poliomyelitis*. StatPearls.

Wolbert, J. G., Rajnik, M., Swinkels, H. M., & Higginbotham, K. (2024). Poliomyelitis. In *StatPearls* [Internet]. StatPearls Publishing., https://www.ncbi.nlm.nih.gov/sites/books/NBK558944/

Wong, W. S. W., Lee, M. W. Y., Dudley, E. G., & Kovac, J. (2020). Prenatal and peripartum exposure to antibiotics and cesarean section delivery are associated with differences in diversity and composition of the infant meconium microbiome. *Microorganisms*, *8*(2), 179. Advance online publication. DOI: 10.3390/microorganisms8020179 PMID: 32012716

Won, S.-M., Oh, K. K., Gupta, H., Ganesan, R., Sharma, S. P., Jeong, J.-J., Yoon, S. J., Jeong, M. K., Min, B. H., Hyun, J. Y., Park, H. J., Eom, J. A., Lee, S. B., Cha, M. G., Kwon, G. H., Choi, M. R., Kim, D. J., & Suk, K. T. (2022). The Link between Gut Microbiota and Hepatic Encephalopathy. *International Journal of Molecular Sciences*, *23*(16), 8999. DOI: 10.3390/ijms23168999 PMID: 36012266

Woodland, D. L. (2019). Hand, Foot, and Mouth Disease. *Viral Immunology*, *32*(4), 159. DOI: 10.1089/vim.2019.29037.dlw PMID: 31038400

World Health O. Disease Outbreak News: 2023-DON469. 2023.

World Health Org. (2023). Enterovirus-Echovirus 11 Infection – European Region. *Disease Outbreak News*, *7*, 2023.

World Health Organization (2018). Rabies vaccines: WHO position paper, April 2018 - Recommendations. Vaccine, 36(37), 5500–5503, [Online]. Available: .DOI: 10.1016/j.vaccine.2018.06.061

World Health Organization. (2003). *Manual for the laboratory identification and antimicrobial susceptibility testing of bacterial pathogens of public health importance in the developing world: Haemophilus influenzae, Neisseria meningitidis, Streptococcus pneumoniae, Neisseria gonorrhoea, Salmonella serotype Typhi, Shigella, and Vibrio cholerae*. https://iris.who.int/handle/10665/68554

World Health Organization. (2005). *The treatment of diarrhoea: A manual for physicians and other senior health workers*. https://iris.who.int/handle/10665/43209

World Health Organization. (2007). *Manual for the laboratory diagnosis of measles and rubella virus infection* (No. WHO/IVB/07.01). World Health Organization.

World Health Organization. (2010). Cholera vaccines: WHO position paper. *Weekly Epidemiological Record*, *85*(13), 117–128. PMID: 20349546

World Health Organization. (2016). *WHO Calls for Early Diagnostic Tests for Lassa Fever*. World Health Organization.

World Health Organization. (2020). *A handbook for integrated vector management.* World Health Organization.

World Health Organization. (2021,August 31) Available from: http://www.who.int

World Health Organization. (2023, September 13). Dengue. https://www.who.int/news-room/fact-sheets/detail/dengue-and-severe-dengue

World Health Organization. (n.d.). Lassa fever. World Health Organization. https://www.who.int/news-room/fact-sheets/detail/lassa-fever

Wright, E. M., Loo, D. D. F., & Hirayama, B. A. (2011). Biology of human sodium glucose transporters. *Physiological Reviews, 91*(2), 733–794. DOI: 10.1152/physrev.00055.2009 PMID: 21527736

Wright, H. T.Jr, Landing, B. H., Lennette, E. H., & Mc, A. R. (1963). Fatal infection in an infant associated with Coxsackie virus group A, type 16. *The New England Journal of Medicine, 268*(19), 1041–1044. DOI: 10.1056/NEJM196305092681904 PMID: 14001956

Wu, Z., Tang, M., Li, X., Jiang, L., Ma, J., Zhou, W., & Shi, W. (2025). Simultaneous detection of Enterovirus 71 and Coxsackievirus A16 based on RT-RPA-CRISPR Cas12a/13a system. *Microchemical Journal, 212*, 113335. DOI: 10.1016/j.microc.2025.113335

Yaeger, R. G. (1996). Protozoa: Structure, Classification, Growth, and Development. In S. Baron (Ed.), *Medical Microbiology*. Galveston (TX): University of Texas Medical Branch at Galveston Copyright © 1996, The University of Texas Medical Branch at Galveston.

Yagovkina, N. V., Zheleznov, L. M., Subbotina, K. A., Tsaan, A. A., Kozlovskaya, L. I., Gordeychuk, I. V., Korduban, A. K., Ivin, Y. Y., Kovpak, A. A., Piniaeva, A. N., Shishova, A. A., Shustova, E. Y., Khapchaev, Y. K., Karganova, G. G., Siniugina, A. A., Pomaskina, T. V., Erovichenkov, A. A., Chumakov, K., & Ishmukhametov, A. A. (2022). Vaccination With Oral Polio Vaccine Reduces COVID-19 Incidence. *Frontiers in Immunology, 13*, 907341. DOI: 10.3389/fimmu.2022.907341 PMID: 35711442

Yamayoshi, S., & Kawaoka, Y. (2019). Current and future influenza vaccines. *Nature Medicine, 25*(2), 212–220. DOI: 10.1038/s41591-018-0340-z PMID: 30692696

Yang, R. (2017). Plague: Recognition, Treatment, and Prevention. Journal of Clinical Microbiology, 56(1). DOI: 10.1128/JCM.01519-17

Yen, C. H. (1964). A recent study of cholera with reference to an outbreak in Taiwan in 1962. *Bulletin of the World Health Organization, 30*(6), 811–825. PMID: 14215187

Yin, J., Wang, L., Jin, Y., He, Q., Li, W., Wang, J., Wang, Y., & Sun, L. (2020). Mechanisms of bactericidal action and resistance of polymyxins for Gram-positive bacteria. *Applied Microbiology and Biotechnology, 104*(9), 3771–3780. DOI: 10.1007/s00253-020-10525-y PMID: 32157424

Yin, Z., Wu, Y., Zhu, R., Xu, L., Lin, Y., Yang, H., Fu, W., Huang, Q., Zhang, D., Wang, J., Wang, W., Wang, Y., Cheng, T., & Xia, N. (2021). Development of A Neonatal Mouse Model for Coxsackievirus B1 Antiviral Evaluation. *Virologica Sinica, 36*(6), 1575–1584. DOI: 10.1007/s12250-021-00444-1 PMID: 34581960

Young, B., Sadarangani, S., Jiang, L., Wilder-Smith, A., & Chen, M. I. (2018). Duration of influenza vaccine effectiveness: A systematic review, meta-analysis, and meta-regression of test-negative design case-control studies. *The Journal of Infectious Diseases, 217*(5), 731–741. DOI: 10.1093/infdis/jix632 PMID: 29220496

Young, N. A. (1973). Polioviruses, coxsackieviruses, and echoviruses comparison of the genomes by RNA hybridization. *Journal of Virology, 11*(6), 832–839. DOI: 10.1128/jvi.11.6.832-839.1973 PMID: 4351457

Yousaf, M. Z., Qasim, M., Zia, S., Khan, M.u, Ashfaq, U. A., & Khan, S. (2012). Rabies molecular virology, diagnosis, prevention and treatment. Virology journal, 9, 50., [Online]. Available: .DOI: 10.1186/1743-422X-9-50

Yu, C. P., Chen, B. C., Chou, Y. C., Hsieh, C. J., & Lin, F. H. (2022, October 28). Epidemiological features and risk factors for measles and rubella in Taiwan during 2011 to 2020. *Medicine, 101*(43), e31254. DOI: 10.1097/MD.0000000000031254 PMID: 36316902

Zachary, J. F. (2017). Mechanisms of Microbial Infections1. *Pathologic Basis of Veterinary Disease*, 132 - 241.e131.

Zanfardino, M., Pane, K., Mirabelli, P., Salvatore, M., & Franzese, M. (2019). TCGA-TCIA impact on radiogenomics cancer research: A systematic review. *International Journal of Molecular Sciences, 20*(23), 6033. Advance online publication. DOI: 10.3390/ijms20236033 PMID: 31795520

Zhang, G., Li, J., Sun, Q., Zhang, K., Xu, W., Zhang, Y., & Wu, G. (2021). Pathological Features of Echovirus-11-Associated Brain Damage in Mice Based on RNA-Seq Analysis. *Viruses, 13*(12), 2477. DOI: 10.3390/v13122477 PMID: 34960747

Zhan, T., & Stremmel, W. (2012). The diagnosis and treatment of minimal hepatic encephalopathy. *Deutsches Ärzteblatt International*, *109*(10), 180–187. DOI: 10.3238/arztebl.2012.0180 PMID: 22470407

Zheng, Y., Jit, M., Wu, J. T., Yang, J., Leung, K., Liao, Q., & Yu, H. (2017). Economic costs and health-related quality of life for hand, foot and mouth disease (HFMD) patients in China. *PLoS One*, *12*(9), e0184266. DOI: 10.1371/journal.pone.0184266 PMID: 28934232

Zhu, P., Ji, W., Li, D., Li, Z., Chen, Y., Dai, B., Han, S., Chen, S., Jin, Y., & Duan, G. (2023). Current status of hand-foot-and-mouth disease. *Journal of Biomedical Science*, *30*(1), 15. DOI: 10.1186/s12929-023-00908-4 PMID: 36829162

Zhu, Y., Huang, W. E., & Yang, Q. (2022). Clinical perspective of antimicrobial resistance in bacteria. *Infection and Drug Resistance*, *15*, 735–746. DOI: 10.2147/IDR.S345574 PMID: 35264857

Zwittink, R. D., Renes, I. B., van Lingen, R. A., van Zoeren-Grobben, D., Konstanti, P., Norbruis, O. F., Martin, R., Knol, J., & Belzer, C. (2018). Association between duration of intravenous antibiotic administration and early-life microbiota development in late-preterm infants. *European Journal of Clinical Microbiology & Infectious Diseases*, *37*(3), 475–483. DOI: 10.1007/s10096-018-3193-y PMID: 29368074

# About the Contributors

**Fatima Mohammed Abbas** is a biophysist graduated from faculty of science, Cairo University in Giza. Interested in neuroscience Biomechanics, microbiology, Nanotechnology and Their research applications in entrepreneurship .

**Abeer Abdalrahman Gendeel Hamid** is a dentist with a strong passion for public health and research excellence. She was born on April 22, 1998, in Khartoum, Sudan. She earned a Bachelor of Dental Surgery (B.D.S) from AL Neelain University, Faculty of Dentistry, Khartoum State in December 2020. Following the outbreak of war, she and her family relocated to Kassala State, where she commenced her role as a Dental House officer at Kassala Teaching Hospital at the end of October 2023. Dr. Abeer actively engaged in community dental health events, workshops, conferences, and research. Her dedication to research is evident in presenting a pre-graduate study on cleft lip and cleft palate as a poster at the 2nd Advanced Dental International Conference (ADIC) - Sudan in November 2019. Throughout her dental education and the early post-graduation period, she served as a dental assistant, supporting numerous general practitioners and specialists while also managing the clinic. Her training encompassed various specialties including oral and maxillofacial surgery, periodontics, orthodontics, pediatric dentistry, conservative dentistry, and fixed and removable prosthodontics. In summary, Dr. Hamid's journey exemplifies a steadfast commitment to excellence, continuous learning, and compassionate patient care.

**Nadia Abd Elmonem Mohammed Hassan** she lives in Helwan. she is student at Faculty of Science, Cairo university, chemistry and Biochemistry department. she is interested in bioinformatics, neuroscience, molecular biology and virus.

**Shahd Gamal Abdelsamad**, a medical university student at Ain Shams university - Egypt

**Ahmad Afyouni** A fifth-year medical student and Neuroscience master's candidate, deeply passionate about research and its implications in the field of medicine. Holding the role of Research Project Manager at MEDICA and serving as the Project Coordinator for the Universal Health Coverage in LeMSIC, he brings his dedication to both education and healthcare policy. His main fields of interest are internal medicine and infectious diseases.

**Sara Khaled Ahmed** was graduated from faculty of science,fayoum university in 2015, obtained MSc in Microbiology Awarded by Next Generation Scholars from (SNG)Academy of Scientific Research and Technology and have experience in scientific research.

**Fillemon Shekutamba Albanus** is a graduate of Bachelor of Nursing Science (Clinical) (Honours) degree in Nursing Science at the University of Namibia, School of Nursing and Public Health, General Nursing department in the Faculty of Health Sciences and Veterinary Medicine (FHSVM) at the University of Namibia, Namibia. He actually has a greater interest of partaking in all the heath care research fields. His research interests would specifically focus, in Primary health Care, Health care services, Nursing education, and Mental health.

**Ali Saad Al-Shammari** s a medical doctor (MbChB, University of Baghdad) with a strong academic record and first-attempt passes on USMLE Steps 1 and 2 CK. He is a member of major professional societies (ACC, HFSA, ASE, AMSA) and focuses his research on cardiovascular medicine and public health. He received global recognition at the 2020 IFMSA meeting in Rwanda. Dr. Al-Shammari is registered with the Iraqi Medical Association and has multiple publications. Outside medicine, he enjoys sports, including soccer and bodybuilding.

**Mohamed Hassan Amer** is a Biophysics student, Faculty of science Cairo universty in Giza. Interested in neuroscience, Nanotechnology, Pathology, Biotechnology, Bioinformatics and their applications in entrepreneurship.

**Daniel Opotamutale Ashipala** (MN Sc) is a senior lecturer and Head of Department for the School of nursing and Public Health (SoNPH), General Nursing Science department in the Faculty of Health Sciences and Veterinary Medicine (FHSVM) at the University of Namibia, Namibia. His research interests include Primary health Care, Health care services and Nursing education, and Mental health. He has published a quite number of peer reviewed articles on the delivery of teaching and learning in higher education studies. He is a doctoral candidate at Stellenbosch University in Cape Town, South Africa. His doctoral work focuses on developing a framework to facilitate the implementation of a task shifting approach for nurses in the Namibia PHC services.

**Hla Dewidar** is a clinical Trial Assistant, with a BSc. in Biotechnology and Genetic Engineering - Cairo University.

**Reem Mohamed Elsapagh** was graduated from faculty of pharmacy, Cairo university in 2019, have experience in scientific research and scientific projects.

**Seif Hussien Eltaweel** is a student in the Chemistry/Biochemistry Department at the Faculty of Science, Cairo University. He also works as a CRM and bioinformatics analyst at i-mole lab, a bioinformatics company in Egypt, Seif has a strong academic background in chemistry and biochemistry.

**Zeina Hisham Gamaleldin Mohamed** is a student at Cairo University's Faculty of Science, studying Biotechnology. She is an undergraduate researcher that worked on a project funded by Cairo University. Her research interests include molecular biology, cancer biology, and stem cells.

**Nourhan Adel Mostafa** graduated from the Faculty of Science, Cairo University with a major in Biochemistry and Chemistry. Nourhan worked as an undergraduate researcher for 3 years in the Chemistry Department. She worked on a research study of the Cu complex spectroscopic properties and its antitumor effect.

**Mariam Ahmed Moustafa Abdou** is currently pursuing a Master's degree in Embryology at Cairo University, where she also earned a Bachelor of Science degree in 2021 in Zoology. Dr. Moustafa's was the team leader of graduation research project on developing a diagnostic liver disease test strip funded by the Academy of Scientific Research and Technology. She has contributed to three published journal articles. In addition to her research work, Ms. Moustafa has taught Cambridge science curriculum for two years. She has prepared digital learning materials and STEM activities for her students. With her strong academic record, research experience, and dedication to science communication and instruction, Ms. Moustafa is well-prepared to continue making meaningful contributions in her field through her ongoing graduate studies and future career.

**Rana Soliman** is an undergraduate student at the department of biotechnology and biomolecular chemistry department, Faculty of Science, Cairo University, and member at student research team (SRT) at Cairo University.

# Index

## A



## C



## D



## E

## T



## V



## W



## Y

www.ingramcontent.com/pod-product-compliance
Lightning Source LLC
LaVergne TN
LVHW080630011026
849160LV00014B/1169
* 9 7 9 8 3 6 9 3 6 6 5 1 6 *